Biomechanics
of
Sport

Editor

Christopher L. Vaughan, Ph.D.
Associate Professor of Bioengineering
Clemson University
Clemson, South Carolina

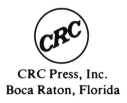

CRC Press, Inc.
Boca Raton, Florida

Library of Congress Cataloging-in-Publication Data

Biomechanics of sport / editor, Christopher L. Vaughan.
   p. cm.

Includes bibliographies and index.   ISBN 0-8493-6820-0
1. Sports — Physiological aspects.   2. Human mechanics.
I. Vaughan, Christopher L.
[DNLM: 1. Biomechanics.   2. Sports. WE 103 B6155]
RC1235.B54 1989
612′.76—dc19
DNLM/DLC   87-34152
                                                                CIP

Direct all inquiries to CRC Press, Inc., 2000 Corporate Blvd., N. W., Boca Raton, Florida, 33431.

© 1989 by CRC Press, Inc.

International Standard Book Number 0-8493-6820-0

Library of Congress Card Number 87-34152
Printed in the United States   3 4 5 6 7 8 9 0
Printed on acid-free paper

PREFACE

Biomechanics may be considered as the science that studies the external forces acting on the human body and the effects produced by these forces. Sport is one area where a knowledge of biomechanics could be of vital importance. This applies both to the improvement of performance and to the etiology and thus prevention of sports-related injuries.

Although biomechanics research, and specifically research on sport, has been carried out for many decades, the formation of national and international bodies is of comparatively recent origin. The *Journal of Biomechanics* was launched in 1968, while the International Society of Biomechanics, after a number of biannual congresses, was officially constituted in 1973. This has been followed by societies being set up in the U.S. (1977), Canada (1980), and Europe (1980). The latest development has been the introduction of the *International Journal of Sport Biomechanics,* which first appeared at the beginning of 1985. All these societies and journals play a major role in disseminating knowledge on biomechanics, and particularly as this knowledge pertains to sport.

The present volume is complementary to the activities of the societies and journals. It is hoped that it will not only provide a basis of knowledge, but also act as a stimulus for further progress. Since there are many different sports practiced worldwide, the volume quite obviously has had to be selective. This has been dictated by two main factors: a sufficient body of research knowledge for a particular sport, and the availability of authors. Thus, a selection of important topics has been chosen. However meaningful the title and their topics seem to be, the eventual value of the volume is to a large extent determined by the value of the separate contributions. I therefore wish to thank and acknowledge all the authors for their hard work, because without their cooperation, this volume would never have been published. It is my fervent hope that their efforts will be rewarded by inspiring those already in the field of sports biomechanics, or perhaps those wishing to join, to extend our knowledge in this exciting field.

In Chapters 1 to 4, the cyclic activities are covered. In Chapter 1, the authors address some of the substantive issues in running. Swimming (in Chapter 2) is discussed from the vantage point of the forces (both propulsive and resistive) acting both on animals and humans. Another aquatic sport, rowing and sculling, is covered in Chapter 3. Subsequently, the biomechanics of speed skating are reviewed in Chapter 4 from a modeling perspective. In Chapters 5 to 9, a variety of different sports activities are covered. In Chapter 5, the use of weights (machines, training, and lifting) is extensively and critically analyzed. The throwing events in track and field (shot, discus, and javelin) are studied in Chapter 6. In Chapter 7, the emphasis is placed on developing training programs for ski-jumping, alpine- and cross-country skiing and also Nordic combination skiing. The mechanics of tennis strokes and equipment are reviewed in Chapter 8, while in Chapter 9, the mechanics of cycling are analyzed.

The publication of this volume could not have been achieved without significant contributions from various individuals and institutions. It therefore gives me great pleasure to acknowledge the following: the authors, without whom the volumes would not exist; CRC Press, and particularly Marsha Baker, for their patience when deadlines were continually being extended: Groote Schuur Hospital and the University of Cape Town for providing me with the necessary facilities and time; the Association of Sports Science and Medical Research Council of South Africa, for providing financial assistance; Carien Coetzee for her substantial secretarial assistance; and my family who endured many hours of work, but provided encouragement when it was most needed.

Kit Vaughan

THE EDITOR

Christopher L. (Kit) Vaughan, Ph.D., is a graduate of Rhodes University, South Africa, with a B.Sc. in Physics and Applied Mathematics (1974). In 1975 he completed the B.Sc. (Hons) degree in these subjects and wrote his thesis on a biomechanical model of running. After working as a research officer at the Applied Physiology Laboratory of the Chamber of Mines in Johannesburg (concentrating on heat-exchange problems in exercise), he enrolled as a student at the University of Iowa. There he majored in biomechanics, anatomy, and exercise physiology, obtaining his Ph.D. degree in 1980 with a dissertation entitled ''An optimization approach to closed-loop problems in biomechanics''. While at Iowa, he acted as a consultant to the Nissen Corporation with emphasis on weight training and trampoline equipment.

Between 1980 and 1986, Dr. Vaughan was on the joint staff of Groote Schuur Hospital and the University of Cape Town Medical School in the Department of Biomedical Engineering. There he held the titles of Specialist Medical Scientist (Biomedical Engineer) and Senior Lecturer. During this period he initiated and taught a course on the biomechanics of sports techniques and injury mechanisms to candidates for the B.Sc. (Medicine) (Hons) degree in Sports Science. In 1983, Dr. Vaughan spent his sabbatical leave as a Research Associate at the University of Oxford Orthopaedic Engineering Centre in England concentrating on joint forces during human walking. Since October 1986 he has been an Associate Professor in Clemson University's Department of Bioengineering, where he is responsible for orthopedic biomechanics as well as being the academic coordinator for the Bioengineering Alliance of South Carolina.

Dr. Vaughan has published in major international journals on a variety of topics. These have included the fields of both orthopedic and sports biomechanics. He is a charter member of the American Society of Biomechanics, and since 1979 he has attended, and presented papers at, the biannual congress of the International Society of Biomechanics.

CONTRIBUTORS

Antonio Dal Monte, M. D.
Head
Department of Physiology and
 Biomechanics
Institute of Sports Science
Italian National Olympic Committee
Rome, Italy

R. W. De Boer, M. Sc.
Department of Exercise
 Physiology and Health
Academic Medical Centre
Amsterdam, The Netherlands

G. De Groot, Ph.D.
Department of Exercise
 Physiology and Health
Academic Medical Centre
Amsterdam, The Netherlands

Bruce C. Elliott, Ph. D.
Senior Lecturer
Department of Human Movement
 and Recreation Studies
University of Western Australia
Perth, Australia

John Garhammer, Ph. D.
Associate Professor
Departmentof Physical Education
California State University
Long Beach, California

Mont Hubbard, Ph. D.
Associate Professor
Department of Mechanical Engineering
University of California at Davis
Davis, California

Andrzej Komor, Ph. D.
Department of Biocybernetics
Institute of Sport
Warsaw, Poland

John W. Kozey, M.Sc.
Director of Research
Orthopaedic and Sports Medicine
 Clinic of Nova Scotia
Halifax, Canada

R. Bruce Martin, Ph.D.
Professor and Director
Orthopaedic Research Laboratory
University of California at Davis
Davis, California

Dirk J. Pons, M. Sc.
Research Associate
Department of Biomedical Engineering
University of Cape Town
 Medical School Observatory
Cape Town, S. Africa

Carol A. Putnam, Ph.D.
Assistant Professor
School of Physical Education
Dalhousie University
Halifax, Canada

Gert J. van Ingen Schenau, Ph. D.
Department of Functional Anatomy
Faculty of Human Movement Sciences
Free University
Amsterdam, The Netherlands

Christopher L. Vaughan, Ph. D.
Associate Professor of Bioengineering
Clemson University
Clemson, South Carolina

Kazuhiko Watanabe, M. D.
Associate Professor
Laboratory of Physiology
 and Sports Biomechanics
University of Hiroshima
Hiroshima, Japan

TABLE OF CONTENTS

Chapter 1

SUBSTANTIVE ISSUES IN RUNNING

Carol A. Putnam and John W. Kozey

TABLE OF CONTENTS

I. INTRODUCTION

Running has received considerable attention from researchers in biomechanics, particularly over the last several decades. The number of publications or presentations at scientific meetings escalates yearly, adding to the more than 600 reported studies dealing with mechanical aspects of running. In addition, biomechanical considerations of running are being featured in popular journals with increased frequency, attempting to satisfy the curiosities of thousands of recreational and competitive runners about the mechanical implications and effects of running.

Consistent with the proliferation of literature in this area, several extensive reviews have been published.[1-4] The present paper is written to augment and update these reviews although some overlap will necessarily exist.

Research into the biomechanics of running is suffering the growing pains of being dominated by descriptive studies. While recognizing the importance of an extensive descriptive foundation, several investigators[2,5-7] have emphasized the importance of addressing more mechanistic issues — What fundamentally dictates the way we run? What forces are responsible for observed running patterns? What criteria dictate optimal performance? What are the mechanisms of injury? — etc. In the present paper we will attempt to review the literature on running mechanics in light of potential answers to these questions.

In the 1920s and 1930s, several papers, considered by many to be classics, were published which dealt with some of the basic, mechanistic aspects of running.[8-11] It is encouraging that the attention of present day researchers is being directed more and more towards these issues. Through these efforts we should start to see the development of a theoretical framework out of which should emerge general biomechanical principles relating to the fundamental mechanisms of human motion.[12]

It is impossible to understand fully the fundamental mechanisms of running from a biomechanical perspective without crossing over into several disciplines, including cardiovascular physiology, neuromuscular physiology, anatomy, and motor control. Space constraints make it impossible to span these areas in the present review so that the discussion will be restricted to a mechanical perspective of running. The reader is directed to an excellent book recently brought out by McMahon[13] entitled *Muscles, Reflexes, and Locomotion*, in which many aspects critical to the fundamental understanding of running are presented in an integrated and lucid manner.

II. RUNNING EFFICIENCY

If one questioned runners or researchers interested in the mechanics of running on what fundamentally dictates the way we run, the answer would probably be efficiency. Efficiency, defined as the ratio of mechanical work done to metabolic energy expended[13,14] is one of the most extensively researched, yet poorly understood concepts of running mechanics. The problem of measuring efficiency is one that requires close cooperation between biomechanists and exercise physiologists, and is complex from both perspectives.[2,15] For the biomechanist, the challenge lies in correctly measuring mechanical work done and interpreting this measure in light of underlying principles which are likely to govern the way we run.

A. Measuring Mechanical Work Done

There is considerable confusion as to how mechanical work done should be measured. Much of this confusion stems from the fact that work done has been quantified in terms of energy changes. As will be pointed out below, this has resulted in both ambiguous and inaccurate measures of mechanical work done in running and consequently running efficiency.

Several investigators have measured mechanical work done in running solely in terms of the work done to cause changes in the energy state of the total body mass center.[16-25] Winter[26] criticized this approach in that it oversimplified the system, and he suggested that the findings of these studies should be regarded with caution. He pointed out that consideration must be given to the mechanical energy changes of individual segments which are collectively responsible for changes in the energy state of the total body mass center. He emphasized that by doing this, the mechanical energy associated with reciprocal actions of body segments, which have no net effect on the motion of the total body center of mass, are not ignored.

One of the first attempts to account for mechanical energy changes of individual segments in running was by Fenn.[10,27] He suggested that the mechanical work done on a runner was the sum of the work done to cause changes in the energy of the total body center of mass (potential energy and kinetic energy due to translation), generally referred to as external work, and the work done to cause mechanical energy changes of individual body segments (potential energy and kinetic energy due to translation and rotation), generally referred to as internal work. This technique has since been employed in several investigations of running.[28-33] This method of analysis treats segment motions as if they were independent of each other and of the movement of the total body mass center, which is clearly inappropriate. The body must be viewed instead as a constrained, linked system. As a result, the work done on the human body cannot be measured by changes in energies of individual segments and/or the total body mass center in the general case.[34]

Measures of mechanical work done on the human body require the identification of individual forces which actually do work on the system and a quantification of the work done by these forces. Forces doing work on the human body system in running include those which arise from both internal and external sources.

1. Work Done by Internal Forces

Internal forces applied to individual body segments include those exerted by muscles (or musculotendinous units), ligaments, joint capsules, and articulating surfaces. Since it is impossible to quantity these forces individually,[35] they are represented by a resultant joint force (RJF) and a resultant joint moment (RJM) associated with each joint of the system. An RJF is the vector sum of all forces applied across or through a joint (including muscle, ligament, joint capsule and bony contact forces), while an RJM is the vector sum of the moments of these forces measured relative to the joint center. Simplified in this manner, the kinetics of the linked segment system can then be solved via an inverse dynamics approach.

The only internal forces that are associated with metabolic energy consumption are those exerted by muscles. The net effect of muscle forces acting on a system of body segments are reflected primarily by the RJMs of the system. It makes sense, therefore, that work done by internal forces be calculated in terms of the work done by the RJMs only. This was done as early as 1940 by Elftman[9] and more recently by Winter[36] and Lin and Dillman[37] to analyze various aspects of the running gait. In each case, the work done by an RJM over a given period of time was quantified by integrating the power-time function of the RJM, where power is the RJM vector multiplied as a dot (or scalar) product with the joint angular velocity vector. This is equivalent to adding the algebraically signed scaler quantities of the work done by a RJM on both segments on which the RJM acts.[38]

Running is periodic in nature, and thus the amount of positive work done by the RJMs will be equal to the amount of negative work done by these moments within any one cycle of constant-velocity-level running in the absence of externally applied forces which do work on the body (e.g., air resistance). From a mechanical perspective, the total work done by the RJMs during each running cycle will be zero. From a physiological perspective, however, both positive and negative work are metabolic-energy-consuming processes. Thus, the total work done by the RJMs is considered to be the sum of the integrals of the absolute value of each RJM power-function during the course of one cycle.[34,36,37]

While it makes sense from a physiological (or biomechanical) perspective that work done by internal forces be calculated in terms of work done by the RJMs of the system, it is important to consider if this also makes sense from a mechanical perspective. If the human body system is viewed as being acted upon internally by a series of RJMs and RJFs, we must consider which of these forces and moments actually do work on the system. The theory of Lagrangian dynamics helps to separate the RJMs and RJFs into forces which do work on the system (nonconstraint forces) and those which do not do work on the system (constraint forces).[39] At any instant of the running stride the degrees of freedom of the human body can be defined in terms of the angular orientations of each body segment relative to a fixed direction in space. Given the initial angular orientations and velocities of these segments, the motion of the system can therefore be completely defined by the RJMs acting at each joint of the system, where the RJMs are defined as the generalized forces associated with each degree of freedom of the system. Onyshko and Winter[40] have demonstrated this for walking. Thus, to quantify work done on the system by forces internal to the system, it is only necessary to account for the work done by the RJMs, i.e., the nonconstraint forces. The RJFs are constraint forces. Although these forces do work on indvidual segments, the work done by equal and opposite force-pairs on adjoining segments, cancel each other out, and no net work is done on the system as a whole.

For a given amount of work done by the internal forces of the system, the resulting mechanical energy can be distributed in a variety of ways to various body segments depending on how the constraint forces are applied to each segment, or the energy can take one of several forms (e.g., potential, kinetic energy of translation, or kinetic energy of rota-tion).[9,34,36] When measuring mechanical work done to arrive at running efficiency, there is no need to be concerned with how energy is transferred between adjacent segments or transformed from one form to another. However, such concerns may lead to a better un-derstanding of running mechanics or interpretations of running efficiency, and will be dealt with in a later section of this review.

In summary, measuring running efficiency requires an accurate quantification of the mechanical work done by internal forces acting on body segments. This cannot be measured by changes in energies of individual segments and/or the total body mass center, but must be quantified in terms of the absolute values of the integrals of the RJM powers. As a result of the confusion in the literature over measuring mechanical work, there has yet to be a study in which running efficiency has been quantified correctly.[41] Williams and Cavanagh[42] showed that measures of mechanical efficiency can differ drastically if mechanical work done is measured incorrectly (e.g., derived by total body and/or segmental energy changes with arbitrary decisions on what energy is transferred or transformed) as has been done in a number of studies.[41,43-50]

2. Work Done by External Forces

External forces applied to the runner include gravity, the ground–reaction force, and air resistance. It is questionable whether the work done by these forces should be included in measures of running efficiency. Nevertheless, work done by external forces becomes an issue when energy changes of the body are considered. Work done by gravitational forces are typically accounted for by potential energy changes in the body. The ground–reaction force in overground running is generally considered to be a force that does no work. Although the friction component of the ground contact force can do work on a runner if the foot slides during the stance phase, the amount of work done is likely to be negligible under normal running conditions. In treadmill running the work done by the frictional component of the ground–reaction force cannot be ignored.[51] Generally, it is not measured, but accounted for indirectly by measuring potential and/or kinetic energy changes of the body relative to a reference frame which moves with the treadmill.[52,53] Air resistance does work on the body in overground running. The effect of this force is generally considered in connection with energy costs of running rather than running efficiency, and will be covered in a later section of this paper.

B. Interpreting Mechanical Efficiency

If the concept of efficiency is to enhance our fundamental understanding of running we must be able to explain why one form of running is more efficient than another. In other words, the factors affecting the relationship between mechanical work done by internal forces and metabolic energy expended must be elucidated.

1. Work Done by RJMs vs. Work Done by Individual Muscles

Metabolic costs are probably more closely linked to work done by individual muscles than work done by RJMs.[38] Unfortunately, the former cannot be quantified easily, so that mechanical work done is generally measured in terms of work done by RJMs. There are several factors which complicate the relationship between work done by an RJM and work done by individual muscle forces contributing to the RJM. The first is related to the uncertainty of how load is shared among muscles capable of performing the same function. The manner in which load is shared among synergistic muscles is likely to depend on the level of force required of the muscle group, the speed of the movement, and the angles of all joints crossed by muscles in the group. As yet, there is no satisfactory solution to the muscle-load sharing problem.[35] Second, when antagonistic muscles are active at the same time as agonistic muscles, the work done by the antagonistic muscles and the equivalent amount of work done by the RJM.[9] Third, multi–joint muscles do work at more than one joint. Thus, it is possible that the same metabolic-energy-consuming process could be counted twice in terms of mechanical work done by RJMs.[9,54] Elftman[9] calculated the rate of work done by muscles during running, accounting for duplicative efforts by two-joint muscles and estimated that this rate would be increased by 52% if only single-joint muscles were concerned. While this is probably a rough approximation, it indicates the extent to which multi-joint muscle involvement could affect the relationship between metabolic energy expended and measures of mechanical work done in running.

2. Type of Muscle Contraction

The type of muscle contraction has a significant effect on the relationship between metabolic costs and mechanical work done.[9,34,42] It is generally assumed that if the RJM power is positive, the muscles crossing the joint are contracting concentrically and doing positive work, while negative RJM powers are associated with eccentric contractions and negative muscle work. Different weighting factors have been assigned to the positive and negative mechanical work phases of the running cycle to reflect the relative metabolic cost of each. Elftman[9] assumed that the energy consumption for a given amount of negative work done in running was 0.4 times that of an equal amount of positive work, while Williams and Cavanagh[42] assumed values ranging from 0.2 to 1.0. As yet, there is no consensus as to what these relative weights should be.[15] Williams[15] has suggested that by examining several simple movements which replicate either a positive or negative work phase of the running action, in isolation, it may be possible to derive appropriate weighting factors. This seems a reasonable direction to take. One does have to consider, however, that while phases of positive (or negative) work for an RJM may coincide with phases of positive (or negative) work for single-joint muscles, the same may not be true for multi-joint muscles.[55,56] The problem of specifying relative energy costs of positive and negative work is further complicated by the fact that the cost of either type of work varies as a function of the rate of lengthening or shortening of the muscle,[57] and the range through which length changes take place relative to the resting length of the muscle.[55] Isometric contractions further complicate the situation, although an energy cost is associated with this type of contraction, no mechanical work is done.

3. Storage and Reutilization of Elastic Energy

Correct interpretation of measures of efficiency also depends on an appreciation of how much energy is stored as potential energy in the elastic components of muscle, tendon, and ligament. It has been postulated that a metabolic-energy saving will be realized if energy so stored is recovered in the form of kinetic energy and not lost as heat.[42,45,57] While the storage and recovery of elastic energy is frequently considered an important factor in running, the extent to which this may influence running efficiency, is not known. It is difficult to quantify energy stored and reutilized as it is likely to depend on the speed and magnitude of stretch, the level of activation of the stretched muscle, the muscle length at the end of the stretch, and the time-lag between the end of the stretch and the onset of the shortening phase of the muscle.[58] The abundance of multi-joint muscles in the leg makes it difficult to quantify many of these parameters during running.[55,56]

Cavagna and Kaneko[19] attributed increased running efficiency with increased running speeds to a greater potential for storage and reutilization of elastic energy at the higher speeds. It should be noted that these authors measured work done during running by considering position and velocity changes of the total body center of mass and not by work done by the RJMs or muscles. Further, while there is some agreement that running efficiency increases with running speed,[29,50] other researchers have found it to remain the same[28,48] or to decrease[28,30,46] with increases in running speed. These differences are almost certainly due to the fact that running efficiency was never quantified in a consistent manner.

Ito et al.[59] defined efficiency in running as the ratio of mechanical work done to integrated EMG, where mechanical work was assumed to be the work done to accelerate the center of mass during stance, and to accelerate the limbs relative to the center of mass during the airborne phase. They found that the integrated EMG recorded from six muscles of the lower extremity during the stance phase did not change as running speed increased from 3.7 m/sec to maximum sprinting speed and running efficiency was higher during stance than swing. These findings were interpreted to be indicative of the importance of elastic energy recoil during the stance phase of running.

Shorten[45] attempted to measure the effect of elastic storage of energy in the knee extensors on the efficiency of running in man. Compliance of the series elastic components of the knee extensors was estimated at various force levels to allow changes in strain energy to be estimated from the magnitude of the RJM at the knee. Significant reductions in apparent running efficiency were found when strain energy was included as part of the total body energy. Shorten pointed out that no account was taken of the possible dissipation of the stored energy, but concluded that despite the approximate nature of his results, they did demonstrate that effects of stored elastic energy on running efficiency should not be overlooked when analyzing even moderate speed running. This being the case, the attention of researchers in biomechanics should be directed towards examining how various kinematic factors might contribute to storage and reutilization of elastic energy and thereby enhance running efficiency.[5]

4. Nonmuscular Force Contributions to RJMs

The relationship between mechanical work done and metabolic energy cost is clouded by the fact that RJMs may be a function of nonmuscular forces (e.g., ligament forces or forces of contact between articulating surfaces) that limit the range of motion of a joint.[15] While the extent to which either may contribute to an RJM is uncertain, it is likely that nonmuscular forces limiting the range of motion play a substantial role during the swing phase of running.[15]

C. Muscular Effort

The above discussion suggests that correct interpretation of mechanical efficiency depends on accurate evaluation of muscular effort. When measures of work done by muscles or RJMs are used to indicate muscular effort, metabolic energy costs of isometric contractions are ignored. While this may not be a major problem for muscle forces which act primarily in the sagittal plane, muscles acting primarily in the frontal or transverse planes are probably fairly active, but do very little mechanical work. Andrews[38] questioned whether work done by muscles or RJMs is the most appropriate indicator of muscular effort. He suggested a variety of alternative techniques, including the sum of the impulses of muscular forces or RJMs where phases of eccentric and concentric contractions are scaled differently. McMahon[13] also suggested that impulses of muscle forces rather than work done may be a better measure of muscular effort. His suggestion was based on the fact that the oxygen consumption of animals trained to run with loads on their backs increased by the same percentage as one would expect the muscular force to increase. He also indicated that some account would have to be taken of the different relationship between the impulse of muscle forces and metabolic energy consumption for concentric and eccentric contractions although he did not suggest how this might be done. Chow and Jacobson[60] suggested that the total mechanical energy expended by muscles is proportional to the time integral of the square of the RJMs.

Quantifying muscular effort in terms of impulses of muscle forces is fraught with many of the problems that complicate the relationship between mechanical work done by muscles and metabolic energy cost. However, it does account for the muscular effort of all types of muscular contractions and warrants further consideration when dealing with the issues of running efficiency.

D. Apparent Efficiency

Apparent efficiency has been defined as the ratio of the rate of work done by an external force to the resulting increment in the rate of metabolic energy expended.[18,53,61,62] External forces considered include gravitational[18,53] (where work done is measured in terms of potential energy changes), air resistance,[18] and externally applied impeding forces.[61,62]

If apparent efficiency is to reflect running efficiency, it must be assumed that the internal work (i.e., work done to move limbs) does not change when external loads are applied.[15,53,61] This assumption is not necessarily valid[18,53] and it is questionable whether apparent efficiency is a good indicator of running efficiency.

E. Summary

Quantifying running efficiency and interpreting measures of running efficiency are clearly difficult and as yet unsolved problems. We are faced with such questions as: How representative is work done by RJMs of work done by individual muscles? How should the relative costs of different types of muscle contraction (concentric, eccentric, and isometric) and different speeds at which the contracting muscles shorten or lengthen be accounted for? How and when should energy stored in elastic components be considered? How should work done by internal nonmuscular forces be accounted for? Answers to these and similar questions should direct us to addressing more fundamental issues such as; Why is one style of running more efficient than another? and, What ultimately dictates the style of running adopted for a given situation?

It is very tempting to assume that with practice we naturally tend to adopt an efficient running style. However, this has never been supported experimentally. Chapman et al.[49] demonstrated that prescribed variations in running style, e.g., exaggerated hip flexion, exaggerated knee flexion, reduced knee flexion, and straight-legged running, resulted in significant differences in mechanical energy costs. Interestingly, the subjects' (only two were studied) natural style was not the one with the lowest mechanical energy cost. These authors therefore questioned the suitability of using mechanical energy cost as an index of efficiency. It is unfortunate that mechanical work done by RJMs was not measured. In any case, the concluding statement by these authors that the search for mechanical variables which reflect the least cost to the metabolism, must be based on muscular properties rather than the kinetic results of muscular contractions, warrants serious consideration.

While efficiency is generally viewed as important in running, it is still not known if running styles are naturally adopted on the basis of efficiency. Further, it is questionable whether the most efficient style of running is the most effective. This has led some researchers to consider running mechanics in light of the metabolic cost of running a certain distance (i.e. running economy) rather than running efficiency.[5,15,57,63]

III. RUNNING ECONOMY

Economy is defined as the metabolic cost of performing a specific task.[57,63] Mass distribution among segments, leg length, the location of muscle origins and insertions relative to joint centers, muscle fiber lengths, and orientations and types, have all been suggested as possible structural factors which could affect the energy required to perform a given task.[57,64] Shoe weight[52] and shoe sole cushioning[65] have also been found to influence running economy. It is unclear whether enhanced economy is reflected in an increase in running efficiency. Frederick[63] suggested that changes in economy probably reflect changes in mechanical work done rather than changes in efficiency. Given that running economy and running efficiency may not be perfectly related, it is possible that we adopt certain styles of running on the basis of economy rather than efficiency.

If minimization of oxygen consumption is a crucial performance criteria for running and one assumes that with practice runners adopt an economical running pattern, then forcing a change in certain aspects of a runner's style should have a predictable effect on running economy. It has been shown that if well-trained runners are forced to alter stride lengths while running at a constant speed (3.8 m/sec) energy costs will change.[66] Runners tend naturally to adopt a stride length which is within 4.2 cm of the stride length at which energy cost is minimized.[66] However, it is questionable how critical stride length is to running economy. Fairly large variations in stride length result in comparatively small changes in oxygen consumption, and day-to-day variations in stride lengths have not been shown to account for day-to-day variations in running economy.[67]

Kaneko et al.[31] also found optimal stride lengths for constant-speed running (3.5 m/sec) based on energy consumption. They went one step further to calculate running efficiency (unfortunately incorrectly) at various stride lengths and found that the most efficient stride length was slightly longer than the optimal stride length based on energy considerations.

Lin and Dillman[37] calculated the work done by the RJMs of the lower extremity for highly skilled runners performing at competitive pace. Variations in each running pattern were then simulated such that the stride length decreased or increased over a range of 42 cm from the subject's freely chosen stride length, but the average running velocity remained the same.

Several assumptions were made regarding the segment kinematic parameters for the simulated trials. They found optimal stride lengths for which the rate of work done by the RJMs was minimized. These varied from the freely chosen stride lengths by an average of 9.7 cm.

Evidence to date suggests that for a given individual and a given running speed, an optimal stride length may exist, but the criteria which ultimately dictate optimal stride lengths are unknown. One would expect optimal stride length to be a function of certain physical parameters. Suprisingly, its does not seem to be a function of leg length.[66] Cavanagh and Kram[57] suggested that it may be a function of the relationship between the efficiency of muscular contractions and the velocity at which muscles contract. The elastic properties of muscle are also likely to play a role in dictating optimal stride length and hence stride frequency. McMahon[13] suggested that the resonant frequency of the elastic component in kangaroo tendon may dictate the hopping speed at which the animal's oxygen consumption rate is minimized. It would be interesting to see if a similar phenomenon occurs in human locomotion. Finally, Kram et al.[68] found that when fatigued, runners tend to adopt longer stride lengths for a given running speed suggesting that the naturally chosen stride lengths may be influenced by changes in muscle function brought on by fatigue.

Williams[15] pointed out that it is difficult to alter one kinematic parameter without affecting several others. It may be for this reason that the effect of performance variations on metabolic costs of running have not been pursued to any great extent. It is also possible that the effect of various mechanical factors on metabolic costs in running may be extremely subtle and therefore difficult to investigate individually. Nonetheless, the challenge exists to understand which kinematic and kinetic patterns lead to greater running economy. More important, our understanding of the mechanisms through which running economy is improved, and how various kinematic factors affect these mechanisms, must be increased.[5]

IV. EXTERNAL FORCES

Fundamental mechanisms of running cannot be fully understood without considering the effect of external forces on the body. In running, external forces which significantly affect body motion are air resistance, the contact force between the ground and the runner's foot, typically called the ground-reaction force, and gravity.

A. Air Resistance

Hill[11] experimented with a model of a runner in a wind tunnel and estimated that the magnitude of the air resistance force acting on a runner moving at maximum speed in still air could be as high as 28 N. Shanebrook and Jaszczak[69] modeled the human body as a series of circular cylinders representing the trunk and appendages and a sphere to simulate the head. With the model orientated in a general position that closely approximated a running posture, they estimated that the total drag on a sprinter running at 10 m/sec would vary from 25 to 36 N for body builds typical of the 2nd and 98th percentile of the adult male American population, respectively.

Comparing the energy costs of an athlete running overground and on a treadmill at 4.4 m/sec, Pugh[70] suggested that the energy cost of overcoming air resistance was approximately 8% of the total cost of running, while additional experimental data[53] collected from athletes running on a treadmill in a wind tunnel, showed that the cost of overcoming air resistance was 7.5% of the total energy cost when running at 6 m/sec, and 13% at sprinting speed. Using a similar experimental technique, Davies[71] found that the cost of overcoming air resistance was 2% of the total cost of running at 5 m/sec, 4% at 6 m/sec, and 7.8% at 10 m/sec. From theoretical considerations involving the balancing of energy derived from metabolic processes and energy expended in the form of thermal energy released, work done to increase the horizontal kinetic energy of the runner's mass center, and work done against air resistance, Ward-Smith[33] found that the latter ranged from 7.5 to 9% of the total energy cost of sprinting. A similar theoretical analysis led Frohlich[72] to conclude that approximately 10% of the total rate of energy expended in sprinting would be used to overcome air resistance, and 3% when running at 5.4 m/sec.

Factors affecting the magnitude of the air resistance force include wind speed, air density, shadowing effects from other runners, clothing and intra-cycle variations in position and speed of body segments.[69] Of these, only the first three have been addressed from experimental or theoretical perspectives. Ward-Smith[73] theorized that if no change in cadence occurred, sprinting into a 5 m/sec headwind would increase the time for the 100 m by 0.62 sec, sprinting with a 5 m/sec tailwind would decrease the time for the 100 m by 0.38 sec, while sprinting in Mexico City where the air density is approximately 75% of that at sea level would reduce the time for the 100 m by about 0.2 sec. Comparable values derived by Frohlich[72] were 0.9, 0.6, and 0.5 sec, respectively. These values are consistently larger than those of Ward-Smith, but this can probably be explained by the fact that Frohlich did not account for the initial acceleration phases of sprinting. Ward-Smith[73] indicated that such an omission would cause the effects of air and wind resistance to be overestimated.

Pugh[53] found that if a runner moving at 4.5 m/sec runs 1 m behind a second runner, the rate of oxygen consumption is decreased by 6.5% thereby abolishing 80% of the energy cost of overcoming air resistance. Kyle[74] showed that running a 1500 m race at 7 m/sec while following 2 m behind another runner would theoretically save enough energy to allow the runner to reduce the time for each lap by 1.7 seconds.

The findings of these studies suggest that air resistance can be a significant factor in running. The effect of this force on body segments could influence calculations of RJMs, and interpretations of running efficiency or economy and should not be overlooked.

B. Ground-Reaction Force

The ground-reaction force exerted against the runner's shoe sole contains a wealth of information on running mechanics. An appreciation of factors affecting specific kinematic or kinetic parameters of the lower extremity segments as well as the linear kinematics of the total body center of mass, is derived from information reflected in the magnitude and/ or impulse of the ground-reaction force. Modifications in running technique which are associated with changes in the ground-reaction force have important implications for running injury (which will be discussed in a later section of this paper) and performance improvement. With regard to the latter, minimizing the impulse of the braking force exerted by the horizontal component of the ground force on the runner's foot during the initial part of the stance, is generally considered important to performance.[36,56,75-79] The magnitude of the braking force is thought to be a function of the foot speed relative to the ground at foot strike and the distance between the foot and the total body center of mass at foot contact, although the relationships between these variables have never been fully tested. Bates et al.[80] presented data which showed that foot speed and position at ground contact could not be used to distinguish between a group of three runners who clearly decelerated at foot strike, and thus experienced a large braking force, and a group of two runners who showed very little deceleration at foot strike and therefore would experience a considerably smaller braking force. It appears, therefore, that the factors responsible for the braking force need to be reconsidered.

It is unknown how the impulse of the braking force is related to other mechanical factors which also affect performance, e.g., the impulses of the forward (propulsive) or vertical components of the ground force, stride length, and stride frequency. Hay[81] has suggested that the apparent virtues of altering performance to decrease the impulse of the braking force may have been too readily accepted in activities such as sprinting or many jumping events in track and field and that careful research directed toward this problem must still be done before we understand the implications of the braking force to performance. The relationship between the braking force impulse and running economy or running efficiency must also be explored in efforts to enhance our fundamental understanding of running.

The nature of the ground force exerted on a runner is affected by the physical properties of the surface across which the runner moves. McMahon and Greene[82] postulated that track surfaces with a spring stiffness considerably less than the stiffness of the leg muscles (e.g. 0.15 times the stiffness of the leg) would greatly reduce running speed, while surfaces with a stiffness 2 to 4 times that of the leg muscle may enhance running speed by decreasing foot contact time and increasing the distance traveled while the foot is on the ground. It is not known how variations in track stiffness affect such variables as running economy or movement efficiency, but these findings suggest certain neuromuscular implications which may dictate how we run and how fast we can run.

There are certain limitations in the information that can be provided by ground-reaction force patterns. From a purely mechanical perspective, this force, along with the other external forces acting on the body, ultimately dictates body motion. However, an analysis of ground-reaction force data on its own, tells us little about the contributions of individual body segments to movement. To this end, Ae et al[83] and Hinrichs[84] adopted an analytical technique first suggested by Miller and East[85] in which the acceleration of the total body center of mass (which is directly related to the ground-reaction force) is expressed as a function of the acceleration of individual body segments. Ae et al.[83] showed that the support leg, and particularly the foot of the support leg, contributed substantially to the whole body momentum in both the forward and vertical directions. The momentum generated by the support leg was found to become increasingly larger relative to the momentum generated by the arms, trunk, and free leg as running speed increased. Hinrichs[84] concentrated on the role played by the arms in running and found that they made a small, but important contribution to the vertical lift of the body which increased with increases in running speed. Surprisingly, the arm actions tended to reduce the changes in forward velocity of the total body rather than increase it, thereby contributing negatively to the forward drive of the runner. The logical extension of this type of analysis is to consider the internal (primarily muscular) forces which cause individual segment motions and ultimately dictate total body movement subject to constraints imposed by the environment.

V. MUSCLE FUNCTION IN RUNNING

A. Resultant Joint Moment Patterns

Execution and control of running lies at the level of the neuromuscular system.[86] Muscular forces are the mechanisms responsible for the motion of segments, but with our present technology it is not possible to measure these forces directly. We must resort, therefore, to quantifying muscle force input in terms of the net moment of all muscles crossing individual joints. Resultant joint moments (RJMs) have been reported by a number of investigators for the full range of running speeds from slow jogging to sprinting.[36,56,76,78,79,87-94]

With some exceptions,[92,93] attention has been focused on the RJMs patterns for the hip, knee, and ankle. The general patterns of these RJM curves are reasonably consistent from subject to subject and across running speeds, although some inconsistencies have been noted close to foot strike[56,79] and during stance.[88,94] Variability in the RJM pattern just before and during the initial part of foot strike are thought to be a function of the variability of the horizontal distance between the foot and the total body mass center at foot strike.[56] It could also be attributed to difficulties in smoothing joint coordinate data through foot contact or locating the center of pressure of the ground force during the initial part of the stance phase.

The magnitudes of these curves generally increase with increases in running speed although not all variability in magnitude can be attributed to running speed. Cavanagh et al.,[89] Mann

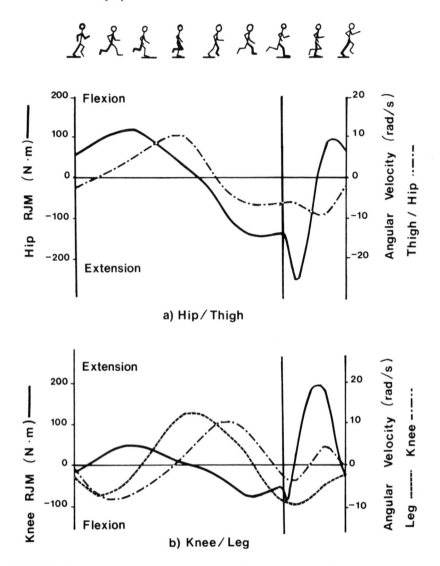

FIGURE 1.   Representative resultant joint moment (RJM) and segment and joint angular velocity
curves for (a) hip and thigh, (b) knee and leg, and (c) ankle and foot. Curves are presented as a
percent of swing time and percent of stance time, and are derived from several sources.[36,56,76,78,79,87,89–91] The angular velocity of the hip can be considered approximately equal to that of the thigh since
the trunk angle rotates through a very small range in the sagittal plane (approximately 4 degrees).[95]

and Sprague,[79] and Winter[36] show considerable variability in the magnitudes of the RJM
curves between subjects running at the same speed. For slow running this variability tends
to be smallest at the ankle and greatest at the hip.[36]

Representative RJM curves for the hip, knee, and ankle are presented in Figure 1 together
with joint and/or segment angular velocity functions. These curves were derived from a
compilation of data presented by several investigators.[36,56,76,78,79,89-91] This was done by
initially expressing each variable presented for the swing phase as a function of percent
swing time and each variable presented for the stance phase as a function of percent stance
time. All curves were then averaged at consecutive points throughout the swing and stance
phases.

When an RJM is in the same direction as the angular velocity of the joint it is sometimes
referred to as a concentric moment, whereas if the directions are opposite, it is referred

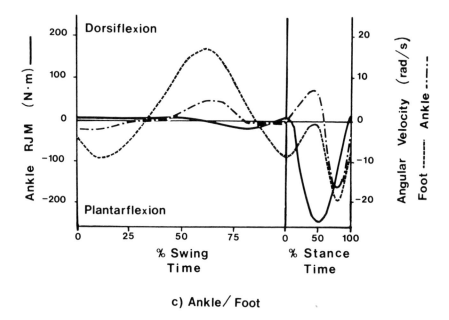

c) Ankle/Foot

as an eccentric moment.[2,78,94] Following this convention, the hip RJM is primarily a concentric moment and the knee RJM is primarily an eccentric moment during swing. During stance, the hip, knee, and ankle RJMs go through both concentric and eccentric phases. While these labels add to our understanding of muscle group functions in running, it should be noted that they are not necessarily consistent with the type of contraction of the multi-joint lower extremity muscles.[55,56] This point will be addressed in further detail in a subsequent section on electromyography.

Analysis of RJM and segment or joint angular velocity patterns of lower extremity segments, leads to an appreciation of the roles played by muscle groups in producing motion of the lower extremity and to some extent the trunk. Such analyses have done much to further our fundamental understanding of running. It should be noted that it is important to view RJM patterns in conjunction with segment angular velocity as opposed to angular displacement patterns, since both the direction of motion and the direction of acceleration of segments must be known to appreciate fully the roles played by muscle groups.

1. Hip Moment

During the first part of the swing phase an eccentric hip flexor moment stops the posterior rotation of the thigh.[79] This is followed by a concentric hip flexor moment which accelerates the thigh forward.[76,79,87,91] During the latter part of the swing phase a concentric hip extensor moment helps to rotate the thigh in the posterior direction in preparation for foot contact.[36,56,76,79,87,91] This concentric hip extensor moment continues throughout the first part of the stance phase and has been interpreted as indicative of an attempt to minimize the braking effect which typically occurs when the foot contacts the ground.[76,78] The eccentric hip flexor moment exerted during the latter part of stance slows down thigh rotation[36] and helps to rotate the trunk forward for take-off.[78] This is consistent with the findings of Thorstensson et al.[95] who showed that the least forward inclination of the trunk occurs at foot strike and the maximum forward inclination coincides with the termination of the support phase.

2. Knee Moment

The first half of the swing phase is dominated by an eccentric knee extensor moment which serves to slow the backward rotation of the leg and foot.[36,79] An eccentric knee flexor moment dominates the latter half of the swing phase, accelerating the leg backward thereby limiting knee extension.[36,79,87,89] Knee extension stops before foot strike so that the knee flexes into the stance phase aided by a concentric knee flexor moment. This has been interpreted as an attempt by the performer to minimize braking at touchdown.[36,76,79] Mann and Sprague[78] found that the magnitude of the knee flexor and hip extensor moment during the initial part of stance in sprinting was inversely related to the loss in horizontal velocity during ground contact, and suggested that high magnitudes of these moments were important to performance, but may implicate hamstring injury.

Following a brief period of concentric knee flexor moment during the initial phase of stance, an eccentric knee extensor moment serves to absorb the shock of landing,[78,79,87,94] then a concentric knee extensor moment propels the body forward.[78,94] The role that the knee extensors play in propulsion has been described as moderate[94] and is usually over before the end of the stance phase. The knee flexor moment at take-off is thought to play a role in resisting the tendency of the extensor moments at the hip and ankle to hyperextend the knee,[94] thereby avoiding injury associated with rapid knee extension.[78]

3. Ankle Moment

The RJM at the ankle is insignificant during the swing phase.[79] A very brief phase of dorsiflexor ankle moment during the initial post-contact phase helps to pull the tibia forward following foot strike.[94] The plantar flexors dominate for the remainder of the stance phase. This moment is initially eccentric and helps to absorb the shock of landing and control the forward rotation of the tibia over the ankle, and is later concentric as it aids in propulsion.[78,94] The decrease in magnitude of this propulsive moment as toe-off is approached, may be due to the rapid rate of shortening of the plantar flexors.[79] The propulsive role of the plantar flexors is considered to be very important in running.[79] Ae et al.[87] found that the positive work done by the plantar flexors was highly correlated with stride length and stride frequency.

4. Summary

RJM patterns, viewed in conjunction with segment angular velocity and/or acceleration data, reveal the roles played by muscle groups to produce a running motion. In the previous sections we have considered the effects of RJMs on the motions of segments upon which these moments act. Our understanding of these effects are still incomplete since it is rare that investigators view RJMs in light of a complete kinematic description of the segment motions. However, the effects of RJMs on individual segment motions are still only part of the kinetic picture. We turn now to a series of investigations in which attempts have been made to understand how RJMs affect the motion of the body as a whole.

B. Functional Significance of RJMs and Segment Interaction

The relationship between the RJMs applied to one segment of a linked segment system and the kinematics of that segment, is dependent on the RJMs applied to all other segments within the system, the resulting segment motions caused by these RJMs, and ultimately the manner in which segments interact. Viewed from a work-energy perspective, the work done by the RJMs will affect the mechanical energy of the system. For a given amount of mechanical work done by the RJMs, energy can be distributed among segments in different ways (transferred between segments) or can take on several different forms (e.g., potential, kinetic due to translation, kinetic due to rotation).[26,96] The distribution of energy among body segments and the form in which energy is expressed in any one segment, is a function of the work done by the RJMs and the RJFs applied to each segment.

In 1980, Robertson and Winter[97] presented a detailed interpretation of work-energy relationships for linked systems. They explained how energy could be transferred between adjacent segments via the work done on each segment by the RJF at the connecting joint. They further explained that if segments rotated in the same direction, energy could be transferred from one segment to the other via the RJM at the connecting joint, whereas if the segments rotated in opposite directions energy could be increased (generated) in each segment if positive work was done by the RJM, or taken away (dissipated or absorbed) from each segment if negative work was done by the RJM.

This interpretation of energy transfer, generation, and dissipation has been used in a number of studies to assess the functional significance of RJM patterns and the interactions between segments in running.[9,36,52,76,87,98,99] The hip RJM was found to be an important generator of energy,[52,76,99] and the energy generated from this source appeared to be a limiting factor in the total amount of energy which could be input to the recovery leg in sprinting.[98] The knee RJM was found to play a primary role in energy absorption.[36,52,76,87,99] The ability of this moment to absorb the energy of the leg toward the end of the swing phase of sprinting, was considered the most important factor limiting stride frequency and therefore sprinting speed.[98] The plantar flexors were found to play an important role in energy dissipation during the initial stance phase and energy generation during the latter part of stance.[36,87] The positive work done by this RJM was about three times that of the knee extensor RJM, indicating the relative importance of these muscles in propeling the body forward and upward.

Energy transferred between segments via RJFs has been used to study interactions between segments of the swing leg.[52,76,98] Martin[52] found that the work done by the RJFs in slow running (3.3 m/sec) dominated the energy transfers between segments of the lower extremity. Martin[52] and Martin and Cavanagh[99] showed that during the first half of the recovery phase, the RJF at the hip did positive work on the thigh thereby increasing the energy level of the thigh. At the same time, the thigh did work on the leg increasing its energy via the RJF at the knee, and the leg did work on the foot via the RJF at the ankle. This segmental interaction represented a transfer of energy from the thigh through the leg and to the foot. During the second half of recovery the direction of energy transfer brought about by the RJFs was reversed. The functional significance of this energy transfer was not addressed.

Chapman and Caldwell[76,98] extended their analysis to include a transfer of energy between limbs. The energy generated and dissipated by the RJF at the hip was considered to be indicative of the energy transfer between the swing leg and the rest of the body, in particular the contralateral leg. They found the RJF at the hip to be an important source of energy for the swing leg during the early part of contralateral stance and an important dissipator of the swing leg energy during the second half of contralateral stance.

The relative amounts of energy transferred between segments and energy generated or dissipated by the musculature is viewed as an indication of running economy.[52] Aleshinsky[100] suggested that in well-coordinated movement, the mechanisms of energy conversion (transfer and transformation) are used as much as possible to minimize the expenditure of energy due to muscle contraction. He developed compensation coefficients which could be used to indicate the degree to which the mechanical expenditure of energy could be minimized, but has yet to quantify these coefficients for human movement. It has been shown that for a given running speed, lower oxygen consumptions tend to be associated with higher-within segment[41] and between-segment[42] energy transfers. In each case the energy transfers were not defined rigorously.[101] It remains to be seen how analyses of energy transfers will enhance our understanding of running efficiency or running economy, or the roles played by muscles in producing a running action.

There are a few problems associated with the work-energy analyses as they have been applied to muscle function in running. First, the transfer of energy between segments is a complex function of the work done by the RJF and the RJM between adjacent segments. Therefore, it is not necessary that muscles (or RJMs) do negative work to transfer energy from one segment to an adjacent segment as has sometimes been implied.[15,42] Second, some researchers refer to RJFs as nonmuscular forces[102] or consider the work done on a segment by an RJF as requiring no muscular activity about the joint at which the RJF acts.[97] These interpretations are incorrect.[34] The RJF is the vector sum of all forces acting on the segment, some of which are muscular. Aleshinsky[34] has derived equations showing that any RJF within a multilink system is determined by the RJMs acting at all articulations and specifically at the one at which the RJF acts.

The work-energy approach is particularly suited to the analysis of running if the performance criterion is viewed as one of minimum energy. However, work and energy are scalar terms and do not uniquely define the kinematics of the system. If the performance criterion or critical aspects of the performance are viewed in kinematic terms this approach may have limited value.

C. Simulation of Running Gait

Much of our understanding of the roles played by muscles in running has come from empirical measurement. More recently, several investigators have developed algorithms to simulate a running action by specifying initial segment angular displacements and velocities and RJM-time patterns.[102-106] This technique has great potential for furthering our understanding of running mechanics as it allows the investigator to examine modifications in technique without requiring repeated performance by a subject. Although models have been developed to simulate the motion of the entire human body in running,[103,105] they have not been used to any great extent. Other models[102,106] have been developed to simulate the motion of the recovery leg. Phillips et al.[102] simulated the motion of the swing leg by reducing the knee RJM to zero over certain phases of the motion. They were able to demonstrate the importance of the knee extensor RJM in stopping knee flexion during the first part of the swing and the knee flexor RJM in slowing down knee extension during the final part of the swing phase. During the time in which the knee RJM was set to zero, the influence of the thigh's motion on the leg via the knee RJF was demonstrated. They showed that this affect served to increase knee flexion during the first part of the swing, and later to facilitate knee extension, playing a substantial role in knee extension during the latter phase of the swing motion. Wood et al.[106] simulated variations in the forward swing of the recovery phase so that recovery time was reduced. They suggested that attempts to increase sprinting speed by reducing the recovery time increased the vulnerability of the hamstring muscle groups to injury.

D. Electromyography

RJM patterns provide limited insights to the involvement of individual muscles in running. To this end a combination of RJM and electromyographic (EMG) data is important. Unfortunately, both sets of data are rarely presented together. A notable exception is the recent publication by Simonsen et al.[56] EMG data are generally reported as the time during which various lower extremity muscles are active or not active throughout the running gait cycle.[55,56,107-114] There is considerable variability in the relative durations and timing of the EMG bursts reported in these studies, due in part to the different methods employed to collect and report the data. Nilsson et al.[113] collected extensive EMG data for 10 subjects running over a range of speeds from 1.0 to 9.0 m/sec. Some irregularities in EMG patterns were found between subjects, particularly for the semitendinosus and semimembranosus muscles. There were also clear differences in both the relative duration and timing of the EMG bursts between running speeds. Nonetheless, the authors felt that the pattern of EMG activity was relatively consistent between subjects and did not change its basic structure over the range of running speeds tested. Simonsen et al.[56] demonstrated distinct differences between subjects in the EMG patterns for the rectus femoris and vasti muscles, but consistent patterns for other lower extremity muscles. In contrast, MacIntyre and Robertson[111] found considerable variability between subjects for gastrocnemius, hamstring, and soleus activity patterns, while the patterns for the vasti muscles were more consistent.

The variability reported in EMG data makes it difficult to summarize the data graphically. Therefore, data from several sources have been presented separately in Figure 2. It is possible to use these data to show how individual muscles contribute to the RJMs, although temporal comparisons between EMG and RJM data are complicated by the delay between the onset of detectable EMG and effective mechanical force, and the cessation of EMG and complete relaxation of the muscle.[56] The following discussion is based on the data presented in Figure 2.

1. Hip Musculature

The phase of dominant hip flexor moment during swing is associated with activity in the rectus femoris. Simonsen et al.[56] found the rectus femoris to be active only during the first part of the hip flexor phase. It is likely that other hip flexors for which EMG data have yet to be collected may contribute substantially to this moment.

The phase of hip extensor RJM during the latter part of swing and the first part of stance roughly coincides with EMG activity in the hamstrings and gluteus maximus, although Nilsson et al.[113] showed that the gluteus maximus tended to be inactive during most of the swing phase for slower running speeds. The final phase of stance is characterized by a hip flexor moment. The rectus femoris was generally found to be inactive during this time, although Simonsen et al.[56] recorded some activity in this muscle for one of their two subjects. These authors considered the hip adductors and iliopsoas to be the more likely prime movers in this instance, but no EMG data were collected for these muscles.

2. Knee Musculature

The dominant knee extensor moment during the first part of the swing phase appears to be caused primarily by the rectus femoris. Activity is generally not seen in the vasti muscles during this phase. When present, it occurs during the final part of the phase, and generally for higher running speeds only. During the phase of knee flexor dominance (latter part of swing and initial part of stance) the hamstrings are generally active. Activity in these muscles lasts much longer during stance than does the knee flexor RJM because these muscles must also serve as hip extensors. Bursts of gastrocnemius activity, although quite variable, are generally found at the end of the swing and throughout the first $^2/_3$ of stance.

Most of the stance phase is dominated by a knee extensor moment. The quadriceps are active for the first half of this phase only, thus, it is not clear how the knee extensor moment is sustained during the latter part of stance. Simonsen et al.[56] suggested that as the knee approached full extension, the gastrocnemius and hamstrings may have paradoxical actions at the knee, acting as knee extensors instead of knee flexors. This could explain why hamstring activity is typically seen during the latter part of stance when there is a dominant knee extensor and hip flexor moment.

3. Ankle Musculature

The ankle RJM is very small during swing. Both the gastrocnemius and soleus are active during most of the swing, but the reported EMG patterns for these muscles are quite variable. The stance phase is dominated by a plantar flexor RJM, and contractions of the gastrocnemius and soleus quite clearly cause this moment. Towards the end of stance, the magnitude of this moment decreases considerably and reverses to a dorsiflexor moment. Activity in the soleus and gastrocnemius generally ceases, while in some studies[55,113] the tibialis anterior becomes active. Despite the importance which is generally attached to the propulsive role of the ankle flexors, it is interesting that in general, there does not appear to be a conscious effort to extend the ankle actively for the completion of the stance phase.

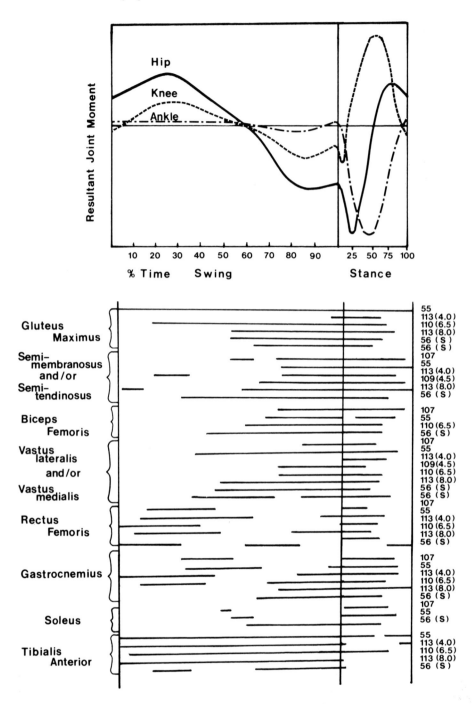

FIGURE 2.   The horizontal bars represent the times (% swing or % stance) during which EMG activity has been recorded. The unbracketed numbers on the right indicate the references from which the data were derived, while the bracketed numbers are the running speeds in m/sec and S refers to sprinting speed. The resultant joint moment data at the top of the diagram have been redrawn from Figure 1 where positive represents the direction of hip flexion, knee extension, and ankle dorsiflexion.

4. Co–contraction

EMG data give a clear indication of periods of co–contraction. During swing there is little evidence of cocontraction of the hip extensors and the hip flexors, while activity is generally seen in both sets of muscles just before foot strike and during stance. This is probably a result of the dual roles played by the hamstrings and rectus femoris at the hip and knee.[56] There is also little evidence of co–contraction of the knee flexors and extensors during swing, except just before foot strike. A notable exception to this is the activity in the vasti muscles which is present during most of the phase in which the knee RJM is in the direction of knee flexion and the hamstrings are active. It appears that the vasti muscles must be called upon to counterbalance partially the effect of the hamstrings at the knee. Throughout most of stance there is co–contraction between the knee flexors and extensors, resulting from the dual roles played by most of these muscles. Activity is generally found in the tibialis anterior during the first half of stance. It is not clear why this muscle should be active since the dominant ankle RJM is in the direction of plantar flexion when both the gastrocnemius and soleus are very active.

Evidence of co–contraction suggests that the roles played by muscles in running can be different than those revealed by RJM patterns alone. It also indicates that measures of muscular effort or work done by muscles based on RJM patterns alone, tend to cause these parameters to be underestimated. On the other hand, measures of muscular effort or work based on RJM patterns are overestimated because of the dual roles played by many of the lower extremity muscles. The dual roles of multijoint muscles appear to have important implications for the organization and coordination of movement. For example, during the early part of swing there is a dominant hip flexor and knee extensor RJM. The rectus femoris, which contributes to both moments, is active, while the vasti muscles are inactive.

E. Muscle Length Changes

Interpretation of muscular involvement is enhanced if EMG data are presented simultaneously with muscle length data as has been done by Frigo et al.[55] and Simonsen et al.[56] In each case, muscles were modeled as a series of straight and curved lines between points of origin and insertion. The lengths of these lines were then calculated as a function of the angle(s) of the joint(s) crossed by the muscles. Frigo et al.[55] showed that muscles were generally active when they were close to their anatomical lengths (i.e., the length of the muscle in a normal standing posture) and that mono–articular muscles work further from their anatomical lengths than multi–articular muscles. Measured as a percent of anatomical length, mono–articular muscles go through greater length changes during the course of one running cycle,[55] while in absolute terms, multi–articular muscles are submitted to larger variations in muscle length.[56] The significance of this has yet to be determined.

Muscle length and EMG data also indicate phases of concentric and eccentric contractions of individual muscles. This is particularly important for multijoint muscles where such information cannot be readily derived from RJM and joint angular velocity data alone. There are several instances where phases of concentric and eccentric RJMs do not coincide with phases of concentric and eccentric activity in the muscles contributing to these moments. (Note that RJMs are typically labeled concentric when they act in the same direction as the joint angular velocity, and eccentric when they act in the opposite direction to the joint angular velocity). First, the rectus femoris switches from eccentric to concentric contraction after approximately 20% of the swing phase.[55,56] The hip flexor RJM makes the same switch after less than 10% of the swing phase, while the knee extensor RJM remains eccentric (Figure 1). Second, the final 40% of the swing is marked by a concentric hip extensor moment and an eccentric knee flexor moment which switches to concentric during the last 5% of the swing phase (Figure 1). The hamstrings, which contribute to both the hip extensor and knee flexor moment, switch from eccentric to concentric during the last 15 to 20% of the swing,[55,56] while the gastrocnemius, which contributes to the knee flexor moment, contracts eccentrically throughout this phase.[56] Third, the concentric knee extensor moment during the latter half of stance coincides with eccentric rectus femoris activity.[56] While these comparisons are based on data which are rather scanty and derived from several sources, they do suggest that the labels ''concentric'' and ''eccentric'' attached to RJMs, should be interpreted with caution.

Muscle length and EMG data also indicate instances where concentric muscle activity is preceded immediately by eccentric muscle activity and thus the potential for storage and reutilization of elastic energy. This occurs during stance in the gastrocnemius[55] and the vasti and soleus muscles.[56,55] The hamstrings work eccentrically during most of the latter half of the swing phase and concentrically during the last 10 to 15% of the swing phase and the first half of the stance phase.[56] Eccentric - concentric phases occur in the rectus femoris during the initial part of the swing phase[55,56] and at the middle of the swing phase for the gluteus maximus.[55,56] In each instance the potential for storage and reutilization of elastic energy may lead to improvements in efficiency and economy of running. However, as indicated in a previous section of this paper, little is known of the extent to which this phenomenon actually occurs in running.

VI. PERFORMANCE IMPROVEMENT

When running is viewed as a competitive event, we are ultimately interested in how performance can be improved. Most of what we know about the differences between good and poor performance is based on descriptive kinematics and ground-reaction force data. These data have been reviewed extensively by Dillman[1] and Williams,[4] and will not be repeated here. In addition, both authors have carefully outlined the problems inherent in determining the factors which characterize good performance. Since the review of Williams,[4] there have been several attempts to determine which structural,[115] muscle strength or joint range of motion[116] and kinematic factors,[75,77] dictate superior performance. Factors found to be characteristic of better performance were (1) those considered to be associated with a reduction in the braking force applied to the foot at contact, namely a short distance between the foot and the total body center of gravity at touchdown,[75,77] an increase in the lower leg angular velocity in the backward direction at touchdown,[77] and an increase in the backward velocity of the foot relative to the forward velocity of the body center of gravity at touchdown;[77] and (2) those resulting in a shorter contact time and therefore a greater stride rate in sprinting,[77] including increased thigh angular velocity during support and decreased leg extension at toe-off.

Cavanagh et al.[117] compiled a series of structural, postural, kinematic, plantar force, and pressure data which they considered to have significant implications for performance, potential for understanding injury mechanisms, and shoe design of elite long-distance runners. Profiles of two elite athletes were presented, not with the intention of distinguishing those factors indicative of elite performance, but rather with the intent of establishing a framework for further studies. They considered that the undesirable features of distance running are those which could result in injury or increased energy cost, but they pointed out that it would be incorrect to convey the impression that these features could be recognized with great certainty at present.

There has been surprisingly little effort directed toward the more fundamental question of what causes differences in kinematic parameters which dictate running performance. To address this question muscle activity or RJM patterns must be examined. Cavanagh et al.[89] did not find significant differences between peak RJMs exerted at the hip or knee by two groups of distance runners categorized as elite and good, running at a speed of 3.8 m/s. There was considerable variability in the magnitudes of the RJMs exhibited by different

Table 1
DISTRIBUTION OF RUNNING
INJURIES BY ANATOMICAL
LOCATIONS

Injury site	Percent of total injuries		
	Clement[118]	James[119]	Maughan[120]
Knee	42	29	32
Leg[a]	28	24	23
Foot/ankle	18	7	25
Thigh	3	—	9
Hip	5	—	3
Other	4	40	8

[a] Includes achilles tendon.

runners. While this may reflect the degree of variability in muscle forces, it probably also reflects the inaccuracies of RJM magnitudes resulting from problems inherent in the elimination of noise from raw displacement data and the estimations of body segment parameters. Perhaps the value of comparing peak magnitudes of RJMs should be questioned. Alternative measures which may be less sensitive to measurement problems might be the work done by RJMs or the impulses of RJM-time functions.

Winter and White[7] presented a series of correlations of kinetic, temporal, and kinematic variables with the intention of finding out what kinetic parameters influenced speed of walking or jogging and what correlations existed between RJMs at different joints, particularly those spanned by multijoint muscles. This sort of analysis warrants serious consideration when addressing some of the more fundamental issues concerning performance in running at the elite level.

VII. RUNNING INJURIES

The worldwide fitness explosion of the 1970's and 1980's has been driven by a desire to improve personal fitness level. This in turn has challenged the previously unfit to exercise regularly, and many times the most convenient form of exercise has been running. One result of this trend has been a large mass of people, ill-prepared for the level of activity they attempt or perhaps not structurally suited for prolonged exposure to exercise, who inevitably suffer pain and injury. Consequently, the new challenge to the runner has meant new challenges to the professionals who treat these injuries as well as those who study the human body in an exercise state.

The final section of this paper is a review of recent publications from the areas of sports medicine and biomechanics which address issues relating to running injuries. We will attempt to examine how the research generated from these two areas has enhanced the understanding of injury mechanisms, and the treatment and rehabilitation of injuries.

A. Sports Medicine

In 1981, Clement and co-workers[118] reported on the injury profile of 1,650 runners who had been treated for over 1,800 injuries in their clinic. Their report identified the anatomical sites of injuries which most frequently required the runner to seek medical attention. Similar studies have been conducted by James et al.[119] on 180 patients and more recently by Maughan and Miller[120] who recorded 358 injuries sustained by 287 athletes training for a marathon. The findings of these studies are summarized in Table 1. There has been some grouping of areas to ease the comparison of the three studies. There is general agreement that the knee is the single most frequently reported site of pain requiring medical attention or interfering with regular training programs. Of interest is the fact that of all the athletes surveyed by Maughan and Miller[120] who reported injuries, only 19% sought medical attention. Approximately 26% sought nonmedical attention, while the majority (55%) of the people sought no help at all even though the injury had affected their training program.

The frequency and type of injuries sustained during different competitions have also been reported. Hutson[121] recorded the injuries occurring during an ultramarathon where competitors attempted to travel as far as possible in a 6-day period around an oval track. The majority of injuries occurred in the foot and ankle region and many were soft tissue in nature.

1. Patello-femoral Syndrome

Pain located in the anterior aspect of the knee has consistently been reported with the highest frequency in most running-injury studies. Clinically, it appears that the majority of the cases are diagnosed as chondromalacia patella (CMP).[118] The clinical signs associated with CMP are pain, crepitus, and swelling during activities in which the patello-femoral forces are increased. In running, the phases of greatest knee extensor moment and therefore patello-femoral forces occur during stance phase (Figure 1). EMG data from most studies indicate activity in the knee extensors commencing prior to heel strike and continuing well into midstance (Figure 2). Therefore, one could expect the patello-femoral joint to be undergoing compressive and shear forces during this time.

An association has been made between the kinematics of both the tibio-femoral and the patello-femoral joint and the function of the foot and ankle.[119] In particular, it is speculated that mechanical abnormalities of the limb such as excessive pronation of the hindfoot contribute to a greater amount of internal rotation of the tibia.[118] This results in a lateral shifting of the patella relative to the femur which leads to higher magnitudes of forces under the lateral facet of the patella. This increase in force presumably contributes to a breakdown in the underlying articular cartilage.

Clinically the treatment of CMP has varied from modified activity to complete rest, control of inflammation and, where deemed necessary, the use of orthotics. Of all of the treatment modalities in use, orthotics would appear to be the only one which has an influence on lower limb alignment, yet the literature available concerning this influence is rather sparse. Smart and Robertson[122] and Taunton et al.[123] used electrogoniometers to examine the motion at the knee joint for treadmill running with and without orthotics. Smart and Robertson[122] reported slight, but nonsignificant decreases in maximum knee flexion and internal rotation of the tibia and a significant increase in maximum knee valgus when the subjects used orthotics. Taunton et al.[123] measured the same variables plus temporal information concerning the time to reach these maximum values and found no significant difference in any of the variables except in the total time during which internal rotation of the tibia occurred.

Therefore, it would seem that the scientific literature does not completely support the clinical assumptions about the biomechanical events which are occurring. However, it may be that the magnitudes of changes required to alter the biomechanical pattern in this case are so small that they are being masked by variability in the measurement techniques. Furthermore, electrogoniometers cannot provide information concerning movement of the patella.

Lafortune and Cavanagh[124] attempted to measure movement of the patella during normal walking by monitoring the motion of intracortical pins inserted into the patella, femur, and tibia of three subjects. Their data, which can be considered to be free of skin motion, demonstrated very small lateral shifts in the patella relative to the femur from its position at heel strike. An estimate of this movement would be in the range of 5 to 6 mm during stance. This magnitude of movement would be difficult to detect with noninvasive cinematographic techniques which must contend with positioning error and skin motion. While this study provides valuable information concerning the kinematics of the knee joint in walking, the technique may not be feasible in more dynamic activities such as running.[125]

2. Achilles Tendinitis

The most common injury in the foot and ankle region is achilles tendinitis accounting for 6 to 11% of all running injuries.[118-120] One proposed mechanism of achilles tendon injury is believed to be associated with an excessive pronation of the hindfoot as the runner moves from heel strike to midstance and toe-off.[119,126] Excessive pronation is thought to produce a bowstring effect of the tendon which increases the stress in the midtendon area. Consequently, this injury is typically treated with orthotics to reduce the excessive pronation of the foot.

Clement et al.[126] reported on the treatment of 109 patients with diagnosed achilles tendinitis over a 2-year period. The treatment regime included exercise for the triceps surae group, control of inflammation and pain, and lastly, the use of orthotics when deemed necessary. They reported a frequency of 67% excellent, 11% good, 21% incomplete, and 1% fair results. Therefore, they suggested this formed an effective treatment regime for achilles tendinitis.

A second proposed mechanism of achilles tendinitis is based on muscle function during the early stance phase of running. It has been suggested by Smart et al.[127] that during this phase, the triceps surae muscles undergo rapid shortening as the foot is plantar flexed, lengthen as the tibia rotates forward over the foot, then shorten again during the forward propulsion phase. During the brief interval of time in which the muscle changes from concentric to eccentric and from eccentric to concentric contraction, the muscle forces may be of sufficient magnitude to cause microtrauma to the tendon.

The limited muscle length and EMG data available[55,56] confirm these clinical observations at least in part. The data of Frigo et al.[55] suggest that the gastrocnemius and soleus go through a rapid lengthening followed by a rapid shortening phase during the early part of stance, while both muscles are active. Simonsen et al.[56] presented similar data for the soleus, but found that the gastrocnemius contracted isometrically during the stance phase of sprinting. Neither study showed an initial shortening phase at the beginning of stance.

Motivated by this proposed mechanism of achilles tendinitis, some clinicians have attempted to treat the injury with heel pads to shorten the achilles tendon during the initial part of stance. Lowden et al.[128] evaluated the effectiveness of heel pads in patients with achilles tendinitis on the basis of a subjective assessment of pain, tenderness, and swelling as well as certain characteristics of the ground-reaction force recorded during normal walking. The parameters chosen were the two peak-force values during the support phase of walking and the total time of foot contact. Their patients were randomly divided into three groups two of which received different heel pads and a third which was not given heel pads. All groups received stretching and strengthening exercises and ultrasound treatments. Remarkably, they reported significant pre- and posttreatment differences in both the subjective and objective measures in all groups, suggesting that heel pads may not be of any greater benefit than exercise and anti-inflammatory programs.

Clinical evidence points to possible mechanisms of achilles tendon injury, but there is insufficient information on muscle-length time histories or muscle force-time histories to verify either of these two mechanisms. The two differing views on the mechanism of achilles tendinitis may stem from the fact that attention has been focused on either the frontal or sagittal plane, whereas a true three-dimensional analysis may be more appropriate.

3. Hamstring Strains

Runners, and particularly sprinters, will often suffer from hamstring strains.[129] The etiology, prevention, and treatment of this injury has recently been reviewed by Agre.[129] He compiled a list of nine etiological factors related to hamstring injuries which were all concerned with either the strength or flexibility of the hamstrings or poor running style. He pointed out, however, that poor running style was not well defined in this context. There is some suggestion that the hamstrings are most susceptible to injury towards the end of the swing phase when the muscles are elongated and change suddenly from concentric to eccentric contraction.[129] Although the data by Frigo et al.[55] and Simonsen et al.[56] show that the hamstrings reach their maximum length (which exceeds the anatomical length of the muscle[55]) approximately 80 to 85% through the swing phase (at which time they switch from concentric to eccentric activity), we have yet to discover where in the running cycle the hamstring musculotendinous unit is most vulnerable to injury.[129]

B. Biomechanical Measurement and Injuries

There have been a number of measurement techniques employed to study injury mechanisms and to identify running patterns which may predispose an individual to injury. The techniques used, either alone or in combination, include force platforms, pressure transducers, cinematography, accelerometry, and electrogoniometry. Cinematography will not be reviewed as a section in this paper because a recent paper by Williams[4] has already provided an extensive review of the area and readers are directed to this work.

1. Force Platform Data

The overwhelming majority of running injuries occur in the lower extremity distal to the knee. This fact has been the main reason for the volume of work which has been done to study the events which occur at the ground-foot interface. Many of the early investigations of ground-reaction force data in running were conducted to establish norms for these parameters. Cavanagh and Lafortune[130] noted that not all runners while running at the same velocity (4.12 to 4.87 m/s) produced similar ground-reaction force (GRF) patterns. They observed a continuum of center of pressure and GRF patterns which they used to categorize runners as heel, midfoot and forefoot (metatarsal) strikers. As they stated, this finding greatly affects the image of a "normal" foot strike from which individual comparisons are made, and has clear implications for the design of running shoes. Equally important it also affects the way one should relate an individual running style to possible injury mechanisms. Intuitively, we may infer that the functional role of muscles and the predisposition of musculotendinous units to injury will probably be different in each of the foot strike types.

Bates et al.[131] selected 30 criterion measures of the vertical and mediolateral GRF curves to assess the variability of these force patterns within and between five runners under ten shod conditions. They found that in order to obtain stable information within a condition for one subject it was necessary to analyze a minimum of 6 to 7 trials depending on the measurement variable and that 10 trials were necessary in order to generate a 95% confidence interval for a particular subject and condition.

These investigators also showed that different subjects responded differently to various types of shoes. Using a rank scoring system on the force measures for each subject and grouping the rank scores by subjects, they clearly demonstrated that no one shoe was most effective in absorbing shock and providing mediolateral control and stability for all five of the runners tested. It remains to be seen whether anatomical and functional parameters might account for these findings.

GRF and center of pressure patterns are specific to conditions of running speed, footwear, ground surface, and gradient.[130] The first two factors have been addressed in a number of recent studies. Hamill et al.[132] examined the changes which occurred to the GRF-time histories during the stance phase of running at different speeds. They limited their study to those subjects who performed a heel-toe running gait over the speeds of 4 to 7 m/s. The vertical GRF patterns were normalized in both time (% total time) and amplitude (% body weight) for intersubject comparisons. The relative magnitudes of the heel-impact portion of the curve increased as the speed of running increased. While the propulsive peak remained the same, the impulse- and average-force values increased significantly with running speed as one would expect.

In the anterior-posterior direction (plane of progression) the relative amplitude of the normalized peak-braking force and the propulsive force both increased significantly as the speed of running increased. The general shape of the force patterns in the mediolateral direction for the first 30% of stance changed phase (positive to negative) between the two slow speeds (4 and 5 m/s) and the two fast speeds (6 and 7 m/s), while the patterns for the remaining portion of the curve were very similar.

Nigg[133] has suggested that it is reasonable to consider the typical GRF curve as a composite of two activities for the runner. The first portion of the curve was originally called the "passive" loading phase, while the second portion was considered the "active" phase. This nomenclature has subsequently been altered to "impact" and "active", respectively. The impact portion of the curve is associated with the initial foot-contact and has been shown to be affected by running speed, surface, running style, and probably fatigue. The active portion is reflective of changes in the muscular activity of the individual during midstance and propulsion. Nigg[134] has recently edited a book on the biomechanics of running shoes, in which he elaborates on his views about how loads acting on the body have the potential to produce adaptive biological changes in the individual.

Clarke et al.[135] compared the effects that varying the midsole hardness had on seven parameters of the vertical GRF for a running speed of 4.5 m/sec. Significant differences were found in the time between the two peaks normally found in heel-strike runners, the local minimum force value seen between the impact peak and the propulsive peak force. No difference was observed in the magnitude of the impact peak, the total contact, time and the total impulse. These authors attributed these findings to the mechanical response of the different midsole materials as well as an adaptive response of the runners.

Lees and McCulloch[136] compared running shoes with and without heel inserts for two heel-toe runners and, like Bates et al,[131] found a marked subject-by-condition interaction. In general, they found that the rate of force application during the heel-impact portion of the curve was affected by the use of inserts more than the peak-force values.

Snel et al.[137] examined three characteristics of the heel-impact portion of the vertical GRF in ten trained runners at a speed of 4 m/sec. They reported no significant differences among ten running conditions (nine shoe types and barefoot) in the peak-force value (expressed as a percent of body weight). The time to these peak values and therefore the average rate of force application showed a greater sensitivity to changes in footwear conditions. All three parameters correlated poorly with mechanical testing of the shoes which had been performed independently. This strongly points to the need for research to rely on biomechanical as opposed to mechanical tests of running shoes.

In summary, it has been demonstrated that differences in footfall patterns and running speed are reflected in the general shape of the GRF curves. It appears that in order to assess a subject adequately by shoe condition, a minimum of eight trials should be used and preferably ten trials in order to obtain representative data for the particular set of trials. Although variations in GRF patterns are evident for different shoe types, midsole hardness and heel lifts, these changes are not necessarily consistent across subjects. This suggests that there are many factors which are acting to alter the gait patterns chosen which in turn affect characteristics of the GRF curves.

2. Pressure Transducer Data

A different approach to the measurement of the foot-shoe-ground interaction is to attach pressure transducers or miniature force transducers to various aspects of the foot or shoe sole. The feasibility and usefulness of this approach in walking and running has been addressed in a number of instances.[138-141] The rationale for this approach is to provide a more detailed description of the force distribution (pressure) across areas of the foot which are actually in contact with the ground or shoe insole during stance.

Scranton et al.[141] used a liquid crystal plate and cinematography to describe the temporal characteristics of the foot-floor contact during walking, jogging, and running. They were able to demonstrate changes in force distribution patterns as individuals progressed from one mode of locomotion to another. However, they were not able to quantify their measures. Cavanagh and Ae[138] accomplished the latter using a commercial device known as the Footprint®. With the aid of high-speed cinematography, force magnitudes were quantified by measuring diameters of circular patterns produced by 500 individual transducer elements. Although considered to be reasonably accurate, this technique proved to be rather labor-intensive.

Hennig et al.[140] developed a piezoelectric method of measuring the vertical stress beneath the foot for which the manual labor involved was considerably reduced. This device has many potential applications in bridging the gap between the scientific and orthopedic domains regarding foot function and injury potential in running. However, it remains to be seen whether this device will gain widespread clinical use.

3. Electrogoniometer Data

As mentioned previously, control of the calcaneous during the stance phase has been implicated in a variety of running-related injuries. Smart and Robertson[122] used electrogoniometers to measure knee and ankle kinematics during treadmill running (average speed of 4.5 m/sec) on groups of runners with and without rigid orthotics. They found that orthotics significantly reduced foot eversion, and increased the knee valgus angle, but did not affect the amount of knee flexion or internal rotation. Taunton et al.[123] reported similar findings for subjects running at 80, 90, and 100% of their best speed of a 10 km run. The results of these studies regarding ankle pronation and supination are in agreement with those in which cinematography was employed to examine the effects of rigid orthotics in running.[4] It is likely that electrogoniometry could be more favorably accepted than cinematography in the clinical setting where facilities for the latter are generally limited.

4. Accelerometer Data

The use of lightweight accelerometers has attracted the attention of researchers for a number of years. Early attempts were made by Morris[142] and Smidt et al.[143] to use accelerometers in the analysis of walking. The initial attraction of these devices was their lightweight, ease of attachment, and on-line signal capabilities. However, their usefulness was limited by the number of transducers necessary to account for their orientation in space. A renewed interest in the use of accelerometers in running research has been directed towards the measurement of the "shock" transmitted along the leg during foot strike. The principle advantages of accelerometry in this case (in addition to the factors already mentioned) is its capability to measure consecutive foot impacts and to be used in treadmill running, both of which are major limitations of the force platform as a measuring device. The limitation of the orientation of the accelerometer is not a problem because the measure of interest is usually relative to the subject's tibia and not to an external reference system per se.

Nigg[133] presented a typical example of a GRF curve and an accelerometer signal collected simultaneously as a subject ran across a force plate. He pointed out that the shapes of the two curves were similar during the initial impact peak. While this might be taken as an indication that the curves are related measurements of the same mechanical event at foot impact, other data have suggested that the two techniques do not always lead to the same results with regard to shoe cushioning. Clarke et al.[144] mounted an acclerometer on the distal-medial surface of the tibia and had a subject run across a force platform at 3.8 m/sec. Five shoe conditions and one barefoot condition were tested. They found a significant difference in both the peak tibial accelerations and the peak vertical ground forces when barefoot running was compared with running in shoes. However, the relative magnitudes of the two measures were not the same within the shoe trials.

Clarke et al.[145] examined the effect of stride rate on leg acceleration at impact. The subjects ran on a treadmill at 3.8 m/sec at five different stride-rates: normal, ± 5% normal, and ± 10% normal. The data were normalized to the peak acceleration found within each subject while running with a "normal" stride rate. They showed that the peak acceleration values increased for the slower stride rates and decreased for the higher stride rates from the normal value.

From an injury perspective, ground-reaction force and/or tibial acceleration data are important in that they provide some indication of the loads sustained by the joints of the lower extremity during running. With known ground-reaction force and segment-kinematic data, forces acting at articulating surfaces can be derived if certain assumptions concerning the distribution of force across all muscles and ligaments surrounding the joint are made. Burdett[146] used this technique to quantify the bony contact force at the ankle for three subjects running at 4.5 m/s. He reported maximum compressive loads of over 12 times body weight during midstance. Denoth[147] showed how the joint forces could be estimated during the foot-impact phase of running from measured shank-acceleration values and a variable called "effective mass". This variable is difficult to grasp conceptually, but is reportedly a function of the body segment masses, the initial conditions at foot strike (particularly the knee angle) and the characteristics of the ground surface (which affect the loading rate).[147] Muscles acting as force generators are ignored when joint forces are measured by this technique and it is recognized that the estimated joint forces will generally be smaller than the real values.[147] Impact loads between 1.0 and 5.3 times body weight for the ankle and 1.6 times body weight for the knee have been reported for various running conditions.[133]

While it is possible to debate the merits of force platform vs. accelerometer measurement techniques, it is clear that either one used in isolation will not provide information regarding joint, ligament, or tendon forces which presumably are necessary in order to relate running mechanics to injuries and injury mechanisms. Consequently, there is a need to combine this information with techniques such as cinematography to measure the kinematic parameters of the runner.

VIII. SUMMARY

If we examine the spectrum of runners from the weekend jogger to the elite sprinter, we find that each faces distinctly different task objectives and meets these objectives in different ways. Each performer must work within his or her inherent physical capabilities. These include biomechanical factors such as muscular strength, joint range of motion, or tissue tolerance; physiological factors related to metabolic processes; and neuromuscular factors related to motor control and mechanical properties of muscle. Of equal importance, the performer also has the capability to adapt, and with repeated performances, adaptations most certainly take place in all of these factors. Presumably performers attempt to optimize each of the functions and their interactions.

The literature reviewed to date shows that we have diligently worked to enhance our ability to measure and describe motion. However, it appears that we have been hampered in our attempts to understand the process of adaptation toward optimal performance by focusing our attention on reasonably skilled runners. By directing our attention towards a broader range of running abilities we may better be able to address some of the fundamental issues concerning the mechanics of running.

REFERENCES

1. **Dillman, C. J.,** Kinematic analysis of running, in *Exercise and Sport Science Reviews,* Vol. 3, Wilmore, J. H. and Keogh, J. F., Eds., Academic Press, New York, 1975, 193.
2. **Miller, D. I.,** Biomechanics of running — What should the future hold?, *Can. J. Appl. Sports Sci.* 3, 229, 1978.
3. **Vaughan, C. L.,** Biomechanics of running gait, *CRC Crit. Rev. Biomed. Eng.,* 12, 1, 1984.
4. **Williams, K. R.,** Biomechanics of running, in *Exercise and Sport Science Reviews,* Vol. 13, Terjung, R. L., Eds., MacMillan New York, 1985, 389.
5. **Frederick, E. C.,** Synthesis, experimentation, and the biomechanics of economical movement, *Medicine and Science in Sports and Exercise,* 17, 44, 1984.
6. **Miller, D. I.,** Signs of the times in sport biomechanics, in *Sport Biomechanics,* Terauds, J., Barthels, K., Kreighbaum, E., Mann, R., and Crakes, J., Eds., Academic Publishers, Del Mar, 1984, 1.
7. **Winter, D. A. and White, S.,** Cause-effect correlation of variable of gait, presented at 10th Congr. Intl. Soc. Biomech. Umea, June 15 to 20, 1985, 294.
8. **Bernstein, N.,** Biodynamics of locomotion, in *Human Motor Actions: Berstein Reassessed,* Whiting, H. T. A., Ed., Elsevier, Amsterdam, 1984. 171.
9. **Elftman, H.,** The work done by muscles in running, *Am. J. Physiol.,* 129, 672, 1940.
10. **Fenn, W. O.,** Frictional and kinetic factors in the work of sprint running, *Am. J. Physiol.,* 92, 583, 1930.
11. **Hill, A. V.,** The air-resistance to a runner, *Proc. R. Soc. London,* B718, 380, 1927.
12. **Norman, R. W.,** Biomechanics: are there substantive issues? *Human Locomotion,* III, Canadian Society for Biomechanics, 1984, 9.
13. **McMahon, T. A.,** in *Muscles, Reflexes, and Locomotion,* Princeton University Press, Princeton, New Jersey, 1984.
14. **Cavanagh, P. R. and Kram, R.,** The efficiency of human movement — a statement of the problem, *Medicine and Sciences in Sports and Exercise,* 17, 304, 1985.
15. **Williams, K. R.,** The relationship between mechanical and physiological energy estimates, *Medicine and Science in Sports and Exercise,* 17, 317, 1985.
16. **Matsuo, A. and Fukunaga, T.,** The effect of age and sex on external mechanical energy in running, in *Biomechanics VIII - B,* Matsui, H. and Kobayashi, K., Eds., Human Kinetics Publishers, Champaign, Ill., 1983, 676.
17. **Matsuo, A., Fukunaga, T., and Asami, T.,** Relationship between external work and running performance in athletes, in *Biomechanics IX - B,* Winter, D. A., Norman, R. W., Wells, R. P., Hayes, K. C., and Patla, A. E., Eds., Human Kinetic Publishers, Champaign, Ill., 1985, 319.
18. **Margaria, R., Cerretelli, P., Aghemo, P., and Sassi, G.,** Energy cost of running, *J. Appl. Physiol.,* 18, 367, 1963.
19. **Cavagna, G. A. and Kaneko, M.,** Mechanical work and efficiency in level walking and running, *J. Physiol.,* 268, 467, 1977.
20. **Cavagna, G. A., Komarek, L., and Mazzoleni, S.,** The mechanics of sprint running, *J. Physiol.,* 217, 709, 1971.
21. **Cavagna, G. A., Saibene, F. P., and Margaria, R.,** Mechanical work in running, *J. Appl. Physiol.,* 19, 249, 1964.
22. **Cavagna, G. A., Thys, H., and Zamboni, A.,** The sources of external work in level walking and running, *J. Physiol.,* 262, 639, 1976.
23. **Fukunaga, T., Matsuo, A., and Ichikawa, M.,** Mechanical energy and joint movements in sprint running, *Ergonomics,* 24, 765, 1981.
24. **Fukunaga, T., Matsuo, A., Yuasa, K., Fujimatsu, H., and Asahina, K.,** Effect of running velocity on external mechanical power output, *Ergonomics,* 23, 123, 1980.
25. **Saito, M., Ohkuwa, T., Ikegami, Y., and Miyamura, M.,** Comparison of sprint running in the trained and untrained runners with respect to chemical and mechanical energy, in *Biomechanics VIII-B,* Matsui, H. and Kobayashi, K., Eds., Human Kinetic Publishers, Champaign, Ill., 1983, 963.
26. **Winter, D. A.,** A new definition of mechanical work done in human movement, *J. Appl. Physiol.,* 46, 79, 1979.
27. **Fenn, W. O.,** Work against gravity and work due to velocity changes in running, *Am. J. Physiol.,* 93, 433, 1930.
28. **Kaneko, M., Fuchimoto, T., Ito, A.,and Toyooka, J.,** Mechanical efficiency of sprinters and distance runners during constant speed running, in *Biomechanics VIII-B,* Matsui, H., and Kobayashi, K., Eds., Human Kinetic Publishers, Champaign, Ill, 1983, 754.
29. **Kaneko, M., Ito, A., Fuchimoto, T., and Toyooka, J.,** Mechanical work and efficiency of young distance runners during level running, in *Biomechanics VII-B,* Morecki, A., Fidelus, K., Kedzior, K., and Wit, A., Eds., University Park Press, Baltimore, Md., 1981, 234.

30. **Kaneko, M., Ito, A., Fuchimoto, T., Shishikura, Y., and Toyooka, J.,** Influence of running speed on the mechanical efficiency of sprinters and distance runners, in *Biomechanics IX-B,* Winter, D. A., Norman, R. W., Wells, R. P., Hayes, K. C., and Patla, A. E., Eds., Human Kinetic Publishers, Champaign, Ill., 1985, 307.

31. **Kaneko, M., Matsumoto, M., Ito, A., and Fuchimoto, T.,** Optimum step frequency in constant speed level running, presented at the 10th *Intl. Congr. Biomech.* Umeå, Sweden, June 15 to 20, 1985, 136.

32. **Ward-Smith, A. J.,** A mathematical theory of running, based on the first law of thermodynamics, and its application to the performance of world-class athletes, *J. Biomech.,* 18, 337, 1985.

33. **Ward-Smith, A. J.,** Air resistance and its influence on the biomechanics and energetics of sprinting at sea level and at altitude, *J. Biomech.,* 17, 339, 1984.

34. **Aleshinsky, S. Y.,** An energy "sources" and "fractions" approach to the mechanical energy expenditure problem. Part 2. Movement of the multi-link chain model, *J. Biochem.,* 19, 295, 1986.

35. **Crowninshield, R. D. and Brand, R. A.,** The prediction of forces in joint structures: distribution of intersegmental resultants, in *Exercise and Sport Science Reviews,* Vol. 9, Miller, D. I., Ed., The Franklin Institute Press, Philadelphia, 1981, 159.

36. **Winter, D. A.,** Moments of force and mechanical power in jogging, *J. Biomech.,* 16, 91, 1983.

37. **Lin, D. C. and Dillman, C. J.,** Optimal stride length in running, in *Biomechanics in Sport,* Terauds, J., Ed., Academic Press, Del Mar, 1982, 317.

38. **Andrews, J. G.,** Biomechanical measures of muscular effort, *Medicine and Science in Sports and Exercise,* 15, 199, 1983.

39. **Wells, D. A.,** *Lagrangian Dynamics,* McGraw-Hill, New York, 1967.

40. **Onyshko, S. and Winter, D. A.,** A mathematical model for the dynamics of human locomotion, *J. Biomech.* 13, 361, 1980.

41. **Shorten, M. R., Wootton, S. A., and Williams, C.,** Mechanical energy changes and the oxygen cost of running, *Eng. Med.,* 10, 213, 1981.

42. **Williams, K. R. and Cavanagh, P. R.,** A model for the calculation of mechanical power during running, *J. Biomech.,* 16, 115, 1983.

43. **Luhtanen, P. and Komi, P. V.,** Mechanical energy states during running, *Eur. J. Appl. Physiol.,* 38, 41, 1978.

44. **Norman, R. W., Sharratt, M. T., Pezzack, J. C., and Noble, E. G.,** Re-examination of the mechanical efficiency of horizontal treadmill running, in *Biomechanics V-B,* Komi, P. V., Ed., University Park Press, Baltimore, Md., 1976, 87.

45. **Shorten, M. R.,** Mechanical energy changes and elastic energy storage during treadmill running, in *Biomechanics IX-B,* Winter, D. A., Norman, R. W., Wells, R. P., Hayes, K. C., and Patla, A. E., Eds., Human Kinetic Publishers, Champaign, Ill, 1985, 313.

46. **Gregor, R. J. and Kirkendall, D.,** Performance efficiency of world class female marathon runners, in *Biomechanics VI-B,* Asmussen, E. and Jorgensen, K., Eds., University Park Press, Baltimore, Md., 1978, 40.

47. **Sakurai, S. and Miyashita, M.,** Mechanical energy changes during treadmill running, *Medicine and Science in Sports and Exercise,* 17, 148, 1985.

48. **Ito, A., Komi, P. V., Sjodin, B., Bosco, C., and Karlsson, J.,** Mechanical efficiency of positive work in running at different speeds, *Medicine and Science in Sports and Exercise,* 15, 299, 1983.

49. **Chapman, A. E., Caldwell, G. E., and Lonergan, R. M.,** Mechanical energy and the preferred style of running, presented at 10th Intl. Congr. Biomech. Umeå, Sweden, June 15-20, 1985, 42.

50. **Ostrowska, E. and Opaszowski, B.,** Mechanical power and efficiency of distance runners in 1000m run, presented at the 10th Intl. Congr. Biomech. Umeå, Sweden June 15 to 20, 1985, 210.

51. **Van Ingen Schenau, G. J.,** Some fundamental aspects of the biomechanics of overground versus treadmill locomotion, *Medicine and Science in Sports and Exercise,* 12, 257, 1980.

52. **Martin, P. E.,** A biomechanical and physiological evaluation of the effect of lower extremity loading on running performance, Unpublished Doctoral Dissertation, Pennsylvania State University, 1983.

53. **Pugh, L. G. C. E.,** The influence of wind resistance in running and walking and the mechanical efficiency of work against horizontal or vertical forces, *J. Physiol.,* 213, 255, 1971.

54. **Aleshinsky, S. Y.,** An energy "sources" and "fractions" approach to the mechanical energy expenditure problem. Part 1. Basic concepts, description of the model, analysis of a one-link system movement, *J. Biochem.,* 19, 287, 1986.

55. **Frigo, C., Pedotti, A., and Santambrogio, G.,** A correlation between muscle length and EMG activities during running, in *Science in Athletics,* Terauds, J. and Dales, G. G., Eds., Academic Publishers, Del Mar, 1979, 61.

56. **Simonsen, E. B., Thomsen, L. and Klausen, K.,** Activity of mono- and biarticular leg muscles during sprint running, *Eur. J. Appl. Physiol.,* 54, 524, 1985.

57. **Cavanagh, P. R. and Kram, R.,** Mechanical and muscular factors affecting the efficiency of human movement, *Medicine and Science in Sports and Exercise,* 17, 326, 1985.

58. **Cavagna, G. A.,** Storage and utilization of elastic energy in skeletal muscle, in *Exercise and Sport Science Reviews,* Vol. 5, Hutton, R. S., Ed., Journal Publishing Affiliates, Santa Barbara, 1978, 89.

59. **Ito, A., Fuchimoto, T., and Kaneko, M.,** Quantitative analysis of EMG during various speeds of running, in *Biomechanics IX-B,* Winter, D. A., Norman, R. W., Wells, R. P., Hayes, K. C., and Patla, A. E., Eds., Human Kinetics Publishers, Champaign, Ill., 1985, 301.

60. **Chow, C. K. and Jacobson, D. H.,** Studies on human locomotion via optimal programming, *Mathematical Biosciences,* 10, 239, 1971.

61. **Lloyd, B. B. and Zacks, R. M.,** The mechanical efficiency of treadmill running against a horizontal impeding force, *J. Physiol.,* 223, 355, 1972.

62. **Zacks, R. M.,** The mechanical efficiencies of running and bicycling against a horizontal impeding force, *Intle. Zeitschr. Angewandte Physiol.,* 31, 249, 1973.

63. **Frederick, E. C.,** Measuring the effects of shoes and surfaces on the economy of locomotion, in *Biomechanical Aspects of Sport Shoes and Playing Surfaces,* Nigg, B. M. and Kerr, B. A., Eds., University Printing, Calgary, Canada, 1983, 93.

64. **Van Der Walt, W. H. and Wyndham, C. H.,** An equation for prediction of energy expenditure of walking and running, *J. Appl. Physiol.,* 34, 559, 1973.

65. **Frederick, E. C., Howley, E. T., and Powers, S. K.,** Lower O_2 costs while running in air cushion type shoes, *Medicine and Science in Sports and Exercise,* 12, 81, 1980.

66. **Cavanagh, P. R. and Williams, K. R.,** The effect of stride length variation on oxygen uptake during distance running, *Medicine and Science in Sports and Exercise,* 14, 30, 1982.

67. **Kram, R. and Cavanagh, P. R.,** Day to day variation in freely chosen running stride length, *Medicine and Science in Sports and Exercise,* 17, 237, 1985.

68. **Kram, R., Cavanagh, P. R. and Kerns, M. M.,** Stride length changes with fatigue in distance running, presented at the 10th Intl. Congr. Biomech., Umeå, Sweden, June 15 to 20, 1985, 149.

69. **Shanebrook, J. R. and Jaszczak, R. D.,** Aerodynamic drag analysis of runners, *Medicine and Science in Sports,* 8, 43, 1976.

70. **Pugh, L. G. C. E.,** Oxygen intake in track and treadmill running with observations on the effect of air resistance, *J. Physiol.,* 207, 823, 1970.

71. **Davies, C. T. M.,** Effects of wind assistance and resistance on the forward motion of a runner, *J. Appl. Physiol.,* 48, 702, 1980.

72. **Frohlich, C.,** Effect of wind and altitude on record performance in foot races, pole vault, and long jump, *Am. J. of Phys.,* 53, 726, 1985.

73. **Ward-Smith, A. J.,** A mathematical analysis of the influence of adverse and favourable winds on sprinting, *J. Biomech.,* 18, 351, 1985.

74. **Kyle, C. R.,** Reduction of wind resistance and power output of racing cyclists and runners travelling in groups, *Ergonomics,* 22, 387, 1979.

75. **Buchalew, D. P., Barlow, D. A., Fischer, J. W., and Richards, J. G.,** Biomechanical profile of elite women marathoners, *Intl. J. Sports Biomech.,* 1, 330, 1985.

76. **Chapman, A. E. and Caldwell, G. E.,** Factors determining changes in lower limb energy during swing in treadmill running, *J. Biomech.,* 16, 69, 1983.

77. **Mann, R. and Herman, J.,** Kinematic analysis of Olympic sprint performance: men's 200 meters, *Intl. J. Sports Biomech.,* 1, 151, 1985.

78. **Mann, R. and Sprague, P.,** A kinetic analysis of the ground leg during sprint running, *Research Quarterly for Exercise and Sport,* 51, 334, 1980.

79. **Mann, R. and Sprague, P.,** Kinetics of sprinting, in *Biomechanics in Sports,* Terauds, J., Eds., Academic Publishers, Del Mar, 1982, 305.

80. **Bates, B. T., Osternig, L. R., and Mason, B. R.,** Variations of velocity within the support phase of running, in *Science in Athletics,* Terauds, J. and Dales, G. G., Eds., Academic Publishers, Del Mar, 1979, 51.

81. **Hay, J. G.,** Biomechanics of the long jump — and some wider implications, presented at the 10t Intl. Congr. of Biomechanics, Umeå, Sweden, June 15 to 20, 1985.

82. **McMahon, T. A. and Greene, P. R.,** The influence of track compliance on running, *J. Biomech.,* 12, 893, 1979.

83. **Ae, M., Miyashita, K., Shibukawa, K., Yokoi, T., and Hashihara, Y.,** Body segment contributions during the support phase while running at different velocities, in *Biomechanics IX-B,* Winter, D. A., Norman, R. W., Wells, R. P., Hayes, K. C., and Patla, A. E., Eds., Human Kinetics Publishers, Champaign, Ill., 1985, 343.

84. **Hinrichs, R. N.,** Upper extremity function in running, Unpublished Doctoral Dissertation, Pennsylvania State University, 1982.

85. **Miller, D. I. and East, D. J.,** Kinematic and kinetic correlates of vertical jumping in women, in *Biomechanics V-B,* Komi, P. V., Ed., University Park Press, Baltimore, Md., 1976, 65.

86. **Miller, D. I.,** Body segment contributions to sport skill performance: Two contrasting approaches, *Research Quarterly for Exercise and Sport,* 51, 219, 1980.

87. **Ae, M., Miyashita, K., Yokoi, T., and Hashihara, Y.,** Mechanical powers and work done by the muscles of the lower limbs during running at different speeds, presented at the 10th Intl. Congr. Biomech., Umeå, June 15 to 20, 1985, 9.

88. **Baumann, W.,** On mechanical loads on the human body during sports activities, in *Biomechanics VII-B,* Morecki, A., Fidelus, K., Kedzior, K., and Wit, A., Eds., University Park Press, Baltimore, Md., 1981, 79.

89. **Cavanagh, P. R., Pollock, M. L., and Landa, J.,** A biomechanical comparison of elite and good distance runners, *Ann. N.Y. Acad. Sci.,* 301, 328, 1977.

90. **Chapman, A. E., Lonergan, R., and Caldwell, G. E.,** Kinetic sources of lower-limb angular displacement in the recovery phase of sprinting, *Medicine and Science in Sports and Exercise,* 16, 382, 1984.

91. **Dillman, C. J.,** A kinetic analysis of the recovery leg during sprint running, in *Selected Topics on Biomechanics,* Cooper, J. M., Ed., The Athletic Institute, Bloomington, 1971, 137.

92. **Hinrichs, R. N.,** A three-dimensional analysis of the net moments at the shoulder and elbow joints in running and their relationship to upper-extremity EMG activity, in *Biomechanics IX-B,* Winter, D. A., Norman, R. W., Wells, R. P., Hayes, K. C. and Patla, A. E., Eds., Human Kinetics Publishers, Champaign, Ill., 1985, 337.

93. **Mann, R. V.,** A kinetic analysis of sprinting, *Medicine and Science in Sports and Exercise,* 13, 325, 1981.

94. **Robertson, D. G. E.,** Functions of the leg muscles in running, presented at the 10th Intl. Congr. Biomech. Umeå, June 15 to 20, 1985, 230.

95. **Thorstensson, A., Nilsson, J., Carlson, H. and Zomlefer, M. R.,** Trunk movements in human locomotion, *Acta Physiol. Scand.,* 121, 9, 1984.

96. **Aleshinsky, S. Y.,** Energy approach to human performance evaluation, presented at the 9th Ann. Meet. Am. Soc. Biomech., Ann Arbor, Mich., October 2 to 4, 1985, 139.

97. **Robertson, D. G. E. and Winter, D. A.,** Mechanical energy generation, absorption and transfer amongst segments during walking, *J. Biomech.,* 13, 845, 1980.

98. **Chapman, A. E. and Caldwell, G. E.,** Kinetic limitations of maximal sprinting speed, *J. Biomech.,* 16, 79, 1983.

99. **Martin, P. E. and Cavanagh, P. R.,** Segmental interactions within the lower extremity during the recovery phase of running, *Medicine and Science in Sports and Exercise,* 17, 223, 1985.

100. **Aleshinsky, S. Y.,** An energy ''sources'' and ''fractions'' approach to the mechanical energy expenditure problem. Part 5. The mechanical energy expenditure reduction during motion of the multi-link system, *J. Biomech.,* 19, 311, 1986.

101. **Aleshinsky, S. Y.,** An energy ''sources'' and ''fractions'' approach to the mechanical energy expenditure problem. Part 4. Criticism of the concept of ''energy transfers within and between links'', *J. Biochem.,* 19, 307, 1986.

102. **Phillips, S. J., Roberts, E. M., and Huang, T. C.,** Quantification of intersegmental reactions during rapid swing motion, *J. Biomech.,* 16, 411, 1983.

103. **Bourassa, P. and Morel, Y.,** A mathematical model for computer simulation of human running, in *Biomechanics IX-B,* Winter, D. A., Norman, R. W., Wells, R. P., Hayes, K. C., Patla, A. E., Eds., Human Kinetics Publishers, Champaign, Ill., 1985, 325.

104. **Marshall, R. N., Jensen, R. K., and Wood, G. A.,** A general Newtonian simulation of an n-segment open chain model, *J. Biomech.,* 18, 359, 1985.

105. **Selbie, W. S. and Chapman, A. E.,** A mathematical simulation of human running, presented at the 10th Intl. Congr. Biomech., Umeå, Sweden, June 15 to 20, 1985, 42.

106. **Wood, G. A., Marshall, R. N., and Jennings, L. S.,.** Optimal requirements and injury propensity of lower limb mechanics in spring running, presented at the 10th Intl. Congr. of Biomech. Umeå, June 15 to 20, 1985, 297.

107. **Brandell, B. R.,** An analysis of muscle coordination in walking and running gaits, in *Biomechanics III,* Cerquiglini, S., Venerando, A., and Wartenweiler, J., Eds., University Park Press, Baltimore, Md., 1973, 278.

108. **Dietz, V., Schmidtbleicher, D., and Noth, J.,** Neuronal mechanisms of human locomotion, *J. Neurophysiol.,* 42, 1212, 1979.

109. **Hanon, P. R., Rasmussen, S. A., and DeRosa, C. P.,** Electromyographic patterns during level and inclined treadmill running and their relationship to step cycle measures, *Research Quarterly for Exercise and Sport,* 56, 334, 1985.

110. **Komi, P. V.,** Biomechanical features of running with special emphasis on load characteristics and mechanical efficiency, in *Biomechanical Aspects of Sport Shoes and Playing Surfaces,* Nigg, B. M. and Kerr, B. A., Eds., University Printing, Calgary, Canada, 1983, 123.

111. **MacIntyre, D. and Robertson, D. G. E.,** EMG profiles of the knee muscles during treadmill running, presented at the 10th Intl. Congr. Biomech., Umeå, Sweden, June 15 to 20, 1985, 167.

112. **Mann, R. A. and Hagy, J.,** Biomechanics of walking, running and sprinting, *Am. J Sports Medicine,* 8, 345, 1980.

113. **Nilsson, J., Thorstensson, A., and Halbertsma, J.,** Changes in leg movements and muscle activity with speed of locomotion and mode of progression in humans, *Acta Physiol. Scand.,* 123, 457, 1985.

114. **Schwab, G. H., Moynes, D. R., Jobe, F. W. and Perry, J.,** Lower extremity electromyographic analysis of running gait, *Clinical Orthopaedics,* 176, 166, 1983.

115. **Yokoi, T., Shibukawa, K., Ae, M., and Hashihara, Y.,** Effects of stature difference on sprint running motion, presented at the 10th Intl. Congr. Biomech. Umeå, Sweden, June 15 to 20, 1985, 305.

116. **Wiklander, J., Lysholm, M., and Lysholm, J.,** The correlation between running movements and muscle strength/joint mobility in the lower extremity, presented at the 10th Intl. Congr. Biomech. Umeå, June 15 to 20, 1985, 290.

117. **Cavanagh, P. R., Andrew, G. C., Kram, R., Rodgers, M. M., Sanderson, D. J. and Hennig, E. M.,** An approach to biomechanical profiling of elite distance runners, *Intl. J. Sports Biomechanics,* 1, 36, 1985.

118. **Clement, D. B., Taunton, J. E., Smart, G. W., and McNicol, K. L.,** A survey of overuse running injuries, *Physician and Sports Medicine,* 9, 47, 1981.

119. **James, S. L., Bates, B. T. and Osternig, L. R.,** Injuries to runners, *Am. J. Sports Medicine,* 6, 40, 1978.

120. **Maughan, R. J. and Miller, J. D. B.,** Incidence of training-related injuries among marathon runners, *Br. J. Sports Medicine,* 17, 162, 1983.

121. **Hutson, M. A.,** Medical implications of ultra marathon running: observations on a six day track race, *Br. J. Sports Medicine,* 18, 44, 1984.

122. **Smart, G. and Robertson, G.,** Triplanar electrogoniometer analysis of running gait, in *Biomechanics IX-B,* Winter, D. A., Norman, R. W., Wells, R. P., Hayes, K. C., and Patla, A. E., Eds., Human Kinetics Pubishers, Champaign, Ill., 1985, 144.

123. **Taunton, J. E., Clement, D. B., Smart, G. W., Wiley, J. P., and McNicol, K. L.,** A triplanar electrogoniometer investigation of running mechanics in runners with compensatory overpronation, *Can. J. Appl. Sports Sci,* 10, 104, 1985.

124. **Lafortune, M. A. and Cavanagh, P. R.,** The measurement of normal knee joint motion during walking using intracortical pins, in *Biomechanics Measurement in Orthopaedic Practice,* Whittle, M. and Harris, D., Eds., Clarendon Press, Oxford, 1985, 234.

125. **Lafortune, M. A., Cavanagh, P. R., Kalenak, A., Skinner, S. M., and Sommer, H. J., III,** The use of intra-cortical pins to measure the kinematics of the knee joint, *Human Locomotion II,* Canadian Society for Biomechanics, 1982, 40.

126. **Clement, D. B., Taunton, J. E., and Smart, G. W.,** Achilles tendinitis and peritendinitis: etiology and treatment, *Am. J. Sports Med.,* 12, 179, 1984.

127. **Smart, G. W., Taunton, J. E. and Clement, D. B.,** Achilles tendon disorders in runners — a review, *Medicine and Science in Sports and Exercise,* 12, 231, 1980.

128. **Lowdon, A., Bader, D. L., and Mowat, A. G.,** The effect of heel pads on the treatment of Achilles tendinitis: A double blind trial, *Am. J. Sports Medicine,* 12, 431, 1984.

129. **Agre, J. C.,** Hamstring injuries, proposed aetiological factors, prevention and treatment, *Sports Medicine,* 2, 21, 1985.

130. **Cavanagh, P. R. and Lafortune, M. A.,** Ground reaction forces in distance running, *J. Biomech.,* 13, 397, 1980.

131. **Bates, B. T., Osternig, L. R., Sawhill, J. A., and James, S. L.,** An assessment of subject variability, subject-shoe interaction, and the evaluation of running shoes using ground reaction force data, *J. Biomech.,* 16, 181, 1983.

132. **Hamill, J., Bates, B. T., Knutzen, K. M., and Sawhill, J. A.,** Variations in ground reaction force parameters at different running speeds, *Human Movement Science,* 2, 47, 1983.

133. **Nigg, B. M.,** Biomechanical aspects of running, in *Biomechanics of Running Shoes,* Nigg, B. M., Ed., Human Kinetics Publishers, Champaign, Ill., 1986, 1.

134. **Nigg, B. M.,** *Biomechanics of Running Shoes,* Human Kinetics Publishers, Champaign, Ill., 1986.

135. **Clarke, T. E., Frederick, E. C., and Cooper, L. B.,** Effect of shoe cushioning upon ground reaction forces in running, *Intl. J. Sports Medicine,* 4, 247, 1983.

136. **Lees, A. and McCulloch, P. J.,** A preliminary investigation into the shock absorbency of running shoes and shoe inserts, *Journal of Human Movement Studies,* 10, 95, 1984.

137. **Snel, J. G., Deleman, N. J., Heerkens, Y. F., and van Ingen Schenau, G. J.,** Shock-absorbing characteristics of running shoes during actual running, in *Biomechanics IX-B,* Winter, D. A., Norman, R. W., Wells, R. P., Hayes, K. C., and Patla, A. E., Eds., Human Kinetics Publishers, Champaign, Ill., 1985, 133.

138. **Cavanagh, P. R. and Ae, M.,** A technique for the display of pressure distributions beneath the foot, *J. Biomech.,* 13, 69, 1980.

139. **Ekstrom, H. and Karlsson, J.,** Direct force measurement in biomechanical investigations, in *Biomechanics IX-B,* Winter, D. A., Norman, R. W., Wells, R. P., Hayes, K. C., and Patla, A. E., Eds., Human Kinetics Publishers, Champaign, Ill., 1985, 201.

140. **Hennig, E. M., Cavanagh, P. R., Albert, H. T., and Macmillan, N. H.,** A piezoelectric method of measuring the vertical contact stress beneath the human foot, *J. Biomed. Eng.,* 4, 213, 1982.

141. **Scranton, P. E., Rutkowski, R., and Brown, T. D.,** Support phase kinematics of the foot, in *The Foot and Ankle,* Bateman, J. E. and Trott, A. W., Eds., Brian E. Decker, New York, 1980, 195.

142. **Morris, J. R. W.,** Accelerometry: a technique for the measurement of human body movements, *J. Biomech.,* 6, 729, 1973.

143. **Smidt, G. L., Arora, J. S., and Johnston, R. C.,** Accelerographic analysis of several types of walking, *Am. J. Phys. Med.,* 50, 285, 1971.

144. **Clarke, T. E., Frederick, E. C., and Cooper, L. B.,** Biomechanical measurement of running shoe cushioning properties, in *Biomechanical Aspects of Sports Shoes and Playing Surfaces,* Nigg, B. M. and Kerr, B. A., Eds., University Printing, Calgary, 1983, 25.

145. **Clarke, T. E., Cooper, L. B., Hamill, C. L., and Clark, D. E.,** The effect of varied stride rate upon shank deceleration in running, *J. Sports Science,* 3, 41, 1985.

146. **Burdett, R. G.,** Forces predicted at the ankle during running, *Medicine and Science in Sports and Exercise,* 14, 308, 1982.

147. **Denoth, J.,** Load on the locomotor system and modelling, *Biomechanics of Running Shoes,* Nigg, B. M., Ed., Human Kinetics Publishers, Champaign, Ill., 1986, 63.

Chapter 2

SWIMMING: FORCES ON AQUATIC ANIMALS AND HUMANS

R. Bruce Martin

TABLE OF CONTENTS

I. INTRODUCTION

The biomechanics of locomotion is a diverse and interesting field involving several aspects of physics and various approaches to mathematical modeling. The study of swimming, however, presents problems which are quite different from those encountered in the analysis of movement on land. Except for creatures without legs, the analysis of locomotion in land animals is essentially similar, whether one is considering a flea, a horse, or a man. One makes assumptions about ground reactions and body segments and develops equations of motion which relate the observed movement patterns to muscle forces. In the case of movement through water, however, the mechanisms and conditions of locomotion become more diverse, and swimming research has proven to be extremely uneven in its progress. In some cases, the analysis has been elegantly executed and highly successful. In others, it has been largely descriptive and little understanding of the involved mechanisms has evolved. In part, this irregular progress is attributable to the fact that fluid dynamics is a less precise discipline than rigid body mechanics. On the other hand, the success achieved in analysis has to some extent correlated with the success achieved by the swimmer. Those animals which swim very well have been the subjects of the more elegant mathematical theories; those which splash about rather clumsily have not been easy to analyze. Human swimmers fall into the latter category, and the situation has not been helped by the fact that most university sport sciences curricula do not include advanced courses in fluid mechanics, or even the necessary prerequisites.

The fastest swimming animal is thought to be the barracuda, which can reach a speed of almost 12 m/sec. Dolphins and whales can swim almost as fast; up to 10 m/sec. or more than 20 mph. Most fish can travel roughly ten times their length per second. By comparison, the fastest human competitive swimmers move along at less than 2 m/sec. thus traveling only one body length per second. Obviously, this is because man has evolved as a land animal, but the special problems arising in his analysis are not readily appreciated by one who only reads the sport science literature. For that reason, this chapter attempts to review the mechanics of human swimming in the context of swimming by aquatic animals so as to illustrate the differences and the similarities, and to encourage sport and biological analysts to join efforts in advancing this intriguing field.

II. FUNDAMENTAL PRINCIPLES

In swimming, propulsive force may be generated by two means. The first is the same in principle as rocket propulsion: water is accelerated and moved in the opposite direction to that in which one wishes to go. Most of us have seen films of an octopus or squid swimming by filling its mantle with water and rapidly ejecting it, and human swimmers achieve the same result when they use their hands to push water to the rear. The second method of propulsion employs lift, the sort of force generated on an airplane wing by virtue of the fact that fluid moves faster along one side than the other. When this happens, the pressure in the faster fluid is decreased, and the wing is pushed in that direction. In an airplane, that direction is primarily up; in a swimming eel, the direction is largely forward. Most creatures, including the eel, seem to employ swimming techniques which utilize both of the afore-mentioned principles.

When swimming by propelling water, one may achieve a given amount of thrust either by accelerating a large mass of water to a small velocity or vice versa. It turns out that the former choice is more efficient. The thrust is equal to the momentum, mv (the product of mass and velocity), of water that is propelled backwards each second. The energy required to accelerate this water is proportional to mv^2. One sees that the thrust is independent of the relationship between m and v, but the energy required is less if v is small. Thus, it is

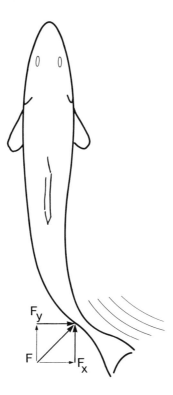

FIGURE 1. A simple view is presented of the propulsive force generated when a fish swims. The motion of the tail propels water back and to the left. The reactive force on the fish's body pushes it forward (component F_x) and to the right (component F_y). The drag of the rest of the body resists both F_x and F_y, and the lateral force F_y is also corrected by an opposite force during the next stroke.

more efficient, mechanically speaking, for a swimmer to move a large tail (or flipper or hand) slowly than a small one rapidly.

III. THE SWIMMING OF AQUATIC ANIMALS

Beginning in the 1930s and 1940s, a number of observational and theoretical papers appeared which elucidated a great deal of scientific information about the swimming of aquatic animals, ranging from microscopic organisms[2-5] to whales.[6] The detailed mathematical analyses of the swimming of various fishes by Wu[7-10] and Lighthill[11-15] are especially noteworthy. Several sections of Alexander's book, *Animal Mechanics,*[16] are devoted to delightful discussions of animal locomotion in water, while Gray's article in *Scientific American,* "How Fishes Swim",[1] is a very lucid introduction to this subject.

Most fish swim by moving their tails from side to side. The simplest view of this mechanism of swimming is shown in Figure 1; the tail pushes water obliquely to the side and backwards, and the reaction to the backward component of the water's motion propels the fish forward. The component of force to the side is corrected on the return stroke of the tail. Whales and dolphins swim in a similar fashion, except that the motion of the tail is in a vertical plane.

Other animals, such as eels, water snakes, and leeches swim by undulating their body so that a wave passes down their length, as shown in Figure 2. In a paper that can only be regarded as a classic, Taylor[4] analyzed this kind of swimming by considering the forces acting on cylindrical elements of the animal's body as they are systematically reoriented relative to the flow of water past them. Using data on the lift and drag acting on cylinders positioned in a wind tunnel, he showed how the animal is able to use both of these forces

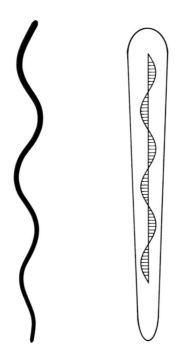

FIGURE 2.   The swimming of long, slender aquatic animals by undulatory motions, is depicted. The animal on the left causes its entire body to move in a continuous wave. Each cyclindrical element of its body produces lateral and forward components of force due to the drag and lift produced by its motion relative to the water. The animal on the right employs a similar mechanism, but only its dorsal fin undulates.

to move forward. Drag is used to set water in a rearward motion, causing the body to accelerate forward. Simultaneously, lift is generated which also pushes the body forward. Taylor successfully compared his theoretical results against films of a water snake and a leech.

Other long, slender fish, including the African, *Gymnarchus* and the South American electric eel, swim by undulating just their dorsal fin, which runs almost the entire length of their body.[17] These animals can swim backward just by reversing the direction of the wave — a significant advantage if the animal is built more like a tanker than a tug boat. On the other hand, most short fish do not actually just wag their tails, but have been shown by cinematography to undulate their shorter bodies in a way similar to eels.[18] It is thus likely that they also actually employ both lift and drag as mechanisms of force generation.

While drag is used to move water about for the purposes of propulsion, it also serves to inhibit the swimmer's motion. One may refer to this inhibiting effect as resistive or body drag. For sustained swimming at a constant velocity, the forces of propulsion must equal the resistive drag forces; thus, resistive drag may be thought of as the factor which limits speed. Resistive drag depends upon many factors, including the size and speed of the swimmer. The fastest swimmers develop ways to minimize it, and whales and dolphins appear to have succeeded at this to an extraordinary degree. Beginning with Gray[19] many investigators have been intrigued with the apparent ability of these marine mammals to sustain speeds which defy the normal limits of mammalian muscle to produce work. For example, Alexander[16] calculated the metabolic power produced by a dolphin (*Tursiops gilli*) swimming at high speed. He assumed that the mechanical power consumed in swimming is equal to the product of resistive drag and velocity, and used standard hydrodynamic formulae for computing the drag from the animal's geometry. He found that the dolphin produces roughly 130 watts/kg of muscle, or three times the maximum power output of a human. Since such a feat seems highly unlikely, a number of scientists have attempted to show that the discrepancy is due to an overestimation of the drag force. Kramer has claimed that these animals are able to maintain a laminar flow over almost their entire body by virtue of their shape and special properties of their skin which cause it to make minute adjustments to the flow when turbulence is imminent.[20,21] However, others have not been able to demonstrate this effect,[22,23] so that the mystery of the dolphin's (and, to an even greater extent, the whale's) enormous speed relative to its body size, remains unsolved.

The swimming of water beetles has been studied by Hughes[24] and Nachtigall[25] and discussed further by Alexander.[16] These papers are of some interest here because this animal swims underwater in a manner quite similar to human swimmers, moving its hind legs in sweeping motions. Unlike humans, however, this animal uses hairs on its legs to increase the drag force propelling water to the rear, and has a mechanism for "feathering" the hairs on the recovery stroke. It is interesting to note that even with this apparent advantage, the mechanical efficiency of the beetle's swimming is only about 0.45, far less than that calculated for undulatory swimmers.

IV. HUMAN SWIMMING

Miller[26] has previously reviewed the biomechanics of human swimming, and Faulker[27] and Holmer[28] have summarized the physiology and metabolic energy requirements of human swimmers. From a coaching perspective, the most significant contributions to swimming biomechanics are those of James Counsilman, whose expertise as a coach and exploits as a distance swimmer are well known. His book, *The Science of Swimming*[29] is unique in that it contains not only the lore of swimming instruction, but also considerable original analysis of swimming biomechanics. It should also be noted that Hay has included a well-referenced chapter on swimming in his textbook, *The Biomechanics of Sports Techniques*.[30]

As Miller[26] has pointed out, one of the reasons that the science of human swimming has progressed rather slowly is that there have been few workers in the field who have devoted a significant proportion of their career to this topic. Much of the literature on the subject consists of unpublished theses and dissertations, and a journal article or two emanating from these works. A great many of these have originated from two sources; Springfield College, Massachusetts, and the University of Iowa at Iowa City. The literature is extensive, but the great majority of the work is descriptive or physiologic in nature, with only a few papers attempting to develop mathematical, biomechanical models, and these contributions stand in contrast to the elegant work of those who studied the swimming mechanics of aquatic animals.

V. RESISTIVE DRAG FORCES

There are three kinds of drag forces which act on an object moving through water; skin friction, head resistance (also known as form drag or viscous pressure drag), and wave drag. Skin friction, as its name implies, is caused by friction between water molecules which are moving relative to the body and those in the boundary layer being carried along with the swimmer. This drag force is proportional to the velocity (V) of the swimmer and the surface area (S) where friction is occurring. Thus,

$$D_s = C_1 \, S \, V \tag{1}$$

where C_1 is a constant. Head resistance, on the other hand, is proportional to the square of the swimmer's velocity and the frontal area of the body (A) as it moves through the water:

$$D_h = C_2 \, A \, V^2 \tag{2}$$

Wave drag occurs when the surface layer of water must be parted to allow the swimmer to pass. It is proportional to a variable known as the Froude number, which is in turn linearly proportional to velocity and inversely proportional to the square root of the length of the body moving through the water. Takamoto et al.[31] measured wave heights produced by swimmers performing the crawl stroke and plotted a wave power function, based on the square of the wave height, against velocity. Contrary to theory, the amount of power wasted in generating the wave increased approximately as the square of velocity. At a given velocity, elite swimmers generated notably less wave power than unskilled swimmers, indicating that adjustment of stroke kinematics to decrease wave production may be an important component of swimming skill. Also, when humans are towed prone through the water, bow waves are observed to develop rather suddenly as the velocity approaches the fastest swimming speeds.[26] For these reasons, this component of drag is thought to be an important determinant of maximum speed, but little is known about its magnitude relative to the other drag components.

As to the comparison between skin friction and head resistance, the balance depends upon a dimensionless variable known as the Reynolds number, N_R. When N_R is less than approximately 2000, the flow of water past the swimmer is likely to be continuous (or laminar) rather than turbulent, and skin friction will be relatively large. However, for human swimmers, the Reynolds number works out to be several million, so that head resistance is certainly the dominant term. Unfortunately, this resistance increases as the square of swimming speed.

This prediction from basic physics is confirmed by experimental data which show that the resistive drag force acting on a person towed through the water is proportional to velocity squared. That is,

$$D = k_B V^2 \tag{3}$$

where k_B may be called the passive body drag coefficient. Its units are $N/m^2/s^2$, which is the same as $kg/m.^3$. As early as 1920, Amar published data showing that $k_B = 25.5$ kg/m.^{3} Later, Karpovich[32] made measurements showing that for male swimmers towed in the prone position $k_B = 30$ Kg/m^3, and Klein[33] published a value of 26.5 kg/m.^{3} Regression analyses have always shown the exponent of V to be very close to 2. Thus, there is good evidence that head resistance is the principal component of the drag force on a human body moving through water at the surface, and that the drag at a given velocity is predictable. As Miller[26] has discussed, these and similar measurements are subject to variations depending upon the subject's body surface area and/or projected frontal area, the position of the body in the water, and whether or not the legs have tended to sink. The fact that k_B is usually found to be less for women than men is not just due to their smaller body size. The buoyant effect of the greater amount of adipose tissue in women, and the smaller proportion of bone mineral among the nonfat components of the body,[34] are thought to reduce drag by causing the body to ride higher in the water. Also, because they have less fat in their hips and thighs, men's legs are more inclined to sink, further increasing passive drag.

In recent years, investigators have come to realize that the many efforts made to measure k_B under various conditions are of little value in the analysis of swimming biomechanics because the drag on a passive body is bound to be quite different from that on a person who is moving both arms and legs in one of the various swimming styles. A few minutes contemplation of this inconsistency, and the problem of trying to overcome it experimentally, will account for the combined frustration and fascination which this topic holds for the biomechanics scientist. If the subject makes swimming motions while being towed, propulsive forces will be introduced so that the drag measured is not accurate. The problem is analogous to Heisenberg's Uncertainty Principle in physics, which states that one cannot simultaneously know both the velocity and the position of an elementary particle (such as

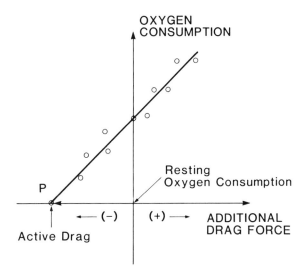

FIGURE 3.   The experimental approach of di Prampero and co-workers[35] is schematically depicted. The oxygen consumption of a swimmer is plotted as a function of "additional drag force" applied with a tether attached to the swimmer's waist. This supplemental "drag" can be negative (i.e., acting forward) as well as positive, and the swimmer's velocity is kept constant with respect to the water. The basic assumption is that if the tether pulled the swimmer forward with a force equaling the active drag, no metabolic energy would be required to swim. Thus, the extrapolated linear regression line is said to pass through a point, P, marking the resting oxygen consumption and a tether force equal to active drag at the velocity tested.

Table 1
COMPARISON OF ACTIVE AND PASSIVE DRAG FORCES

Velocity m/sec	Active drag force, N	Passive drag force, N	Active drag/ passive drag
0.54	28.7	8.7	3.30
0.91	62.3	24.8	2.51

an electron), because the act of measuring one variable introduces an error in the measurement of the other. How can this dilemma be resolved?

An ingenious solution was presented a decade ago by di Prampero, and co-workers.[35] Using methods originated by Webb[36] for studying the swimming of trout, they employed a circular pool equipped with an apparatus which allowed an additional drag force to be applied to the swimmer via a belt and tether line. The additional drag force could be positive or negative, depending upon the direction of pull applied to the belt around the swimmer's waist. Stroke rate was adjusted so that a constant swimming velocity was achieved, and the swimmer's oxygen consumption was measured as a function of the additional drag force. The experimental approach rests on the assertion that if one plots oxygen consumption vs. additional drag force and extrapolates the data to be resting oxygen consumption, the additional drag force intercept should be the drag force experienced during free swimming (cf. Figure 3). It was found that oxygen consumption was linearly proportional to additional drag force with correlation coefficients ranging from 0.80 to 0.99. Table 1 shows how the results compared to the drag forces calculated form Karpovich's passive towing equation. It is seen that the "active drag forces" are more than double those obtained in passive drag experiments. Subsequently, this research group[37] has determined active drag values for swimming velocities ranging from 0.4 to 2.0 m/sec. and they report that the data for both active and passive drag can be expressed by the empirical equation:

$$D = k\, V^n \tag{4}$$

where k depends on the body geometry and n depends on the technical ability of the individual swimmer. The exponent varies from 1.35 to 2.11, and seems to be larger and less variable for passive towing and smaller and more sensitive to individual variations for active swimming. Both k and the actual drag tend to be larger for active swimming, however. In general, both active and passive drag are significantly less for women than for men.

This work must be regarded as among the best in the swimming literature, for it resolves a fundamental predicament, at least to a first approximation. It should be noted that additional support for the postulate that active drag exceeds passive drag, is provided by Lighthill[15] and Webb[36] for fish, and by Holmer[38] and Clarys,[39] who did experiments which confirmed the results of di Prampero et al.[35] in most respects.

Finally, we may note that the proportionality constants in equations concerned with various forms of drag, reflect, among other things, the viscosity and density of the water. These in turn are influenced by water temperature and the presence of dissolved salts and surfactants. Clarys[40] has shown that an increase in water temperature of 6°C can notably diminish passive drag. While water purity and temperature are usually not controlled in experiments or in competitive swimming, they may have a subtle but important effect on swimming performance.

VI. PROPULSIVE FORCES

The study of the propulsive aspect of human swimming has proven to be as challenging as the study of resistive drag forces. One historical hypothesis was that propulsive force is provided by the backward ejection of water when the swimmer draws (adducts) his legs together, much the same as a bellows forces air out when its sides are pulled together. Cureton[41] and Counsilman[42] showed that this concept was an oversimplification, and it was replaced in the minds of most investigators by the hypothesis that propulsive force is produced by using drag to move water backwards as the arms and legs are moved through a stroke cycle. This hypothesis has been studied in some detail by a number of investigators, and has been shown to explain many experimental observations. Later, however, Counsilman[43,44] and Brown and Counsilman,[45] introduced the additional hypothesis that lift as well as drag acts (especially on the swimmer's hands) to provide propulsive force. Thus, the analysts of human swimming have invoked the same two basic propulsive mechanisms as the investigators of animal swimming. The literature related to these two aspects of propulsion in human swimming will now be surveyed in some detail.

A. Propulsive Force Due to Drag

The generation of propulsive force by virtue of drag may be analyzed using the same concepts introduced above in the section on body drag; basically, one assumes that the force produced by each limb segment is proportional to the square of the velocity of the segment relative to the water, and acts in the opposite direction to the relative velocity vector, as shown in Figure 4. One faces the problem of determining the drag coefficient and the relative velocity of each segment as the swimmer strokes through the water, but the analysis of this model is reasonably straightforward. It has been essayed in various forms by several investigators, including Seireg et al.,[46] Seireg and Baz,[47] Gallenstein and Huston,[48] Jensen and Blanksby,[49] Bourgeois and Lewillie,[50] and Martin et al.[51]

Seireg and Baz[47] were the first to make a serious attempt to model a human swimmer, mathematically. They used a five-segment model consisting of a head-torso, two arms, and two legs. The arms remained straight, and rotated about the shoulders to simulate the crawl stroke, while the legs also remained straight and executed a flutter kick. By making as-

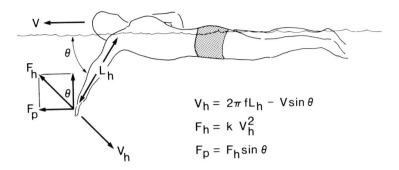

$$V_h = 2\pi f L_h - V \sin \theta$$

$$F_h = k\, V_h^2$$

$$F_p = F_h \sin \theta$$

FIGURE 4. A simple model of the crawl stroke is shown which is similar to that used by several analysts of human swimming. The arm is assumed to be a rigid conic frustrum or cylinder, and the hand a plate located a distance L_h from the shoulder. As the swimmer moves through the water with stroke rate f and average velocity V, his hand has velocity v_h relative to the water when the arm makes an angle θ with the horizontal. The drag of the water on the hand produces a force F_h, which has a propulsive component F_p acting in the forward direction.

sumptions about the drag coefficients of the limbs and exercising the model at appropriate stroke rates, such variables as velocity, rotations about the center of mass, and mechanical efficiency, could be predicted. Gallenstein and Huston[48] used similar methods to produce a more elaborate model having 15 segments. Their results indicated that a bent leg flutter kick is more effective than the straight leg kick of Seireg and Baz's model. They also predicted that the velocity obtained in the complete breast stroke would be slightly less than the sum of those resulting when the model swam using the kick and arm strokes separately.

Following Gallenstein and Huston, Jensen and Blanksby[49] analyzed the effects of elbow flexion on the dynamics of swimming the front crawl. They also used a simple conic frustrum for the two segments of the arm and flat plates for hands, and wrote equations of motion based on simple hydrodynamic drag, but assumed variable elbow flexion angles. The moments required to move the arms were similar to those experimentally measured by Jensen and Bellow.[52] As one might expect, elbow flexion reduced the shoulder moment; it also tended to delay the greatest moments (and propulsive forces) until the arm was further along in the stroke. The authors suggested that the former effect increases swimming efficiency; however this is not obvious, since *both* muscle force *and* propulsive force were reduced simultaneously. It seems more likely that the change in the timing of the propulsive force as the arm is pulled through the water improves efficiency, but this possibility was not pursued.

Yet another model of the crawl stroke was developed by Bourgeois and Lewillie,[50] who used Lagrangian methods to derive the equations of motion for a crawl stroke model composed of cylindrical segments. Their analysis points out the significance of inertial factors in the stroke cycle, and also suggests that the kick is important since it maintains the rest of the body in a horizontal position, a conclusion reached intuitively by Counsilman.[29]

B. Propulsive Force Due to Lift

Hydrodynamic lift forces may be mathematically formulated in a manner similar to that employed for drag, resulting in an equation of the form

$$L = C_L V^2 \tag{5}$$

where L is the lift force, V is the velocity of the body segment relative to the water, and C_L is a lift coefficient which depends upon the density of water and the geometry of the body segment. Both drag and lift forces depend upon V^2, but they act in different directions relative to the flow of water past the body segment. Lift acts perpendicular to the flow, while drag acts opposite to the flow, and the total propulsive force will act in a direction given by the resultant of these two vectors.

Counsilman's proposal[29,44] that lift is employed in generating swimming propulsion applies primarily to the hand because it is the most maneuverable body segment and has the most appropriate geometry for producing lift. The proposal also suggests that the best swimmers would constantly adjust their hands so as to optimize the resultant of the lift and drag vectors. This would seem to be an extremely difficult task, but proprioception of the force acting on the hand may enable the swimmer to respond to the resultant itself rather than all the variables which control it. By studying hand motions in the butterfly stroke, Barthels[53] determined that the hand moves at an angle to the flow of water throughout the stroke, but that lift seems to be the predominant force during the insweep and drag the major force during the push stroke. Schleihauf[54] conducted a detailed study of the lift and drag characteristics of castings of the human hand in a swimming configuration. He found that the lift force was maximized at an ''angle of attack'' of approximately 40°. The lift coefficient for the hand was similar to that of a flat plate having the same aspect ratio; the drag coefficient was found to be slightly larger than that of a plate. He went on to study in detail the lift and drag characteristics of swimmers' hands in the principal swimming styles. His discussion emphasized the fact that there is no unique hand path and position combination which maximizes the resultant force. Individual elite swimmers were found to choose techniques which balanced lift and drag in different ways. These experimental results confirm in a qualitative way the postulate that in each style of swimming, the expert athlete learns to optimize the balance between lift and drag forces within the bounds of joint kinematics and the intricacies of water flow patterns near his or her body during the course of a stroke.

C. Experimental Measurement of Propulsive Force

Regardless of the balance between lift and drag in producing propulsive force, the latter is clearly a function of the velocity of the swimmer, just as body drag was seen to be. This causes problems for the researcher because a favorite technique for studying propulsive force has been to tether the swimmer to the edge of the pool and measure the force in the tether line. This produces a record of the forces produced by the swimmer's motions; Figure 5 shows typical curves for the front crawl, breast, and back strokes. These curves are of considerable value for comparing swimming styles and individual athletes, but the propulsive force, F_p, will not be the same in a stationary swimmer as in a moving one; F_p will be a function of the velocity of the swimmer's hand (and other limb segments) relative to the water, and this will decrease as the swimmer's speed increases.

In the face of this problem, several variations of the tethered-swimmer experiment have been devised. Alley,[55] Counsilman,[56] and more recently Adams et al.,[57] partially restrained the swimmer by paying out the tether line at various velocities, and measuring the tether force. Craig and Boomer,[58] on the other hand, let their subjects swim against a variable tether force and recorded the resulting velocity. Magel[59] introduced another variation when he varied the tether force and had the swimmer adjust his stroke rate for zero velocity. The results of such tethered swimming experiments may be displayed graphically as shown in Figure 6A. As the tether force is relaxed, the swimmer quite naturally goes faster, and the relationship is usually almost linear. The problem is that the propulsive force during free swimming cannot be found on this graph; it is not the fully tethered force (FTF, i.e., the ordinate intercept, or the average tether force when the tether is held fast) because the swimmer's velocity is zero for that point, and it is obviously not the tether force during free swimming (i.e., zero). Thus, one is faced with a conundrum similar to the one posed by the need to measure active swimming drag.

This problem has not been solved experimentally as yet. The nearest approach to a solution appears to be a theoretical analysis of the problem by Martin and co-workers.[51] Their analysis

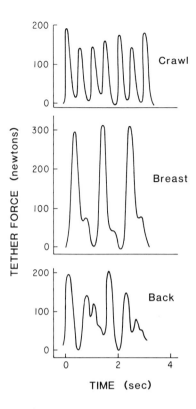

FIGURE 5. Typical tether force vs. time patterns are shown for three styles of swimming. The crawl produces the most regular pattern; the breast stroke produces the highest forces, but may contain slightly backward (negative) forces during the recovery stroke.

employed a model similar to that used by Seireg and Baz,[47] but in this case the behavior of the model in a partially tethered swimming experiment was investigated. First the parameters of the model were adjusted so that it behaved like a real swimmer in terms of such variables as FTF, free-swimming velocity, and stroke rate. It was then subjected to the partial tethering experiment, and the results are shown in Figure 6B. The graph illustrates the relationship between the tether force (F_T), the body drag force (F_D), and the propulsive force (F_P) as velocity is increased. During free swimming, F_T is zero and $F_P = F_D$. An FTF value of 129 N corresponds to a free swimming propulsive force of only 41 N. One approach to estimating F_P from the FTF in a human experiment would be to assume that the F_P/FTF ratio is constant, but it was found that this force ratio was sensitive to variations in the model parameters. An alternative would be to have the subject swim with the tether released at the speed for which $F_T = F_P$; this turned out to be approximately $^2/_3$ of the free-swimming velocity over a wide range of model parameters. Thus, the model provides useful insights regarding the interpretation of the experimental data, but it needs to be improved in several respects: for example, the active drag results were not good when the model was subjected to the di Prampero experiment, and the body segments should include legs and be made more realistic.

Indeed, significant improvement of the analytical models used to study swimming would not be difficult. The most obvious points of improvement would be to extend the work of Jensen and Blanksby[49] by using arms with multiple articulations, and to compute lift generated by the hands. Today, these refinements could be easily handled by a desk-top personal computer.

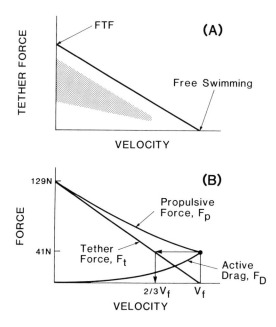

FIGURE 6. The results of the analysis of tethered swimming performed by Martin et al.[51] are depicted. (A) The model predicts a linear relationship between tether force and velocity, and the model parameters are adjusted so that the line passes through experimentally determined fully tethered force (FTF) and free-swimming-velocity intercepts. Data obtained by Counsilman[56] and Craig and Boomer[58] for partially tethered swimming fall in the shaded area somewhat below this line. (B) The predicted relationships between tether force (F_T), propulsive force (F_P), and active drag (F_D), are shown. F_T was found to equal the free-swimming propulsive force when the tethered swimming velocity was $2/3$ of the free-swimming velocity.

D. Tethered Swimming as a Coach's Aid

Even though tether force measurements do not represent actual propulsive force during free swimming, it is still possible that such measurements may correlate with swimming speed or performance in competition. This possibility is of considerable interest to swimming coaches who would like to evaluate or compare their athletes. Craig and Boomer[60] compared FTF measurements with maximum swimming speed for a group of collegiate swimmers and found linear correlation coefficients of 0.81 for males and 0.82 for females. Yeater et al.[61] found that the five best and worst swimmers on a collegiate swimming team (based on competitive times) exhibited a significant difference in their mean FTF measurements. Thus, there is a statistically significant, and probably useful, relationship between this kind of test result and performance, but the correlation does not seem strong enough to be highly selective. This is reasonable given the fact that FTF does not assess active drag or the relationship between velocity and propulsive force in individual swimmers.

It should also be mentioned that many coaches use tethered swimming as a training aid. That is, the athlete swims against a line attached to the end of the pool. The tether is sometimes made of rubber or another elastic material so that the swimmer's maximum progress down the pool is essentially a measure of his or her FTF. Given the above discussion regarding the dependency of both FTF and active drag on swimming speed, it seems clear that while this exercise should build strength, it may not offer an appropriate opportunity for the swimmer to hone his or her skills in a manner related to the hydrodynamics of swimming. In fact, it is conceivable that it may teach poor or undesirable habits.

E. Contribution of the Kick to Propulsion

The relative contribution of the kick to propulsion in various swimming strokes has been a matter of interest and debate for coaches for many years. Counsilman[29] has suggested that the kick contributes little propulsive force in the crawl stroke, serving instead to keep the legs elevated and thereby reduce drag. Mosterd and Jongbloed[62] maintained that the flutter kick could potentially produce only half the thrust of the arms in the front crawl, but Yeater et al.[61] found that the flutter kick could actually produce more FTF than the crawl arm stroke. However, in testing the kick and arm stroke as separate components of swimming propulsion, Alley[55] found that the kick force fell more rapidly than the arm force as velocity increased in a tethered swimming experiment. Thus, there may be no inconsistency between these seemingly divergent views. (The previously discussed tethered swimming analysis of Martin et al.[51] did not include a kick, and thus had no predictions on this point). Karpovich and Sinning[63] analyzed the relationship between the propulsive forces and velocities associated with arms only, legs only, and combined swimming. They assumed that

$$F_W = F_A + F_L \qquad (6)$$

where F denotes propulsive force and the subscripts W, A, and L refer to the whole stroke, arms only, and legs only, respectively. They then assumed that each of these forces must equal the product of an active body drag coefficient and the square of the velocity obtained under that condition. Furthermore, they assumed that the active drag coefficient was the same for each condition - arms only, legs only, and the whole stroke. This leads directly to the result

$$V_W = (V_A + V_L)^{1/2} \qquad (7)$$

There would appear to be two potential problems with this result. First, it seems unlikely that the active drag coefficient is the same for arms only, legs only, and combined swimming. There is also some doubt that the propulsive force produced, say, by the legs alone, would be the same as that produced by the legs during the whole stroke, because the velocity would be greater, and therefore F_L must be velocity dependent. In fact, MacDonald and Stearns[64] found that for the breast stroke, the left side of the above velocity equation was only approximately $3/4$ as great as the right side. It may also be recalled that the theoretical model of Gallenstein and Huston[48] predicted a similar result.

An important determinant of the contribution of the kick to propulsion not considered in the above analyses is its timing relative to the arm stroke. Propulsive forces supplied by the arms are intermittent, producing a repeated cycle of acceleration and deceleration (cf. Figure 5). If the kick is timed so that it occurs when the propulsive force from the arms is at a minimum, then it may improve performance by preventing the body from decelerating too much between strokes.[48,65] Since resistive drag is exponentially proportional to velocity, it is in principle more efficient to increase average speed by increasing minimum velocity rather than maximum velocity.

VII. ENERGY EXPENDITURE AND EFFICIENCY

The physiology of swimming is beyond the scope of this review, but some note should be made of the metabolic and mechanical energy requirements of human swimming. In order to estimate the mechanical power P expended while swimming, it is common to use the product of resistive drag and velocity, as previously mentioned in the case of the dolphin. Thus, if D_a represents active drag on the swimmer's body,

$$P = D_a V \qquad (8)$$

If the rate of metabolic energy production (P') is then determined from oxygen consumption measurements, one may estimate the overall or *total efficiency* of the swimmer as

$$e_T = P/P' \tag{9}$$

Holmer[28] estimates this efficiency to be 15% for the front crawl stroke. Pendergast et al.[37] cite values ranging from 2 to 18% based on data in the literature. These numbers stand in contrast to earlier reports (such as those given in Miller's review[26]), which were in the neighborhood of 2 to 3%. This is least partly due to the fact that many earlier computations employed passive drag rather than active drag.

Consider now the *mechanical efficiency* of the human swimmer. This would be the power used to overcome drag (P) divided by the total mechanical power expended in executing swimming motions (P_S). *Metabolic efficiency,* on the other hand, may be defined as P_S divided by the metabolic power consumed by the swimmer (P'). The total efficiency must equal the product of the mechanical efficiency and the metabolic efficiency. Thus,

$$e_T = \frac{P \; P_S}{P_S \; P'} \tag{10}$$

Since the metabolic efficiency of human muscle for a sustained activity is approximately 20%, a total efficiency of 15% implies that the mechanical efficiency of human swimmers is 0.15/0.20 or approximately 75%. This is considerably better than the 45% efficiency of the water beetle (referred to above); indeed, it is suspiciously high. An overall efficiency of 10% (mechanical efficiency approximatly 50%) seems a more reasonable figure for human swimmers, and would not be inconsistent with most of the available data. Efficiency figures should be regarded as *estimates* because they depend upon knowledge of active drag, and in spite of the work of di Prampero and others, the measurement of this variable cannot be considered to be on a solid footing.

The energy expenditure for swimming increases disproportionately with velocity, probably due in large measure to increased drag.[28] The energy required for the front and back crawl strokes is only half that needed for the breast and butterfly strokes, and the kick consumes more than the arm stroke. Women are 1.3 to 2 times more efficient swimmers than men in terms of oxygen consumption/unit distance, and skilled swimmers are 1.5 to 2 times more efficient than untrained swimmers.[66] For humans, swimming a given distance consumes 7 times as much metabolic energy as walking, and 3.5 times as much energy as running.[28] It is interesting, however, that the estimates of dolphin and whale energy consumption lead to the conclusion that these animals swim with approximately the same metabolic cost that humans run — approximately 300 J/m.

VIII. OTHER MATHEMATICAL ANALYSES

An interesting start-to-finish model of a generalized swimming race was presented by Francis and Dean.[67] Equations describing the projectile (i.e., starting dive), glide, and constant velocity swimming phases of the race were combined and solved numerically by seeking the best fit to 1973 world freestyle records for men and women. The model was able to duplicate the results of both sprints and distance races closely, with residual mean square errors of 1.6 and 1.2% for men and women, respectively. However, the best fits were obtained when it was assumed that incredibly large differences existed between the basic parameters of men and women. For example, the body drag coefficient for women was less than $1/3$ that of men, and women were also superior in terms of the initial amount of anaerobic energy available (twice as great), the rate of aerobic energy conversion (3 times greater), and the starting dive velocity (twice as great). The magnitude of these differences leads one to suspect that the model has a fundamental flaw in terms of accurately representing swimming biomechanics.

Finally, it is noteworthy that nearly all the literature on human swimming reflects an interest in achieving maximum velocity. There are, however, circumstances (e.g., man overboard of a vessel) where maximum distance achievable, or minimum metabolic energy required per distance traveled, are of much greater importance, but optimization analyses directed in this way seem not to have been done.

IX. SUMMARY

The swimming of aquatic animals which generate propulsive forces by undulatory body motions may seem more complicated than that of humans, but it is actually more amenable to mathematical analyses having closed form solutions. The study of human swimming has encountered fundamental experimental problems related to the fact that it has been impossible to measure propulsive or resistive swimming forces experimentally during free swimming. Some success has been achieved in circumventing these problems using analytical techniques, despite the fact that the theoretical analyses to date have used greatly simplified models. Perhaps the greatest opportunity for a significant contribution to the biomechanics of swimming is in the development of a segmented analytical model which incorporates lift as a propulsive mechanism and has arms with multiple articulations. These innovations are entirely within the capabilities of computer-based analysis techniques, and sufficient experimental data exist to set up and test such models.

ACKNOWLEDGMENTS

I wish to thank Dr. Michael Madison for his help in reviewing the literature, and both Dr. Madison and Dr. Mont Hubbard for their critical reading of this work.

REFERENCES

1. **Gray, J.,** How fishes swim, *Scientific American,* 197, 48, 1957.
2. **Hancock, G. J.,** The self propulsion of microscopic organisms through liquids, *Proc. R. Soc.,* 217a, 96, 1953.
3. **Taylor, G.,** Analysis of the swimming of microscopic organisms, *Proc. R. Soc.,* 209a, 447, 1951.
4. **Taylor, G.,** Analysis of the swimming of long and narrow animals, *Proc. R. Soc.,* 214, 158, 1952.
5. **Taylor, G.,** The action of waving cylindrical tails in propelling microscopic organisms, *Proc. R. Soc.,* 211, 225, 1952.
6. **Gray, J.,** Aspects of the locomotion of whales, *Nature, (London),* 161, 199, 1948.
7. **Wu, T. Y. T.,** Accelerated swimming of a waving plate, in Proc. 4th Symp. Nav. Hydrodyn., U.S. Government Printing Office, Washington, D.C., 1962.
8. **Wu, T. Y. T.,** The mechanics of swimming, in *Biomechanics,* Fung, Y. C., Ed., American Society of Mechanical Engineers, New York, 1966.
9. **Wu, T. Y. T.,** Hydromechanics of swimming propulsion, I., *J. Fluid Mech.,* 46, 337, 1971.
10. **Wu, T. Y. T.,** Hydromechanics of swimming propulsion, II. *J. Fluid Mech.,* 46, 521, 1971.
11. **Lighthill, M. J.,** On the squirming motion of nearly spherical deformable bodies through liquids at very small Reynolds numbers. *Communic. Pure and Appl. Math.,* 5, 109, 1952.
12. **Lighthill, M. J.,** Note on the swimming of slender fish, *J. Fluid Mech.,* 9, 305, 1960.
13. **Lighthill, M. J.,** Hydromechanics of aquatic animal propulsion, *Ann. Rev. Fluid Mech.,* 1, 413, 1969.
14. **Lighthill, M. J.,** Aquatic animal propulsion of high mechanical efficiency, *J. Fluid Mech.,* 44, 265, 1970.
15. **Lighthill, M. J.,** Large amplitude elongated body theory of fish locomotion, *Proc. R. Soc.,* 179B, 125, 1971.
16. **Alexander, R. M.,** *Animal Mechanics,* University of Washington Press, Seattle, 1968.

17. **Tricker, R. A. R., and Tricker, B. J. K.,** *The Science of Movement,* Elsevier, New York 1967.
18. **Gray, J.,** Studies in animal locomotion, I. The movement of fish with special reference to the eel, *J. Exp. Biol.,* 10, 88, 1933.
19. **Gray, J.,** Studies in animal locomotion, VI. The propulsive powers of the dolphin, *J. Exp. Biol.,* 13, 192, 1936.
20. **Kramer, M. O.,** The dolphin's secret, *New Scientist,* 7, 118, 1960.
21. **Kramer, M. O.,** Hydrodynamics of the dolphin, *Adv. Hydrosci.,* 2, 111, 1965.
22. **Gadd, G. P.,** Some hydrodynamic aspects of swimming, National Physics Laboratory, (Ship Division) Ship Report, 45, 1, 1963.
23. **Lang, T. G., and Pryor, K.,** Hydrodynamic performance of porpoises, *Science,* 152, 531, 1966.
24. **Hughes, G. M.,** The co-ordination of insect movements. III. Swimming in *Dytiscus, Hydrophilus,* and a dragonfly nymph, *J. Exp. Biol.,* 35, 567, 1958.
25. **Nachtigall, G.,** Über Kinematik, Dynamik, und Energetik des Schwimmens ein Heimischer, *Dytisciden, Zeitschr. Vergl. Physiol.,* 43, 48, 1960.
26. **Miller, D. I.,** Biomechanics of swimming, in *Exercise and Sport Sci. Rev.,* Wilmore, J. H. and Keogh, J. F., Eds., Academic Press, New York, 1979, 219.
27. **Faulkner, J. A.,** Physiology of swimming and diving, in *Exercise Physiology,* Falls, H. B., Ed., Academic Press, New York, 1968, 415.
28. **Holmer, I.,** The physiology of swimming man, in *Exercise and Sport Sci. Rev.,* Hutton, R. S. and Miller, D. I., Eds., Academic Press, New York, 1979, 87.
29. **Counsilman, J. E.,** *The Science of Swimming,* Prentice-Hall, Englewood Cliffs, N.J., 1978.
30. **Hay, J.,** *The Biomechanics of Sports Techniques,* Prentice-Hall, Englewood Cliffs, N.J., 1978.
31. **Takamoto, M., Ohmichi, H., and Miyashita, M.,** Wave height in relation to swimming velocity and proficiency in the front crawl stroke, in *Biomechanics IX-B,* Winter, D. A., Norman, R. W., Wells, R. P., Hayes, K. C., and Patla, A. E., Eds., Human Kinetics Publishers, Champaign, Ill., 1985.
32. **Karpovich, P. V.,** Water resistance in swimming, *Res. Quart.,* 4, 21, 1933.
33. **Klein, W. C.,** Tests for the prediction of body resistance in water, Masters' thesis, State University of Iowa, Iowa City, 1939.
34. **Lohman, T. G., Slaughter, M. H., Boileau, R. A., and Lussier, L.,** Bone mineral measurements and their relation to body density, *Human Biol.,* 56, 667, 1984.
35. **di Prampero, P. E., Pendergast, D. R., Wilson, D. W., and Rennie, D. W.,** Energetics of swimming man, *J. Appl. Physiol.,* 37, 1, 1974.
36. **Webb, P. W.,** The swimming energetics of trout, *J. Exp. Biol.,* 55, 489, 1971.
37. **Pendergast, D. R., di Prampero, P. E., Craig, A. B., and Rennie, D. W.,** The influence of selected biomechanical factors on the energy cost of swimming, in *Swimming Medicine IV,* Eriksson, B., Furberg, B., Nelson, R. C., and Morehouse, C. A., Eds., University Park Press, Baltimore, 1978, 367.
38. **Holmer, I.,** Propulsive efficiency of breaststroke and freestyle swimming, *Eur. J. Appl. Physiol.,* 33, 95, 1974.
39. **Clarys, J. P.,** Onderzoek naar de hydronynamische en morfologischeaspekten het menselijk lichaam, Vrije Universiteit Brussel, Brussels, 1976.
40. **Clarys, J. P.,** Morphological data for the hydrodynamic investigation, unpublished manuscript, 25pp., 1978.
41. **Cureton, T. K.,** Mechanics and kinesiology of swimming, *Res. Quart.,* 1, 87, 1930.
42. **Counsilman, J. E.,** A cinematographic analysis of the butterfly breaststroke, Unpublished Masters' thesis, University of Illinois, Urbana, 1948.
43. **Counsilman, J. E.,** The role of sculling movements in the arm pull, *Swimming World,* 10, 6, 1969.
44. **Counsilman, J. E.,** The application of Bernoulli's principle to human propulsion in water, in *Biomechanics in Swimming,* Lewille, L. and Clarys, J. P., Eds., Université Libre de Bruxelles, Brussels, 1971, 57.
45. **Brown, R. M., and Counsilman, J. E.,** The role of lift in propelling the swimmer, in *Selected Topics in Biomechanics,* Cooper, J. M., Ed., Chicago Athletic Institute, Chicago, 1971.
46. **Seireg, A., Baz, A., and Patel, D.,** Supportive forces on the human body during underwater activities, *J. Biomech.,* 4, 23, 1971.
47. **Seireg, A. and Baz, A.,** A mathematical model for swimming mechanics, in *Biomechanics in Swimming,* Lewille, L. and Clarys, J. P., Eds., Université Libre de Bruxelles, Brussels, 1971, 81.
48. **Gallenstein, J. and Huston, R. L.,** Analysis of swimming motions, *Human Factors,* 15, 91, 1973.
49. **Jensen, R. K. and Blanksby, B.,** A model for upper extremity forces during the underwater phase of the front crawl, in *Swimming,* II, Lewille, L. and Clarys, J. P., Eds., University Park Press, Baltimore, 1975, 143.
50. **Bourgeois, M. A. and Lewille, L.,** Mathematical model and Lagrangian analysis for the dynamics of the human body in the crawl stroke, in *Biomechanics VIII-B,* Matsui, H. and Kobayashi, K., Eds., Human Kinetics Publishers, Champaign, Ill., 1983, 978.
51. **Martin, R. B., Yeater, R. A., White, M. K.,** A simple analytical model for the crawl stroke, *J. Biomech.,* 14, 539, 1981.

52. **Jensen, R. K., and Bellows, D. G.,** Impulse and work output curves for swimmers, in *Biomechanics,* IV, Nelson, R. C. and Morehouse, C. A., Eds., University Park Press, Baltimore, 1974, 198.
53. **Barthels, K. M.,** The mechanism for body propulsion in swimming, in *Biomechanics,* IV, Nelson, R. C. and Morehouse, C. A., Eds., University Park Press, Baltimore, 1974, 45.
54. **Schleihauf, R. E.,** A hydrodynamic analysis of swimming propulsion, in *Swimming,* III, Terauds, J. and Bedingfield, E. W., Eds., University Park Press, Baltimore, 1979, 70.
55. **Alley, L. E.,** An analysis of water resistance and propulsion in swimming the crawl stroke, *Res. Quart.,* 25, 253, 1952.
56. **Counsilman, J. E.,** Forces in swimming two types of crawl strokes, *Res. Quart.,* 26, 127, 1955.
57. **Adams, T. A., Martin, R. B., Yeater, R. A., and Gilson, K.,** Tethered force and velocity relationships, *Swimming Technique,* 221, November 1983.
58. **Craig, A.B. and Boomer, W. F.,** Relationships between tethered and free swimming the front crawl stroke, *J. Biomech.,* 13, 194, 1980.
59. **Magel, J. R.,** Propelling force measured during tethered swimming in the four competitive swimming styles, *Res. Quart.,* 41, 68, 1970.
60. **Craig, A. B., Boomer, W. L., and Gibbons, J. F.,** Use of stroke rate, distance per stroke, and velocity relationships during training for competitive swimming, in *Swimming,* III, Terauds, J. and Bedingfield, E. W., Eds., University Park Press, Baltimore, 1979.
61. **Yeater, R. A., Martin, R. B., White, M. K., and Gilson, K. H.,** Tethered swimming forces in the crawl, breast, and back strokes and their relationship to competitive performance, *J. Biomech.,* 14, 527, 1981.
62. **Mosterd, W. L. and Jongbloed, J.,** Analysis of the stroke of highly trained swimmers, *Intle. Z. Angew. Physiol. Einsch. Arheitsphysiol.,* 20, 288, 1964.
63. **Karpovich, P. V. and Sinning, W. E.,** *Physiology of Muscular Activity,* W. B. Saunders, Philadelphia, 1971.
64. **MacDonald, F. W. and Stearns, W. J.,** A mathematical analysis of the dolphin, butterfly, and breast strokes, unpublished Masters' thesis, Springfield College, Springfield, Mass., 1969.
65. **Persyn, U., Vervaeke, H., and Verhetsel, D.,** Factors influencing stroke mechanics and speed in swimming the butterfly, in *Biomechanics VIII-B,* Matsui, H. and Kobayashi, K., Eds., Human Kinetics Publishers, Champaign, Ill., 1983, 833.
66. **Pendergast, D. R., di Prampero, P. E., Craig, A. B., Wilson, D. R., and Rennie, D. W.,** Quantitative analysis of the front crawl in men and women, *J. Appl. Physiol. Respir. Envir. Exercise Physiol.,* 43, 475, 1977.
67. **Francis, P. R. and Dean, N.,** A biomechanical model for swimming performance, in *Swimming,* II, Lewille, L. and Clarys, J. P., Eds., University Park Press, Baltimore, 1975, 118.

Chapter 3

ROWING AND SCULLING MECHANICS

Antonio Dal Monte and Andrzej Komor

TABLE OF CONTENTS

I. INTRODUCTION

Of all the well-known modern sport disciplines there are few which can be distinguished from others in some special way, and which have particular value and nobility. It can be said, and it is not only the authors' opinion, that rowing, together with track-and-field, swimming, and cycling, represents this long-term tradition and popularity. Here the opinion of Marchesi,[1] though somewhat controversial, can be cited " . . . that however the programme of the Olympic Games constantly grows, the revolutionary reduction of acknowledged disciplines can be assumed, but neither track-and-field nor rowing will ever be touched . . . "

Although rowing had been a practiced and competitive sport for 5,000 years, it was not until 1900 that Baron Pierre de Coubertin personally endorsed the sport as an Olympic discipline. Rowing by means of long oars, was well known as an effective way of moving boats in ancient Egypt. First signs of rowing activity can be found on frescas and graphics from the Vth Dynasty of the Pharoahs in 2600 B.C. (Figure 1). Rowing races, using various kinds of boats, were very popular in ancient Greece and during the whole Roman period as well. The famous Naumachi games organized by Emperor Augustus or enormous races founded by Emperor Claudius (more than 100 boats and 1900 oarsmen), are the highlights of ancient rowing history.

It is usually assumed that the first race of the famous rowing teams of Oxford and Cambridge Universities of 1829 began modern rowing history and stimulated significant technological development. The period from the Paris Olympic Games in 1900 until the last Olympic competitions at Lake Casitas in 1984, represents the continuous growth in popularity of rowing as a sport discipline. During this short period, the sport of rowing has been considerably changed and developed. Materials for making oars and boat shells have become lighter and better from the hydrodynamic viewpoint, and new ideas like sliding seats have enabled the athlete to perform more effectively.

Nowadays, while a split second or a centimeter plays a big part in success or failure, we should consider the outstanding result or record not only as an individual achievement, but as a result of complex organization, scientific, and training efforts which are focused on a top-level-sport training process. Nowadays, it is really more and more difficult to obtain peak physical fitness in exact time, to break a record, or to win in any discipline without permanent, extended studies and investigations performed on athletes and the equipment they use, and this is done by researchers who represent a variety of scientific disciplines.

Due to the complexity of the rowing pattern, where optimum human action combined with high-quality equipment guarantee top performance, only a wide and extended scientific approach enables both the further technological development on the one hand and protection of top-level athletes against health hazards on the other. However, many coaches and athletes still doubt the practical application of research done in rowing. Some reasons for this were wittily pointed out by Pope[2] " . . . we seriously doubt that any oarsman anywhere will pull a bit harder during a "Big 10" simply because he is aware that the solution of a differential equation somewhere suggests that he ought to be able to . . . "

Many of the old hand-rowing practitioners and experts are really convinced that rowing is an art and not a science, so the application of scientific principles does not fit into this sport discipline. This "argument" was perfectly answered by Williams[3] " . . . of course rowing is an art—who denies it? Almost any human activity is capable of elevation to artistic status and there can be very little from which no esthetic value can be wrung . . . to the oarsman, if he is fortunate, will come one or more of those moments of truth when somehow man, oars, boat, and water are perfectly integrated and rowing transcends for a brief spell all normal experience. It is surely reasonable to suggest that such moments will be more frequent, and rowing in general more effective, if to it is brought a scientific approach . . . "

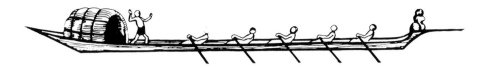

FIGURE 1. An Egyptian rowing boat, dating back almost 5,000 years.

Coming back to rowing reality, in the last investigations on spinal deformities and their pathology in top-level oarsmen (Endler et al.[4]) it was found that the frequency of peak stress in active rowing may lead to early and augmented degenerative changes in the vertebral bodies. The clinical and radiological investigations of 45 top Australian oarsmen made it clear that 68% of them showed signs of previous Scheuermann's disease, while degenerative changes of vertebral bodies were found in 48%.

Among many science branches, such as physiology and psychology, mechanical engineering, and computer science, the biomechanical investigations have a big influence in modern top-level oarsmen training both from the point of view of maximization of sport result and the athletes' protection against health hazards. These investigations combine simultaneously the biological aspects of athletes' activity during rowing (muscle activity and musculo-skeletal system loads) and the mechanics of oars and boats and their interaction with the oarsmen as a propulsive unit.

Some of the very first pioneers in the biomechanics of rowing were: Atkinson[5,6] (whose major works were done at the end of 19th century), Lefeuvre and Pailliotte,[7] and Alexander.[8] The first biomechanical approach to rowing focused on objective measurements of forces applied to the oar and a preliminary evaluation of the efficiency of rowing motion. In the last two decades, approximately 150 papers have been presented, among them a few general (Edwards,[9] Herberger,[10] Schroeder,[11]) and detailed, comprehensive review publications (Nolte,[12] Schneider,[13] Williams,[14] Zatziorski[15]) can be distinguished. It is really difficult now to follow all biomechanics projects and papers dedicated to rowing, due to the fact that many scientific projects have been conducted not only in biomechanical departments and laboratories, but also because several successful attempts were undertaken even in rowing clubs and national rowing centers. These were performed with the help of a variety of engineers, sometimes remote from the direct sport sciences, but nevertheless enthusiasts of rowing. The present review is not intended as a comprehensive overview of the subject matter, and therefore only the most significant references have been included.

If one intends to summarize very briefly the history of the development of biomechanical research in rowing, it can be said that if the first works were dedicated to pure measurements of basic kinematic and dynamic parameters of the rowing pattern, the later projects focused on more complex analyses of limiting factors in rowing and on objective evaluation of athletes' rowing technique. Several papers dealing with the optimum crew selection have been presented, as well as a considerable number of more fundamental works concerning hydrodynamic analysis and improvement of oars and boats. More recently, the computer-technology revolution has resulted in many studies dealing with mathematical modeling and computer simulation of the rowing pattern. A few sophisticated computer-aided measurement systems, and simulators for rowing, have also been developed and introduced in biomechanical research and rowing training.

II. GENERAL CHARACTERISTICS OF MODERN ROWING AND EQUIPMENT USED

A. Main Rules

Modern Olympic competition occurs in eight classes: from the smallest one (skiff), to the largest and fastest (eight). The dimensions and minimum weight allowed by FISA are

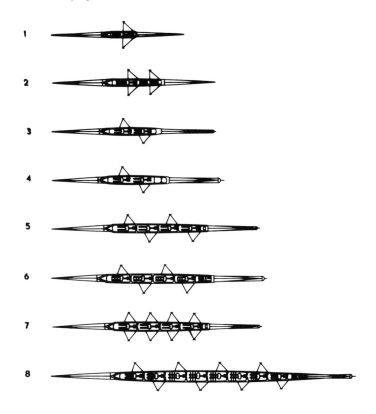

No.	TYPE OF BOAT	L (m)	W (m)	M (kg)
1	SINGLE SCULL	8.20	0.40	14
2	DOUBLE SCULLS	10.00	0.45	26
3	PAIR-OARED SHELL WITHOUT COXWAIN	10.30	0.47	27
4	PAIR-OARED SHELL WITH COXWAIN	10.50	0.50	32
5	FOUR-OARED SHELL WITHOUT COXWAIN	12.60	0.50	50
6	FOUR-OARED SHELL WITH COXWAIN	13.00	0.55	51
7	FOUR (QUADRUPLE SCULLS)	13.00	0.55	52
8	EIGHT	17.50	0.65	93

FIGURE 2.   Modern Olympic boat types.

presented in Figure 2. The race distances are 1000 m for women in categories: $1\times$, $2\times$, $2-$, $4\times+$, $4+$, $8+$, and 2000 m for men in categories: $1\times$, $2\times$, $2-$, $2+$, $4\times$, $4-$, $4+$, $8+$ ($+$ with coxwain, $-$ without coxwain, $\times$ scull). The races are carried out on 6 lines of the minimum water depth of 4 m. As an example, the approximate final times (the best results at the Moscow Olympic Games) are presented in Table 1.

B. Athletes

Athletes are generally tall, powerful individuals. According to Pope[2] they represent tall ectomorphs/mesomorphs, with the latter attribute predominating. The elementary anthropometric and kinesiological characteristics of international, national, and club male oarsmen are presented in Table 2.

Table 1
THE BEST RESULTS AT THE MOSCOW
OLYMPIC GAMES IN HOURS,
MINUTES, AND SECONDS

Category	Women — 1000 m	Men — 2000 m
1x	3'40''69	7'09''69
2x	3'16''27	6'24''33
2 −	3'30''49	6'48''01
2 +		7'02''54
4 −		6'08''17
4 +	3'19''27	6'14''51
4 ×	3'15''32	5'49''81
8 +		5'49''05

Note: See explanation in text for different categories.

Table 2
COMPARISON OF SELECTED
ANTHROPOMETRIC PARAMETERS FOR
INTERNATIONAL (GROUP I), NATIONAL
(GROUP II), AND CLUB (GROUP III)
OARSMEN[42]

Parameter	Group I	Group II	Group III
Age (yr)	26	24	24.2
Height (cm)	189	187	183
Mass (kg)	89	83	78
Handgrip force (Kp)	76	67	67
Arm force (pull) (Kp)	65	61	55
Elbow flexion (Kp)	48	43	44
Trunk extension (Kp)	112	104	107

C. Equipment

Modern boats have the hull cross-section as a slightly flattened circle. The draft of the boat with oarsmen varies from 20 to 25 cm depending on hull configuration. The riggers are usually made of stainless steel or hard alloy tubes of approximately 16 mm diameter spread from the shell centerline by approximately 0.8 m. The position of the oarlocks can be adjusted according to a given oarsman requirement. The oars are prevented from sliding overboard by a ridge, or button, on the shaft. The oarsmen are located on moveable seats with the range of slide being approximately 65 to 75 cm. The feet are placed in the adjustable stretchers fixed in the hull.

The classic top-level boats are made of high-performance laminated sheets of red cedar. However, there have been attempts to use new composites as a shell structure, due to their mechanical features and easy maintenance. The typical oars are approximately 3.75 m long and weigh from 3.5 to 4 kg. The standard oars are made of laminated spruce and ironwood. However, there is growing popularity for oars made of Kevlar® or various composites with carbon fibers.

New materials allow a better weight/stiffness ratio in comparison to standard wooden oars. The blades are double curved and there are many variations in the size and shape of the single blade. The typical shape and dimensions are presented in Figure 3.

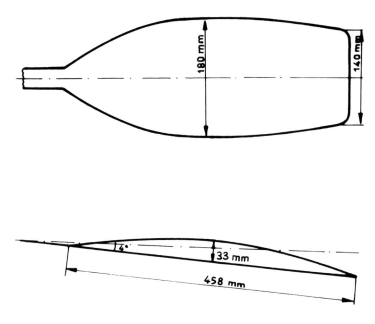

FIGURE 3.   Typical blade dimensions.

D. Motion Technique

The boat motion is executed by the oars pulled during the stroke. The whole stroke cycle consists of a drive (pull) or active phase and a recovery or passive phase (Figure 4). The pulling of the oar is executed by the extensors of lower extremities and trunk, and the flexors of the upper extremities. It is necessary that precise synchronization of muscle action occurs in order to exert a smooth, continuous flow of power to the shell. There exist several styles of rowing technique (more precisely discussed in Section IV.), but generally, the pull is initiated by lower-extremity action and then the trunk and arms. The approximate distance covered by the oar handle varies from 1.4 to 1.6 m. The oar is feathered during the recovery and is carried with the blade horizontal during the run of the boat between strokes in order to reduce air drag. The stroke rate varies from 30 to 40 beats per minute depending on style, training level, and the race distance.

The complexity of the men-boat-oars system — the peculiar motion technique with sliding body, the hydrodynamic and, to some extent aerodynamic effects — make rowing a unique sports discipline. This complexity also creates a lot of problems for biomechanists and engineers alike. Extensive studies of kinematics, dynamics, and hydrodynamics of the rower-boat-oars system are necessary to measure top-level competition and to carry out further development in this fascinating discipline.

III. BOAT OARSMAN SYSTEM AS AN OBJECT OF BIOMECHANICAL RESEARCH

A. Main Goals

To formulate the main goals of biomechanics research in rowing it is necessary to present briefly the basic field of interest of biomechanics as a science particularly involved in sport. Various definitions of biomechanics already exist[16,17] and it seems that the best explanation will be through presentation of its object of studies, functions, and goals.

A man's mechanical structure, his motion, both natural and specific, interaction with environment, equipment or implements and the influence of external conditions, determine the main object of biomechanics.

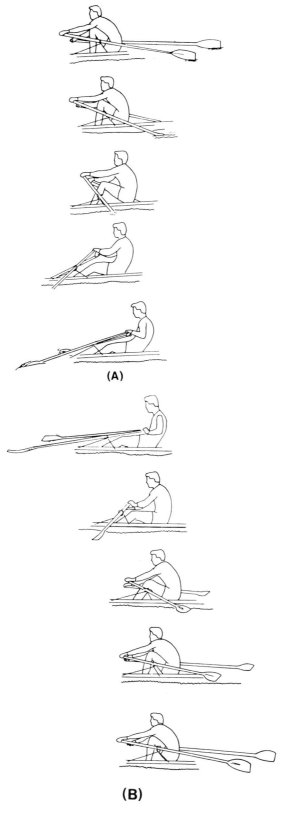

(A)

(B)

FIGURE 4.   Rowing cycle: (A) pull phase, (B) recovery phase.

The functions biomechanics is "obliged" to fulfill can be presented as follows:

- quantitative description of man's mechanical system i.e., geometry, static, and dynamic characteristics of its passive (skeleton, joints, tendons and ligaments) and active (muscles) elements.
- objective and quantitative analysis of: kinematic parameters of a human motion pattern (i.e., trajectories, velocities, and accelerations of selected points of the human body); dynamic parameters (i.e., internal and external forces the man exerts or is influenced by during this motion); environmental influences on human motion (aerodynamic and hydrodynamic aspects, ground floor structure, etc.); interaction of the human body with various types of additional equipment and implements (shoes, bicycles, poles, javelins, boats, oars, etc.).

The gaining of new knowledge of human behavior as a mechanical system by use of objective and quantitative analysis, represents a valuable goal in the field of research. The more practical goals of biomechanics, particularly in sport, can also be formulated, i.e.:

- identifying the limiting factors of athletes' performance[16,18,19]
- searching for the best available motion technique for a given sport discipline or exercise[20-25]
- identifying the factors causing injuries and damage to man's motion system from sports activity, and searching for effective ways of prevention[4,17]

All these functions and goals are strictly related to biomechanical studies in rowing. Most of them are concentrated on searching for factors influencing and limiting rowing performance.

Performance in sport has many aspects. In rowing, the determinant of performance is clearly defined — it is the final time of the boat for a given race. This final index is determined by many parameters which are related to each other. The relationship of the most important factors from which final time results can be seen is illustrated in Figure 5. The final time depends firstly on the average velocity of the boat and the distance to be covered. The average velocity is calculated as the mean of all strokes over the whole distance. The velocity for one stroke is determined by the distance covered during one stroke and the number of strokes exerted during a given time, i.e., stroke rate. The whole stroke distance can be divided into two parts, the pull and the recovery distance. The pull distance is the distance covered during the active motion of the athlete (pulling the oar with the blade in the water). The recovery distance is covered during the passive phase, while the boat moves due to the inertial forces, and the oarsmen move the oars back over the water to the starting position of the next stroke.

The factors determining the pull distance are:

- force applied by the rower on the oar handle
- blade hydrodynamic characteristics and resulting force on the blade
- angle the oar is moved from initial to final position in the water
- the timing of the pull
- air drag affecting athletes, oars, and part of the shell over the water
- hydrodynamic drag affecting the part of the shell under the water

The recovery distance is determined by:

- the initial forces acting on boat-crew system
- the masses of the boat and the crew
- the time of the recovery phase
- the aerodynamic and hydrodynamic drag

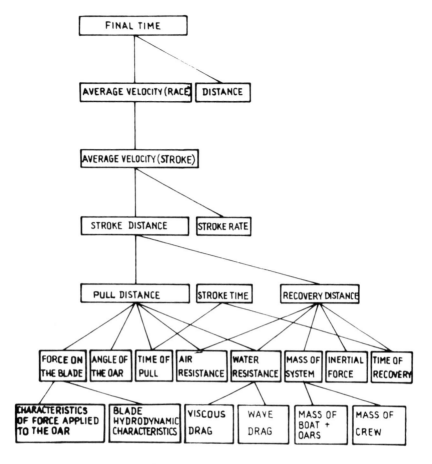

FIGURE 5. Basic factors in rowing (Adapted from Schneider.[50])

B. Main Methods

Biomechanics has introduced a wide variety of methods for rowing motion investigation. A somewhat daunting scientific approach to rowing was drawn by Dal Monte[27] (Figure 6).

The biomechanical analysis of rowing can be divided into two categories to determine what kind of parameters are to be measured:

(a)   analysis of kinematics of boat-oars-rowers system and its separate components, and
(b)   analysis of dynamics

Technically, the effort of rowers can usually be explored in three different ways:

- with the athlete working on a rowing competition boat
- with the athlete working at the training pool
- with the athlete working directly in the laboratory on an ergometer

Kinematic analysis consists of measurement, recording, and processing of the kinematic parameters of boat, oars, and athletes' motion. The following parameters are taken into consideration:

- boat — velocity of boat V_B
- oars — the angular range of displacement $\Delta\alpha$,

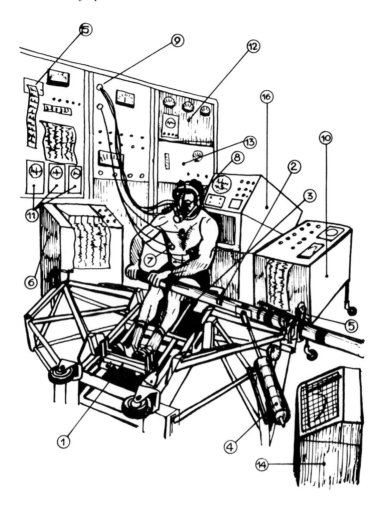

FIGURE 6.   Scientific studies of rowing can become very complex.[27]

— angular velocity $\dot{\alpha}$
— trajectory of handgrip
— oar blade angle of attack α_f
- athletes   — trajectories (x_i, y_i, z_i) of centers of gravity and selected points of body (joints, hands)
— linear velocities $(\dot{x}_i, \dot{y}_i, \dot{z}_i)$ and accelerations $(\ddot{x}_i, \ddot{y}_i, \ddot{z}_i)$
— angular displacements, velocities, and accelerations of selected body points and segments $(\phi_i, \dot{\phi}_i, \ddot{\phi}_i)$.

Various types of goniometry systems and cinematography are used as a measurement method.[12,18,27-35]

Dynamic measurements are subjected to analysis of internal and external forces. With respect to the boat, the fluctuation of hydrodynamic drag D_t and its components — viscous (D_v) and wave (D_w) drag are analyzed, as well as inertial forces acting on the boat-oars-crew center of gravity.

The hydrodynamic drag is measured directly by towing the boat in natural conditions[36] or in special pools with forced water flow.[6,37-39] Several evaluations of drag forces were made in an indirect way from the whole system dynamics analysis.[12,36]

The reaction forces at the oarlocks (F_o) resulting from the oars' action are the least significant components of forces acting on a boat. Usually the existing upward lift force (F_u) is neglected in biomechanical investigations due to its quite constant value.

Oars as the main propulsive units are investigated in a highly selective manner. The following forces are commonly measured:

- force exerted on a handgrip (F_h)
- components of forces acting on the blade i.e., longitudinal (F_{bx}) and transverse (F_{by}) to the main boat axis.

The athlete as an active dynamic system of joined masses is identified by measurements of:

- inertial forces acting on athlete's center of gravity
- forces exerted on the handgrip
- reaction force on the saddle (F_{RS})
- reaction forces on feet stretchers (F_S).

As an important factor, the "timing" of transient forces have been frequently studied i.e., time instances and periods of selected cycles, phases, and the appearance of peaks.[13,25,27,29,32,34] Several studies have also been dedicated to the evaluation of isometric strength of the athlete's main muscular groups.[13,32,41,42]

Measurement methods applied in dynamic studies vary from strain-gauge units attached to the oar bar,[12,13] or to the oarlock elements, to piezoelectric force transducers applied to the seat, and feet support.[32,43] The data are transmitted directly via multichannel telemetry systems or are recorded by use of onboard installed recording systems.[4,12,27,30,31,40] Numerous works have also been dedicated to the measurement of forces appearing during "rowing" on various types of ergometers.[12,13,29,32,43,46,47] In some cases, ergometers were installed on piezoelectric force platforms in order to measure resultant horizontal (F_{RX}) and vertical (F_{RZ}) forces. Inertial forces are usually obtained in an indirect way through processing the cinematographic data (double differentiation of center of gravity trajectory components).[12,32,43]

It should also be mentioned that there have been a limited number of researchers who studied the EMG activity of selected muscles or muscle groups which play a main role in an athlete's rowing pattern.[27,48] However, the methods were presented separately and most of the research done in rowing biomechanics combines all the methods. Despite the scientific value of a comprehensive analysis, there is also the significant practical aspect of clear presentation of parameters and timing of the rowing cycle.

Due to the definition of classic methodology, the methods presented above represent a direct experimental approach. It should also be said that notwithstanding the modern technology used in these studies (telemetry, recording systems), they are not far off the research philosophy of Atkinson[6] or Alexander,[8] who performed their work at the end of the 19th and beginning of the 20th centuries.

The significant step forward in the modern scientific approach to rowing and biomechanics, results from the introduction of computers in research investigations. Modeling, computer simulation, and optimization are the key words of modern science, and their application in biomechanics constantly grows. Even in rowing, several significant papers have been written which deal with prediction of motion and complex dynamic optimization.[2,12,14,32,49-53]

Despite some reservations regarding the direct applications of computer modeling and simulation in rowing practice, the few leading models and results of computer simulation presented later in this chapter, will strongly support the high value of this new approach both from a scientific and a practical point of view.

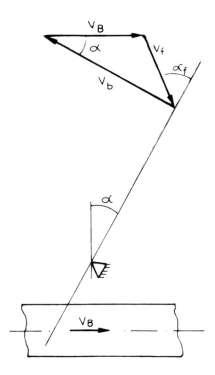

FIGURE 7.   Oar kinematics (Adapted from Alexander[8]).

C. Kinematics of Rowing

Kinematic parameters represent the ''external'' view (i.e., the output) describing the rowing pattern. The first comprehensive studies concerning boat and oar kinematics were done by Alexander[8] and extended by Gutschow.[54] The first schema of oar kinematics done by Alexander is presented in Figure 7. He obtained the following values:

- maximum blade velocity V_b was approximately 2 to 3 m/sec
- maximum blade velocity relative to the boat was approximately 1 m/sec

The one stroke velocity transients were recorded by Gutschow and are presented in Figure 8.

Several papers[55-58] were dedicated to the evaluation of boat velocity (V_B), fluctuation ΔV_B, and its dependence on stroke frequency (f).

The mean $\bar{V}_B$ as a function of stroke frequency for an Olympic two-oared shell with coxwain, was experimentally studied by Celentano et al.,[29] and the results are presented in Figure 9. The function $\bar{V}_B$ = function (f) has a nonlinear form which can be approximated by a second-order polynomial and $\bar{V}_B$ increases with the increase of stroke ratio. This shape of the $\bar{V}_B$ function is valid for all Olympic shells and was theoretically proven by comprehensive studies of Pope[2] and Senator[52] dealing with the optimum stroke rate.

The fluctuation of boat velocity ΔV_B represents an important factor for quantitative analysis of rowing performance and depends on:

- the mean velocity of the boat - one example of stroke velocity transient versus mean velocity is presented in Figure 10.
- strokes per minute (f) in Figure 11
- longitudinal slide of rower(s).

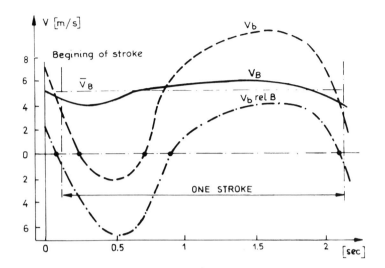

FIGURE 8.   An example of boat velocities (Adapted from Gutschow[54]).

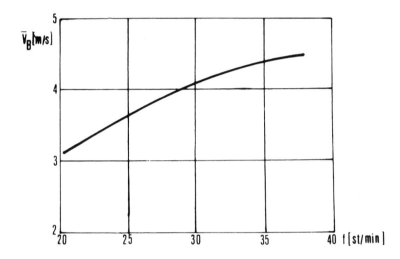

FIGURE 9.   Mean boat velocity as a function of rowing frequency (Adapted from Celentano et al.[29]).

For evaluation of ΔV_B several indexes were formulated: (a) absolute result of subtraction of maximum and minimum velocities in one stroke, or divided by mean velocity[10,59]:

$$K = |V_{Bmax} - V_{Bmin}|$$

or

$$K' = [0.5(V_{Bmax} - V_{Bmin})/\overline{V}B] \, 100 \qquad (1)$$

The value of K varies from 2.4 m/sec for a single scull to 4.5 m/sec for the eight. The value of K′ equals approximately 0.3 for a single scull; (b) subtraction of local (temporary) V_{BL} and mean velocity divided by the mean[29]

$$K_L = [(V_{BL} - \overline{V}_B)/\overline{V}_V)] \, 100 \qquad (2)$$

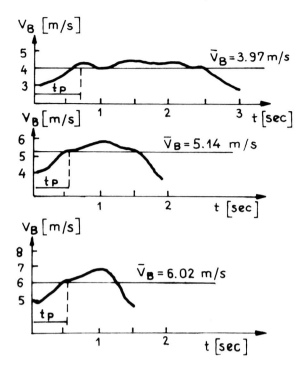

FIGURE 10.   Boat velocity transients relative to mean values (Adapted from Herberger[10]).

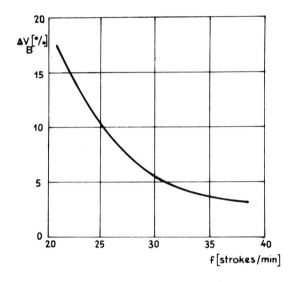

FIGURE 11.   Fluctuation of boat velocity as a function of rowing frequency (Adapted from Celentano et al.[29]).

For eight or a pair-oared shell with coxwain, K_L varies from 9.5 to 12%; (c) the integral of ΔV_B in the form[26]:

$$K_I = \int_o^{t_s} \Delta V_B(t) \, dt \approx 0.15 \tag{3}$$

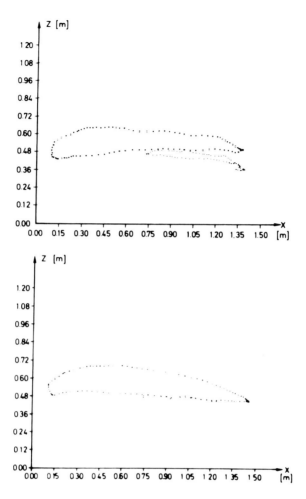

FIGURE 12. Examples of handgrip (top) and oarsman gravity center (bottom) trajectories (Adapted from Nolte[12]).

The fluctuation of V_B is one of the most important factors for evaluating rowing-motion performance. Generally speaking, the lower the value of ΔV_B, the more efficient the rowing technique. This fact results from the hydrodynamic drag function which depends on V_B to the power of two (detailed analysis of hydrodynamic drag will be presented later in this chapter).

A number of studies have also been dedicated to oar kinematics which are considered as:

- handgrip motion[12,35,60,61]
- oar blade motion[12,62-66]
- angular displacement of oar bar[12,29,63,66]

For this purpose, cinematography has mainly been used (handgrip and blade trajectories analysis) as well as goniometry systems (angular oar bar motion).

The wide experimental studies of handgrip kinematics were mainly done by Nolte[12] (examples of experimental data of handgrip trajectories vs. body center of gravity are presented in Figure 12).

The total horizontal displacement of the handgrip varies from 0.85 up to 1.5 m (mean value of all subjects was about 1.4 m), while the vertical displacement varies from 0.18 to 0.29 m (mean value was 0.24 m).

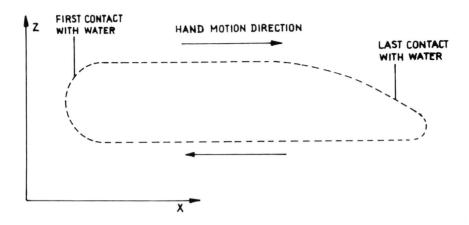

FIGURE 13.   "Ideal" handgrip trajectory.[12]

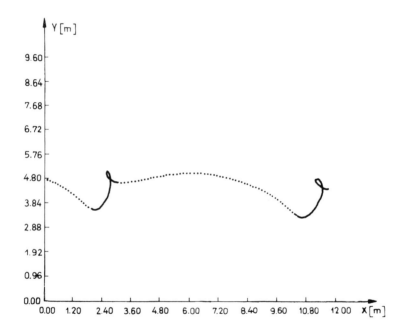

FIGURE 14.   An example of blade trajectory.[12]

Despite the presentation of comprehensive experimental results, only a qualitative analysis of the results has been attempted. General conclusions were related to a so-called "ideal" trajectory (Figure 13) which should be flat and horizontal both during the pull and recovery phase. All vertical fluctuations during the cycle create additional disturbances of water flow around the blade and reduce the pull efficiency.

Handgrip trajectory shape represents a significant factor to be analyzed in crew selection. The athletes who have the identical handgrip curves should be selected as a crew. The handgrip motion and the oar blade trajectory are strictly related, due to pure kinematic constraints. The first cinematographic studies of blade trajectory were done by Gutschow.[54] An example of blade trajectory is presented in Figure 14. Similar studies were also done by Nolte[12], but both works present only brief qualitative analyses. It seems that present knowledge of blade hydrodynamics should make it possible to begin more complex and quantitative studies concerning optimum blade shape and blade trajectory.

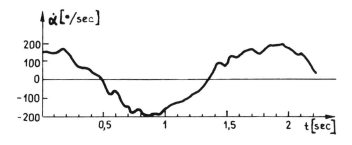

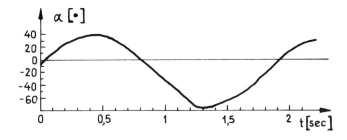

FIGURE 15.   An example of oar angle and angular velocity transients.[12]

Table 3
VALUES OF SELECTED KINEMATIC PARAMETERS OF ROWER MOTION[a]

Parameter	Min. value	Max. Value	Difference
Horizontal displacement of athlete CG vs. boat CG (m)	0.22	0.70	0.48
Horizontal velocity of athlete CG vs. total CG velocity (m/sec)	− 0.18	0.15	0.33
Knee angle (°)	55	160	105
Hip angle (°)	26	116	90
Arm angle (°)	95	172	77
Trunk angle (°)	− 26	26	52
Shank angle (°)	4	69	65

[a]   Adapted From Nolte.[12]

The final aspect of oar kinematics relates to angular motion of the oar, and it is usually combined with other kinematic and dynamic parameters. Typical oar angle and angular velocity transients are presented in Figure 15. For the top level oarsman the α range is approximately 80°.

The last aspect of kinematics concerns the man's motion. Rower kinematics were widely studied by Nolte,[12,67,68] and valuable data for top-level international athletes were obtained by means of cinematographic analysis. These data are summarized in Table 3.

Although kinematics represents the overall "shape" of motion, it is only the result of internal and external forces acting on the system. A detailed analysis of the dynamics of the boat, oars and rower, the forces, and their relation to the main kinematic parameters, will follow in the next section.

D. Dynamics of Rowing

The boat-oars-rowers system, as a complex mechanical system, should be considered in the context of classical dynamic and hydrodynamic principles. This part of the review stresses analysis of internal and external forces and their influence on kinematics and the performance of rowing, that is the final time for a given distance.

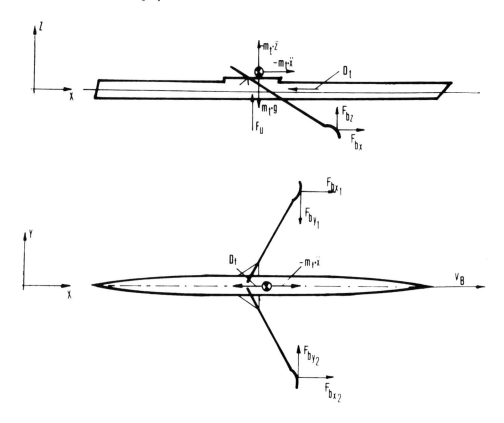

FIGURE 16.   Free-body diagrams showing the main forces acting on the boat-oar-rower system.[12]

Although each rowing researcher has tried to measure at least one of the forces appearing in our system, it is difficult to find a comprehensive study which gives answers to "simple" questions; what should be the "shape" of the force applied to the oar (Fh), or what should be the overall motion of rowers to generate the fastest possible motion of the boat and to cover a set distance in the shortest time? The peculiarity of this system of men, boat, and oars, the effect of sliding masses, the interaction of the oar with the water, all affected by the physiology of the athletes and their endurance, contribute to one of the most fascinating problems in biomechanics.

It is obvious that a brief presentation cannot pretend to provide the final answer to the optimum dynamics of rowing. However, from the first experiments of Atkinson,[6] to recent comprehensive reports of Cameron,[56] Celentano et al.,[29] Dal Monte et al.,[27,31,32] Nolte,[12,33,40,67-69] Pope,[2] and Williams,[3,14] a lot of valuable data have been obtained. This makes it a little bit easier to understand the phenomenon of rowing and to conduct further investigations.

Due to the complexity of the hydrodynamics of rowing, the analysis of factors influencing the hydrodynamic performance of the boat and oars, will be presented separately in the next section, while the overall analysis of forces acting on the whole system will be given now.

In order to simplify the discussion, a single-scull boat will be analyzed dynamically. However, the equations and conclusions are valid for the other rowing categories.

Due to the main mechanical principles, the system can be defined as in the simplified form of Figure 16, and can be described by the equations:

$$\sum F_x = F_{bx} - D_t - m_t\ddot{x} \qquad = 0$$

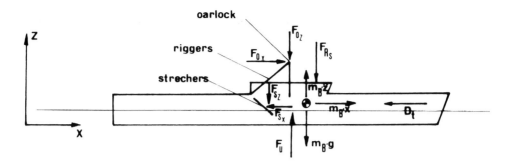

FIGURE 17.   Forces acting on the boat.

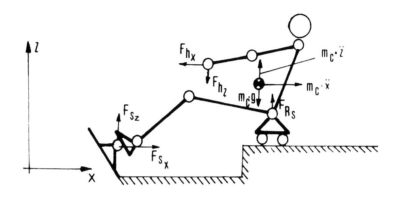

FIGURE 18.   Forces acting on the rower.[12]

$$\sum F_y = F_{by2} - F_{by1} - m_t\ddot{y} \quad = 0$$

$$\sum F_z = F_u + F_{bz} - m_t(g - \ddot{z}) = 0 \qquad (4)$$

These expressions describe the pull phase while the oars are in the water ($F_{bx} \neq O$, $F_{by} \neq O$, $F_{bz} \neq O$).

The recovery phase simplifies the form of Equation 4 to:

$$\sum F_x = -D_t - m_t\ddot{x} \quad = 0$$

$$\sum F_y \qquad\qquad\qquad = 0$$

$$\sum F_z = F_u - m_t(g - \ddot{z}) = 0 \qquad (5)$$

The dynamics of the boat as a part of the system (Figure 17) can be satisfactorily described by the following set of equations:

$$\sum F_x = F_{ox} - F_{sx} + m_B\ddot{x} - D_t = 0$$

$$\sum F_z = F_u - F_{oz} - F_{RS} - F_{SZ} + m_B(\ddot{z} - g) = 0 \qquad (6)$$

The dynamics of the athlete can be presented in many ways, depending on assumed simplification of his body structure. Usually a simple mass representation is used.[2,12,14,15,43] However, several studies of kinematics and dynamics of multisegment structures have also been done (Dal Monte et al.[32]). According to Nolte,[12] the dynamics of the rower can be defined as follows (Figure 18):

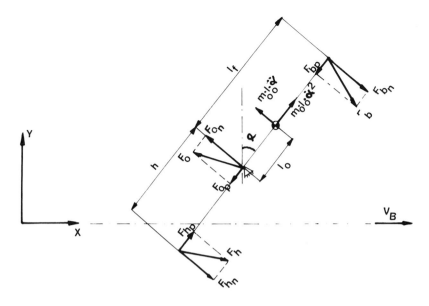

FIGURE 19.   Forces acting on the oars.[12]

$$\sum F_x = F_{sx} - F_{hx} + m_c \ddot{x} = 0$$

$$\sum F_z = F_{sz} - F_{hz} - m_c(g + \ddot{z}) + F_{RS} = 0 \qquad (7)$$

Focusing attention on the oars, their dynamics can be presented as in Figure 19, while the full force acting on the blade is as in Figure 20. The components can be described by the following formulae:

$$F_b = F_p \sin \gamma$$

$$F_d = F_b \cos \gamma$$

$$F_{bn} = F_b \cos \epsilon'$$

$$F_{bp} = F_b \sin \epsilon'$$

$$F_{bx} = F_b \sin \psi$$

$$(8)$$

where γ = arc tan (F_p/F_d) and results from blade propulsion (ζ_p) and drag (ζ_d) coefficients (further analysis in a later section).

$\epsilon' = \epsilon - 90°$
ϵ = arc tan $(F_p/F_d) + \alpha_f - \tau$
α_f = angular position of the oar blade
τ = angle between longitudinal axes of blade and oar bar

All the forces appearing in the dynamic Equations 4 to 8 can be measured in a direct or indirect way. The attention of researchers has focused mainly on external forces acting on the oars as the main propulsive units of the system.[5,12,28,61]

A variety of instrumentation was used in these measurements. The 80 years of history of oarlock forces (F_o) and measurement techniques is presented in Figure 21, where the first

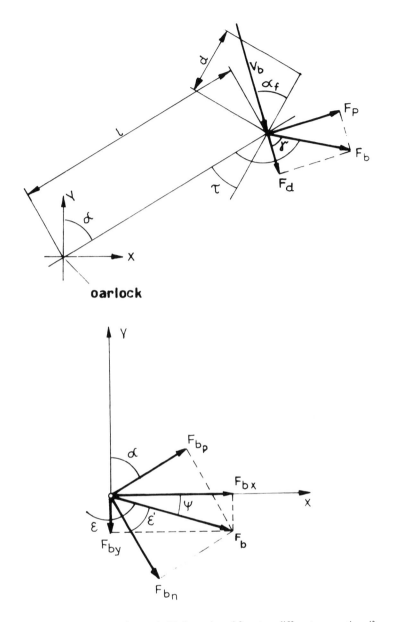

FIGURE 20.   Forces acting on the blade as viewed from two different perspectives.[12]

unit represents the mechanical system used by Leufeuvre and Paillotte[7] in 1904, and the second a complex measurement unit used by Nolte[12] in 1980. The typical shapes of external forces acting on the oar (according to the force system presented in Figure 19) is shown in Figure 22.

A particular problem related to forces applied to the oar, concerns the reproducibility of the given shape during the whole race. This aspect, maintaining the same motion technique and resulting propulsive impulse, was widely studied by Dal Monte et al.,[27] Nolte,[12] Schneider,[34] and others.

The experimental results obtained by Dal Monte, of force F_h vs. angle of oar pattern during a 6-min test, provided evidence for both the effect of fatigue and the individual differences between oarsmen. Similar results were also observed while measuring the forces applied to the stretchers (F_s). The results for four rowers are presented in Figure 23. In

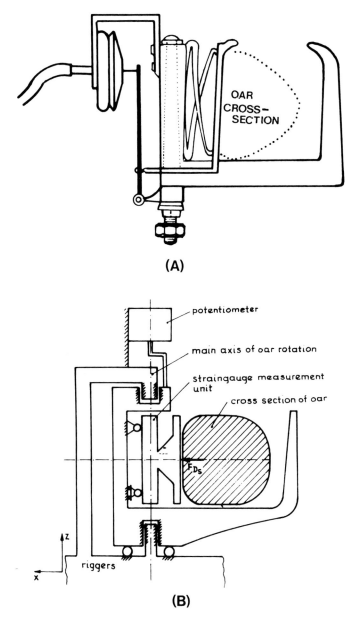

FIGURE 21. Oarlock force measurement units: (A) Lefeuvre and Pailliotte[7] in 1904; (B) Nolte[12] in 1980.

Figure 23 a one can see the first loop on the left side marked with a 1 that represents the force/angle pattern in the first minute of the simulated competition. With a 2 in the center, the curves representing the pattern of effort at the second, third, fourth, and fifth minutes of the effort are indicated, while a 3 in the right shows the force/angle pattern taken at the very last moment of the test. In Figures 23b, c, and d one can observe the variations in timing and the area of the force curves. In Figure 23b, an athlete with a comparatively high force capability in the first minute, can be observed. He is quite able to maintain a fairly high level of strength in the whole simulated competition, but is not able to increase his power in the last minute. Figure 23c presents an athlete with a force profile with the maximum value in the first minute during the competition. This athlete has a marked reduction of his power and only at the very last moment is he able to increase his strength.

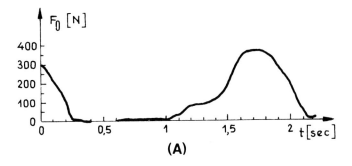

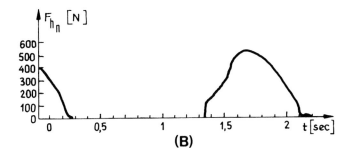

FIGURE 22. Examples of force transients acting on the oar: (A) transient of oarlock force; (B) transient of handgrip force (norman component according to Figure 15); (C) transients of angle of water flow around the blade and main force components acting on the blade (Adapted from experimental data of Nolte[12]).

The last athlete, seen in Figure 23d, is quite poor in performance in the first minute; he changes his force/angle pattern in a dramatic way during the test, and at the last minute is able to perform at a level with a similar shape of force curve as in the first minute of competition.

Interesting three-dimensional computer elaboration of force vs. length of stroke and time of stroke, are presented in Figure 24. It is clearly shown that even top-level athletes cannot repeat their movements with absolute regularity. The "ideal", but unreachable dream of any rower and coach is presented in Figure 25; however, the author's serious opinion was " . . . it could be obtained if the athlete was a robot . . . ".[27] A similar problem together with the timing aspect, was studied by Schneider.[13,34] The same shape reproducibility during the whole race and by all the members of the crew, was found crucial in winning a given race. An example of force reproducibility and timing (time of pull phase, t_p) and time of gaining the maximum force (t_m) vs. stroke rate is shown in Figure 26. It was observed that the force curve and timing changes significantly for some athletes, particularly for rower number 2. Such details seem to have some practical value and should be considered by coaches as a way of improving the training of selected teams and to control their efficiency. Overall stroke timing related to the force on a blade (force exerted by the water perpendicular to the oar blade, F_b) is strictly related to the previous point. Figure 27 shows typical timing vs. stroke rate. It was previously shown during a kinematic analysis that the time of the stroke (t_s) decreases a hyperbolic function of time, while the stroke ratio increases. Time of pull (t_p) remains almost the same, and this means that a higher rate of rowing is achieved by shortening the period of the recovery phase (t_r).

The dynamic pattern of motion is closely related to the EMG activity of main muscle groups. A simple explanation of the action of selected muscles of the rower and a visualization

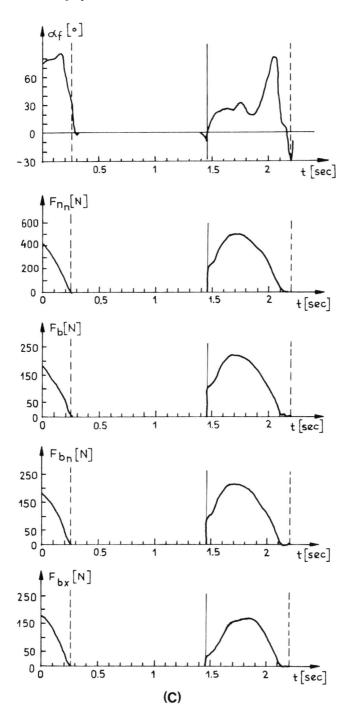

(C)

of the concentric, eccentric, and isometric action is shown in Figure 28. Due to the complexity of motion and the technical problems, associated with transmitting the EMG signals during rowing in natural conditions, only a few papers exist which touch on this problem. A comprehensive study of the EMG activity of well-trained oarsmen and beginners was done by Kabsch and Dworak.[48] A comparison of the EMG pattern of the main muscles "responsible" for the rowing action, for two top-level oarsmen and one beginner, is presented in Figure 29. The authors concluded, and it is evident from the illustration, that the well-

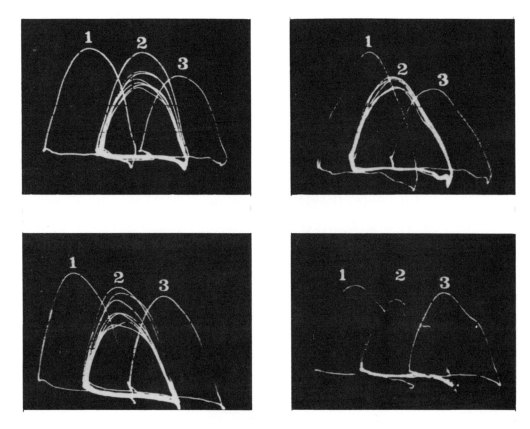

FIGURE 23. An example of fatigue effects on force/angle patterns during a 6-min test (Adapted from Dal Monte[27]).

trained competitors demonstrated significantly more-thrifty muscle activity. A comparison of subjects 1 and 2 also shows a high uniformity which confirms the well-known phenomenon of muscle coordination developed in the course of the training process. Although technical problems limit the wide use of electromyography in rowing, it seems evident that such data have a high diagnostic value in crew-member selection and training.

E. Hydrodynamic Aspects of Rowing

The primary performance criterion in rowing is the minimization of the final time. Therefore, the main goal of rowers is to overcome, and, if at all possible, to utilize all external resistance forces in order to move their boats and bodies with the highest possible velocity. With regards to rowing practice and training, as well as the improvement of boat and oar design, the following questions should be addressed by biomechanics research:

- what kind of external resistance forces act on the boat and oarsmen during rowing?
- what are the factors these forces depend on?
- what are the values and characteristics of the resistance forces?

Hydrodynamic drag forces result from two sources. The first is a viscous drag (D_v) which depends on Reynolds number and the smoothness of the hull. The second one, the wave drag (D_w), arises while the boat has to pass the waves generated on the water level. Wave drag is a function of Froude number. The total drag (D_t) as a sum of D_v and D_w, can be measured in many ways. Usually, two methods are the most common. The first one applies to the natural conditions of the race or training and is based on cinematography.[12,36] Analysis of the film enables us to calculate trajectories of gravity centers of the boat and body segments

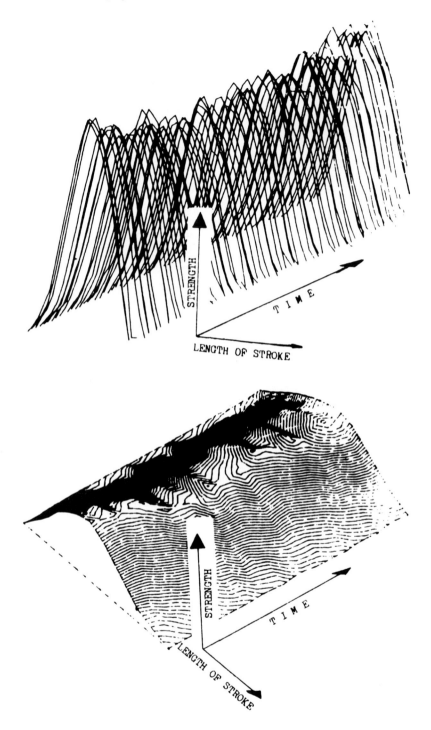

FIGURE 24.   Two forms of three-dimensional representation of real force exerted by a rower
vs. time and length of stroke.[27]

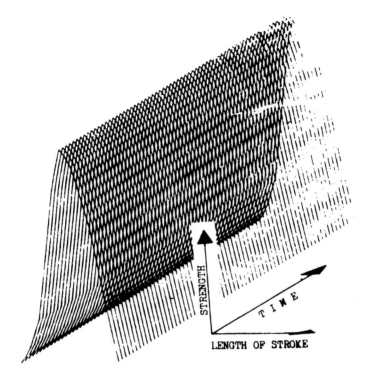

FIGURE 25. An "ideal shape" of force vs. time and length of stroke pattern.[27]

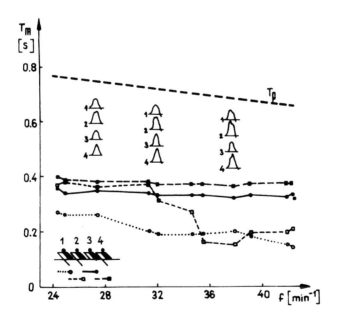

FIGURE 26. Force reproducibility vs. stroke rate (Adapted from Schneider[34]).

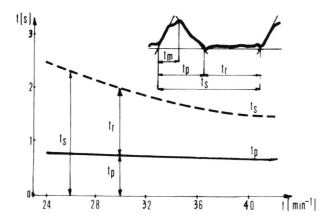

FIGURE 27.   Timing of stroke vs. stroke rate (Adapted from Schneider[34]).

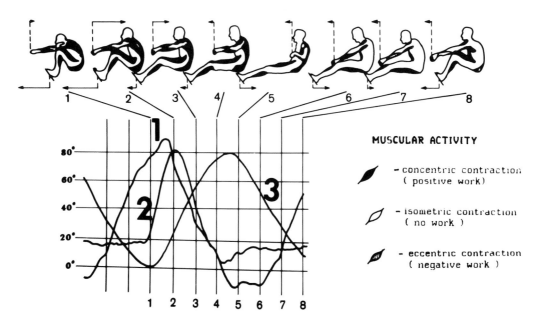

FIGURE 28.   Muscular activity during rowing.

of the oarsmen, and then the velocities and accelerations of the whole system. Knowing the mass of the boat, oars, and crew it is possible to calculate forces acting on the oarsmen (F_R), boat (F_B), and the whole system (F_S) (Figure 30). While F_B approximately $= 0$ then $F_S = F_R = D_t$. On the basis of the example presented in Figure 30, the evaluated total drag D was equal to 70 N for a velocity equal to 4.68 m/sec (single scull). Similar values were obtained by Celentano et al.[29] by measuring the overall propulsive force F_P and then calculating the mean value of the total drag i.e.,:

$$D_t = (\overline{V}_B/L_S) \int_o^{t_s} F_p \, dt \qquad (9)$$

where $\overline{V}_B$ = mean velocity of boat during one stroke,

L_S = distance covered by boat in one stroke,

t_s = time duration of one stroke.

81

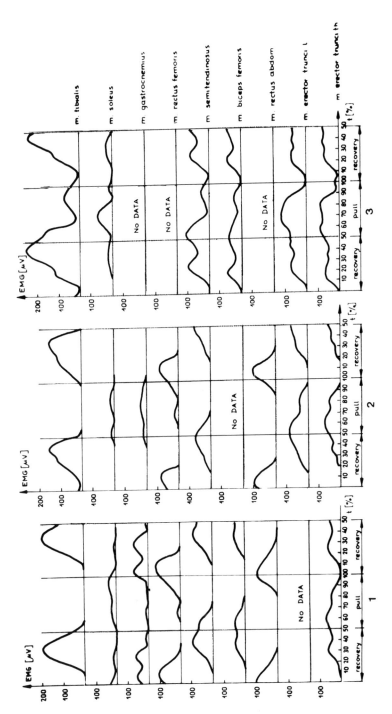

FIGURE 29. EMG activity of main muscles during rowing; 1 and 2 are experimental data of top-level oarsmen, while 3 is of beginners (Adapted from Kabsch and Dworak[48]).

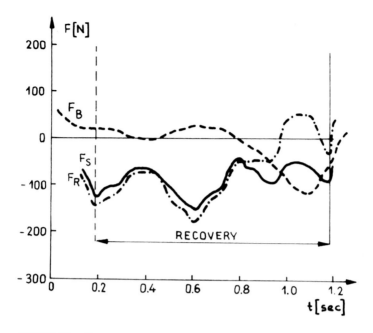

FIGURE 30.   Forces acting on the boat (F_B), rower (F_R), and the whole system (F_S) during the recovery phase (Adapted from Wyganowska[36]).

The D_t function of $\bar{V}_B$ for a pair-oared shell with coxwain is presented in Figure 31.

The second method is based on the measurement of reaction force, while towing the boat at a constant speed, or during experiments in pools with a forced water flow.[36,39,57] Examples of data for an eight show the following values of D_t:

$$V_B = 5 \text{ m/sec} \qquad D_t = 310 \quad \text{to} \quad 340 \text{ N}$$

$$V_B = 6 \text{ m/sec} \qquad D_t = 428 \quad \text{to} \quad 458 \text{ N}$$

However, it is necessary to mention that such an approach is limited due to the fact that measurements are made for a constant boat velocity or water flow. A fluctuation in velocity results in significant changes of D_t and its components.

Viscous drag measurements have been widely studied. A comprehsnsive discussion was presented among others by Marchaj,[70] Wellicome,[39] and Wyganowska.[36]

Viscous drag results form transferring the kinetic energy of the boat to the water surrounding the shell. This drag arises in the boundary layer, the thickness (H_{bL}) of which can reach 2% of the shell length (L_B) at the water level. Using the example of the single scull and eight, the thickness of the boundary layer at the stern can be:

$$\text{Single scull} - L_B = 8 \text{ m} \qquad H_{bL} = 16 \text{ cm}$$

$$\text{eight} \quad - \quad L_B = 18 \text{ m} \qquad H_{bL} = 36 \text{ cm}$$

The flow in the boundary layer depends on the Reynolds number:

$$Re = V_B L_B / \nu \tag{10}$$

where ν = viscous coefficient of water ($\nu = 1.2 \times 10^{-6}$ m/sec for a temperature of 15°C).

While Re is comparatively small, the flow in the boundary layer is laminar and D_v is proportional to V_B. If Re is greater than some critical value (according to Marchaj,[70] $Re_{crit} = 5 \times 10^5 / 5 \times 10^6$) the flow becomes turbulent and D_v increases significantly and is proportional to $V_b^{1.75} \div V_b^2$.

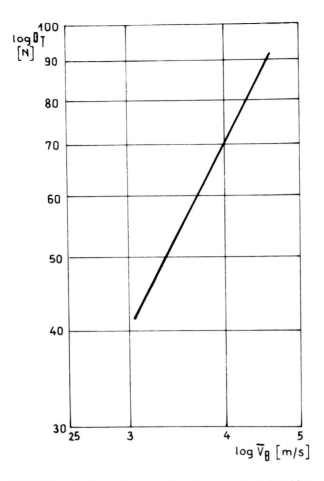

FIGURE 31.   Total drag D_T as a function of boat velocity (Adapted from Wyganowska[36]).

Based on Equation 9 the point on the shell where turbulent flow appears can be calculated as follows:

$$L_{crit} = Re \ \nu/V_B \qquad (11)$$

For $Re = 5 \times 10^6$ the values of L_{crit} are as follows:

$$V_B = 3 \text{ m/sec} \qquad L_{crit} = 2 \text{ m}$$

$$V_B = 4 \text{ m/sec} \qquad L_{crit} = 1.5 \text{ m}$$

$$V_B = 5 \text{ m/sec} \qquad L_{crit} = 1.2 \text{ m}$$

$$V_B = 6 \text{ m/sec} \qquad L_{crit} = 1 \text{ m}$$

Taking the standard lengths of boats and mean race velocities it can be seen that approximately 90% of shell length is usually covered by turbulent flow.

The viscous drag D_v is defined by the equation:

$$D_v = 0.5 \ C_{vs} \ V_B^2 \ A \qquad (12)$$

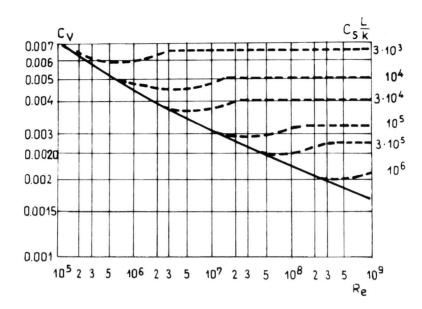

FIGURE 32.   Smoothness of shell vs. Reynolds number.

where

$$C_v = \text{coefficient of viscous drag}$$

$$\rho = \text{water density}$$

$$A = \text{wetted area of boat}$$

The C_v coefficient is proportional to Re and is also a function of the smoothness of the shell. This smoothness is defined as follows:

$$C_s = L_B/k \tag{13}$$

where k = height of surface irregularities

Typical values of k are:

surface absolutely smooth (theoretical)   k = 0

surface polished and varnished   k = 0.005 mm

surface painted   k = 0.05 mm

pure wood   k = 0.5 mm

The function $C_v = f(Re,C_s)$ is presented in Figure 32.

If we assume k = 0.005 then for the single shell $0 = 1.6 \times 10^6$ and for eight, $C_s = 36 \times 10^6$.

For higher velocities, Re increases and the requirements concerning the shell smoothness are more rigorous. Assuming that $V_B = 6$ m/sec and k = 0.005 for eight, the value of C_v will be 0.0023 and $D_v = 410$ N (Wygarowska[36]). However, the same boat with k = 0.55 has $C_v = 0.04$ and then the viscous drag reaches a value of 714 N.

The viscous drag, according to Equation 12, depends also on the wetted surface. This surface can be estimated by using the following equation:

$$A = \sqrt{2\pi L_B V} \qquad (14)$$

where V = volume (uplift) of the boat

Taking the eight as an example, the total weight can be evaluated as follows:

$$8 \text{ rowers} \times 800 \text{ N} = 6400 \text{ N}$$

$$\text{oars} = 320 \text{ N}$$

$$\text{coxwain} = 500 \text{ N}$$

$$\text{boat} = 1150 \text{ N}$$

$$\text{Total} = 8370 \text{ N}$$

Then the volume is equal to 0.837 m³ and the wetted surface A = 9.72 m². Assuming the weight of each rower equals 800 N, the wetted surface for all categories varies from 2.25 for a single scull to 9.72 for an eight.[36]

According to Equation 12 the viscous drag is proportional to A and thus to the weight of the rowers. The higher the mass of the rowers the greater is the wetted area and the resulting viscous drag. Gerdes[37,38,64] estimated that if the weight of the oarsmen decreased by 10% then the D_v would be reduced by approximately 5%. Having the same crew but a boat which was lighter by 5%, velocity would increase by approximately 0.9% and there would be an advantage of 18 m in a 2000 m distance.

The viscous drag represents 88% (single scull) to 93.5% (eight) of total hydrodynamic drag.[36] Similar values were obtained by Wellicome[39] during a test made at the National Physical Laboratory in England. A brief mention concerning the effect of water temperature on D_v should also be made. The viscosity of water depends on temperature, that is the higher the temperature the lower the viscosity and the higher the value of Re. Gerdes[38] estimated that an increase in water temperature of approximately 5% results in a reduction in D_v of approximately 3%, and gives an advantage of 14 m over a 2000 m distance (for eight). Another component of the total hydrodynamic drag, but to a lesser extent, is wave drag D_w. The wave drag, as a function of the Froude number, exhibits the shape of the maxima and minima, which results from the interference of the bow and stern on the wave pattern. It therefore depends on the hull shape in a complex way.

According to Marchaj,[70] the wave drag can be approximated by the equation:

$$D_w \approx h^2 \lambda$$

where   h = height of the wave

λ = length of the wave   (15)

Given these considerations, Pope[2] suggested that the total hydrodynamic drag could be modeled as:

$$D_t = 0.5(1.07) V_B^2 L_B A = k_o V_B^2 \qquad (16)$$

where the factor 1.07 was included to account for the effect of wave drag.

The last aspect concerning the effect of depth of water on the wave drag should also be briefly mentioned. Shallow water increases the value of D_w significantly. It results from critical wave velocities V_{wc} which depend on the depth of the water as:

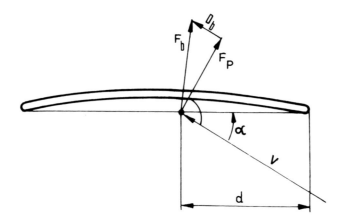

FIGURE 33.   Forces on the blade (Adapted from Foppl[62]).

$$V_{wc} = \sqrt{gh}$$

where   h = depth of the water

g = gravity coefficient   (17)

If $V_B = V_{wc}$ then a local increase of D_w appears.
According to Marchaj[70] for:

$$h = 2 \text{ m} \quad V_{wc} = 4.42 \text{ m/sec}$$

$$h = 3 \text{ m} \quad V_{wc} = 5.43 \text{ m/sec}$$

$$h = 4 \text{ m} \quad V_{wc} = 6.27 \text{ m/sec}$$

$$h = 5 \text{ m} \quad V_{wc} = 7.1 \text{ m/sec}$$

The highest wave drag for a boat moving with a velocity equal to 4.42 m/sec appears on water of 2 m depth. It also appears that the faster the boat the deeper the water should be.

These considerations have significant practical implications in rowing races. Generally, the rowing line should have a depth of 4 m, but the fluctuation in depth, depending on the line, affects the changes for a given boat. For example, if line 1 has a depth of 4 m and lines 4 to 6 have a depth of 9 m, the boat racing on line 1 is slightly handicapped.

Attention should also be given to the oar blade hydrodynamics. Unfortunately, only very few papers dealing with this subject are available. The first experimental analysis of blade hydrodynamics was done by Foppl.[62] The total force on blade F_b and its components (drag D_b and the propulsive component F_p) were evaluated as seen in Figure 33.

The propulsive efficiency of the blade was defined as:

$$\zeta_p = F_p/(S\gamma V_b^2/g)   (18)$$

and the drag coefficient as:

$$\zeta_d = D_b/(S\gamma V_b^2/g)   (19)$$

where S = surface area of the blade

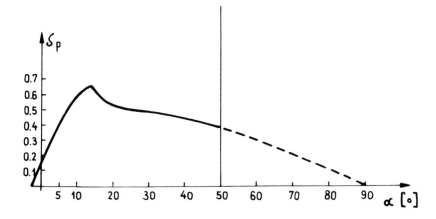

FIGURE 34. Propulsive efficiency of the blade as a function of angle of water flow.[62]

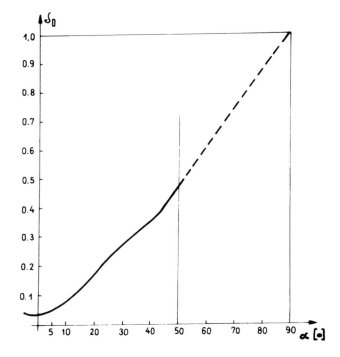

FIGURE 35. Blade drag as a function of angle of water flow.[62]

These coefficients were evaluated as a function of the angle of water flow around the blade, α_f. The example of ζ_p = function (α_f) and ζ_d = function (α_f) are presented in Figures 34 and 35, respectively.

IV. MAIN PERFORMANCE INDICES FOR EVALUATING ROWING TECHNIQUE

The previous sections were focused mainly on fundamental studies of the mechanics of rowing. It would also seem to be appropriate to present some aspects of biomechanical research which are directly applied to rowing practice and training. Generally, the qualitative

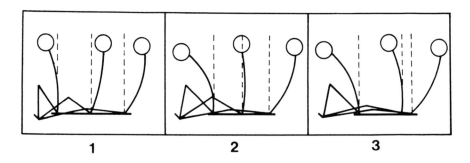

FIGURE 36.   Schematic representation of Adam (1), DDR (2), and Rosenberg (3) rowing styles.[96]

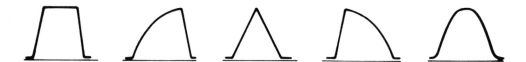

FIGURE 37.   Classification of force shapes applied to the oargrip (adapted from Szapkov[79]).

and quantitative approaches to rowing technique, its evaluation, and athlete selection, can be emphasized.[13,15,22,25,34,71-74]

The first refers mainly to classification of the variations in rowing technique, called "rowing styles". Several authors and practitioners have attempted to standardize this classification based on kinematic or dynamic patterns of rowing. The first attempt Klavora[96] defines the following three main styles of rowing (Figure 36).

- Adam[76] — comparatively long-lasting activity of lower extremities, a limited lowering of the trunk at the beginning of the stroke, and simultaneous activity of legs and trunk during the stroke.
- DDR — large, forward declination of the trunk at the beginning of the stroke without a significant press on the stretchers, followed by simultaneous activity of the legs and trunk extensors.
- Rosenberg — large, forward declination of the trunk at the beginning of the stroke, then strong leg extension without significant trunk activation. At the end of the cycle the trunk stops in the deep backward position.

Several authors have also mentioned the so-called "Tsukuba" style.[13,77,78]

Another classification of rowing styles is based on an analysis of the shape of the force that is applied to the oargrip, or the forces on the oarlocks. A peculiarity of this shape was used as a basis for style differentiation by Dworak,[71] Schneider,[13] and Szapkov.[79] The shape analysis done by Szapkov is presented in Figure 37. It was assumed that shape No. 1, the "idealistic" one, represents the optimum form from a mechanical viewpoint. However, due to the kinematic structure of the human body and characteristics of the muscle actuators, this shape seems practically impossible to realize.

A comprehensive study of force shapes which was more quantitative was done by Korner.[25] Based on the oarlock force shape, and velocity of the boat and blade transients during the pull phase, he defined three main styles of rowing pattern (Figure 38):

- style A — fast increase of force in the initial phase of the pull (Δt_1) and later a smooth decrease

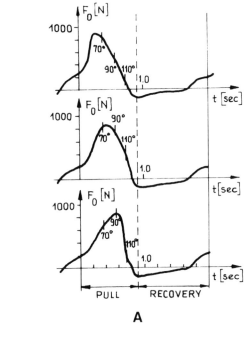

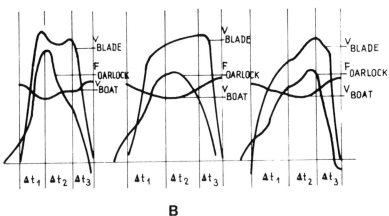

FIGURE 38. Kinematic and dynamic characteristics of A, B, and C rowing styles; (A) forces F_O, (B) transients of blade velocity, V_b, boat velocity, V_B, and oarlock reaction, F_o (Adapted from Korner[25]).

- style B — the pulling force grows steadily and attains its maximum value in the middle of the stroke (Δt_2) then symmetrically decreases in the final part of the pull
- style C — opposite of style A — the maximum pulling force is attained in the final part of the pull (Δt_3)

It was assumed that style B was the optimum one. However, several additional conditions like horizontal and linear blade motion should also be satisfied. Although the above qualitative classification is significant and important, it represents a subjective analysis, and therefore cannot be used as a precise and objective tool for evaluating rowing performance. This was also noticed by Schneider[13] while analyzing the Klavora classification. He felt that the more objective and quantitative criteria concerning kinematics and dynamics should be defined

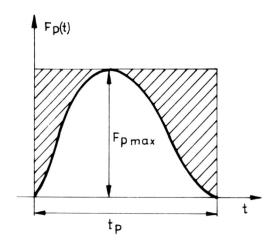

FIGURE 39. Graphic representation of efficiency index (Adapted from Dworak[44]).

and then used in rowing practice in order to maintain effective oarsmen selection, and to perform exact control of training.

In the biomechanics literature, several quantitative criteria directed at rowing performance evaluation can be found, but they still do not present a uniform and unequivocal system of evaluation.

Generally, these criteria can be divided into two categories:

●   indices related to the forces and timing
●   indices related to work, power, and overall efficiency

The first category can be represented by the following indices[71]

$$I_{Fh} = \int_o^{t_s} F_h(t) \, dt \rightarrow max \qquad (20)$$

where I_{Fh} = impulse of force applied to the handle, or Figure 39:

$$\eta_I = \int_o^{t_p} F_h(t) \, dt / F_{hmax} \, t_p \rightarrow max \qquad (21)$$

where η_I = dynamic efficiency index, and represents the relationship between real force impulses developed by the athlete an the "ideal" rectangular shape.

According to Dworak's[44] studies of 32 top Polish oarsmen, the following classification was obtained:

very high efficiency	—	80 to 100%, 2 subjects
high efficiency	—	70 to 80%, 3 subjects
average efficiency	—	60 to 70%, 12 subjects
low efficiency	—	50 to 60%, 14 subjects
very low efficiency	—	< 50%, 1 subject

The force impulse index was also widely used by Schneider[32] in rower selection from the point of view of uniformity of the impulse shape and value. Examples of a four without a coxwain (Figure 40) show that there are rather big differences in impulses between the

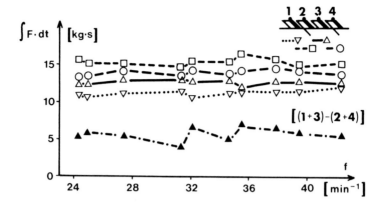

FIGURE 40.   Force impulse per stroke for four without coxwain vs. stroke rate.[32]

members of the tested crew. Since the oars of the two stronger rowers were positioned on the same side of the boat the crew was obliged to steer. Steering, however, consumes a part of the propulsive energy and reduces the speed of the boat. In order to achieve a better-balanced crew the coach changed the position of rowers with the resulting difference between the sides approximately zero. According to Schneider[13] this might be one of the reasons why this crew won the championship.

The criteria related to work and power usually have a very simple form:

$$W_{7min} \rightarrow max \text{ (where } W_{7min} = \text{ work done during a 7-min test)}$$

and

$$\bar{P} \rightarrow max$$

The values of W_{7min} and $\bar{P}$ give the simple stratification of physical fitness of athletes and are frequently used as a main selection criterion.

Several criteria have also been developed to evaluate overall rowing efficiency. According to Zatziorski[15] they can be defined as follows:

(1) relative boat and oar blade velocities index:

$$\eta_1 = \bar{V}_B/(\bar{V}_B + \bar{V}_b)/2$$

the value of η_1 reaches 0.6135   (22)

(2) relative velocities coefficient including blade drag:

$$\eta_2 = (V_B/V_{bre1B})(D_{bp} - D_{br})/(D_{bp} + D_{br})$$

where V_{bre1B} = velocity of blade relative to the boat

D_{bp} = mean hydrodynamic drag on the blade during the pull

D_{br} = mean aerodynamic drag on the blade during the recovery   (23)

(3) overall propulsion coefficient

$$\eta_3 = \eta_b \eta_f$$

where η_b = coefficient representing hydrodynamic efficiency of the blade   (24)

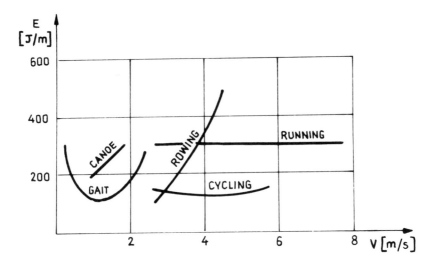

FIGURE 41.   Energy cost of selected parameters vs. time (Adapted from Asami[82]).

$$\eta_f = 1 \Big/ \int_o^{t_s} (1 + \overline{V}_B)^3 \, dt \tag{25}$$

and is the coefficient representing energy cost resulting from the velocity of the boat fluctuation ($\eta_f \approx 0.94$)

(4) overall mechanical efficiency

$$\eta_4 = \eta_m \, \eta_h \tag{26}$$

where η_m = mechanical efficiency coefficient representing energy cost related to interaction of rower and oar, and angular motion of the oar in the oarlock (friction) ($\eta_m \approx 0.9$); η_h = hydrodynamic efficiency coefficient (for boat and oars); for a single scull $\eta_h \approx 0.67$. The value of η_4 varies from 0.585 to 0.603.

V. ENERGY, WORK, AND POWER

Due to the fact that rowing represents a limited type of motion, the problem of global energy efficiency is crucial for maximum rowing results. A 7-min race results in a heart rate of more than a 200 beats/min and an oxygen uptake of more than 700 mℓ/kg/min. Rowing is one of the sports where the highest energy expenditure is attained. It has also been found that absolute maximum aerobic power is definitely higher for rowers than for other athletes performing aerobic exercises (Di Pampero et al.,[80] Cerretelli and Padovani[81]).

The brief comparison of energy cost for various sport disciplines is presented in Figure 41. According to Vaughan[24] " . . . of all different topics on the biomechanics of running gait, this one on mechanical energy, work, and power is undoubtedly the one where least agreement exists . . . ". The same can be said of biomechanics studies of work and power in rowing. Instead of long-winded discussion and analysis of the correctness of existing work and power definitions, authors are summarized in Tables 4 and 5 including the definitions of these mechanical factors in rowing biomechanics.

Generally, the work or power calculations are related to oarsmen activity (work exerted

Table 4
THE MECHANICAL WORK EVALUATION OF ONE STROKE[a]

Formula	Evaluated value (kJ)	Comment	Ref.
$W = \bar{F}_h \cdot l_h$	387.6	$\bar{F}_h$ — mean force applied to oar handle	75
		l_h — distance covered by the handle	
$W = \int_0^{t_s} F_h \, dt \cdot l_h/t_s$	$627.6 \div 711.2$	t_p — time of the pull blade	84
$W = \bar{F}_b \cdot (V_B \cdot t_p + r)$	610.0	$\bar{F}_b$ — mean force on the blade	29
		$\bar{V}_B$ — mean velocity of the boat	
		r — oar blade regression	
$W = m \cdot \omega \cdot V_b \cdot t_p + m \cdot \dfrac{\omega^2}{2} \cdot t_p$	—	m — mass of water pushed by the blade	92
		ω — additional velocity of the water gained during the pull phase	
$W = \kappa \cdot V_B^2 \cdot L_B$	539.9	κ — coefficient characteristic for a given boat ($\kappa \approx 1.3$)	93
		L_B — distance the boat covers during one stroke	
$W = \sum_{i=1}^{n} F_{bi} \cdot \Delta S_i \cdot \cos\alpha_i$	—	F_{bi} — temporary force on the blade in respect to ΔS_i distance covered by the blade vs. boat	94
		α_i — temporary angle between blade and boat longitudinal axis	
$W = \int_0^{t_s} F_{bx}(t) \cdot \dot{x}_t(t) \, dt$	—	F_{bx} — longitudinal component of force on the blade	12
		$\dot{x}_t$ — velocity of total boat and oarsmen center of gravity	

[a] Adapted from Zatziorski.[15]

Table 5
MECHANICAL-POWER EVALUATION

Formula	Evaluated value (W)	Comment	Ref.
$P = d(u + V_B) + D_t \cdot V_B + d(u - V_B)$	—	d — hydrodynamic drag force acting on blades during the pull	95
		u — velocity of blades in respect to the boat	
$P = 2.8 \cdot V_B^{3.2}$	310.0	for $V_B = 4.5$ m/sec	84
$P_t = P_{Fh} + P_{mx} + P_{mz}$	373.8	P_t — total power; P_{Fh} — power exerted on the handle; P_{mx}, P_{mz} — power components necessary for move the inertial masses in x and z directions	12
$P_{Fh} = \int_{t_s} F_{hx}(t) \cdot h \cdot \dot{\alpha}(t) \, dt/t_s$	292.9	m_t — mass of the system	
$P_{mx} = \int_{t_s} m_c \cdot \ddot{x}_{c\text{-}t} \cdot \dot{x}_{c\text{-}t} \cdot dt/t_s$	25.0	m_c — mass of the crew	
$P_{mz} = \int_{t_s} m_t \cdot \ddot{z}_t \cdot \dot{z}_t \, dt/t_s$	55.9	Index$_{c\text{-}t}$ — parameter of crew relative to system	
or: $P_p = W/t_s$	249.3	P_p — propulsive power	
$P_{Fh} = F_{hx} \cdot h \cdot \alpha$	—	P_b — power developed on the blade	13
$\bar{P}_{Fh} = \int_{t_s} F_{hx}(t) \cdot h \cdot F\dot{\alpha}(t) \cdot dt/t_s$	—		
$P_b = F_b(1 \cdot \dot{\alpha} - V_B \cdot \cos\alpha)$	—		
$P_p = \bar{P}_{Fn} - P_b = F_b \cdot V_B \cdot \cos\alpha$	—		
or: $\bar{P}_p = \int_{t_s} F_b(t) \cdot V_B(t) \cdot \cos\alpha(t) \, dt/t_s$	—		

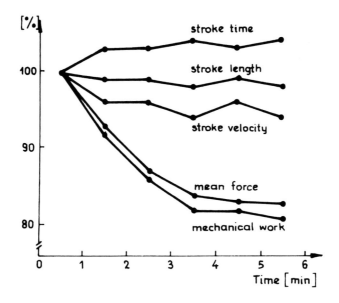

FIGURE 42.   Variability of selected parameters versus time (Adapted from Asami[82]).

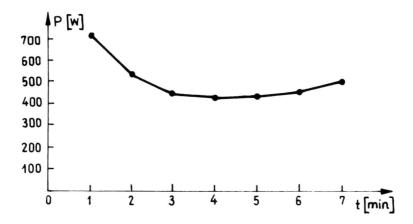

FIGURE 43.   Mean power exerted by oarsman vs. time.[12]

on the oargrip) or to an evaluation of the work necessary to overcome the hydrodynamic drag. Several papers have also been devoted to measuring the work done by the oar blades. A comprehensive analysis of mechanical work and various parameters of rowing, was done by Asami et al.[82] The mechanical work, stroke time, stroke velocity, mean force, and force impulse values were measured in 6 min of vigorous rowing in a pool with controlled flow of water. Their results are presented in Figure 42. Mechanical work was derived from mean force and stroke length and therefore these parameters were not independent. It was calculated that the low correlation with the peak force ($r = 0.16$) suggests that the strain curve pattern of the oar was not like a triangle with a sharp peak, but somewhat trapezoidal in shape. Several studies were also done to evaluate the power curve as a function of important rowing parameters.[2,13,30,83] The relationship between power exerted by athletes and time was widely studied by Nolte[12] and Schneider.[13] Typically, increased power is exerted in the first minute of the race (gaining speed), then a level of approximately 500 W is maintained for the next 5 min, and a small increase in power is observed at the very end of the race (Figure 43).

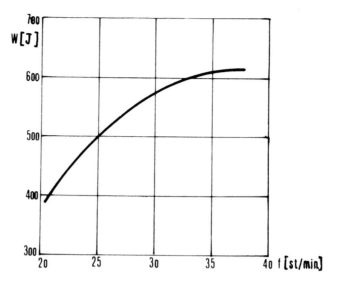

FIGURE 44.   Power as a function of stroke rate.[29]

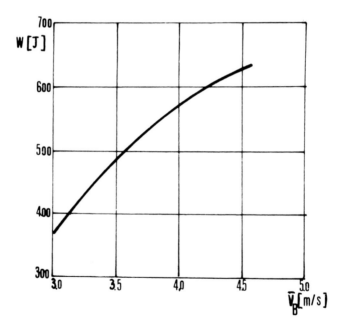

FIGURE 45.   Power vs. boat velocity.[29]

The power as a function of stroke rate and mean velocity of the boat, was measured by Celentano et al.[29] Examples of their results are presented in Figures 44 and 45.

An important problem arises if one attempts to compare work done in natural conditions and "rowing" on various types of ergometers or in training pools. It is obvious the ergometers or pool conditions should simulate as precisely as possible the functional relationship between power exerted and stroke rate typical for natural conditions. However, significant discrepancies are usually found when the same rowers perform the motion in natural vs. "ergometer" conditions. Comparisons of such differences are presented in Figure 46. Substantial differences can be observed in the range from 20 to 30 strokes/min. This fact should be of

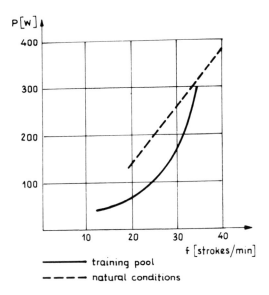

FIGURE 46.   Comparison of power exerted during rowing in a training pool and in natural conditons.[84]

significance to coaches testing the rowers' fitness on ergometers and for designers of new ergometer systems.

The last problem in rowing when considering time and aerobic factors, is efficiency. Only a fraction of the total work performed by the subject is utilized for forward progression. The measurement of this fraction is defined by the efficiency coefficient.

Efficiency, using mechanical terms, represents the relationship between input (energy exerted) and output (resultant mechanical work). The input reflects the physiological work done by a man. The mechanical efficiency coefficient is defined as:

$$\eta = W_d/W_o$$

where

$$W_d = \text{work done}$$

$$W_o = \text{work output} \tag{27}$$

Based on the last evaluation, the efficiency appears to be of the order of 20%, tending to increase slightly with an increasing workload.[12,13,29,84] The overall mechanical efficiency shape vs. stroke frequency is shown in Figure 47. It appears to be of the order of 0.18 at a low rowing stroke ratio, increasing to a constant value of approximately 0.23 for a range of frequencies between 25 and 37. Similar values were obtained by Asami et al.[82] while a direct method was applied to determine total oxygen requirement and total mechanical work during a 6-min exhaustive test. Their results are presented in Figure 48. This brief analysis leads one to a simple conclusion about the limited energy sources of man. One of the ways of optimizing performance is by improvement of the fitness level and motion technique, not neglecting the possible improvement in boat and oar design. The physiological energy is limited, but a higher efficiency (let us say an increase from 0.12 to 0.18) gives an advantage of a 50% work achievement.

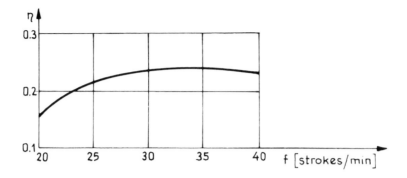

FIGURE 47. Overall efficiency vs. stroke rate.[84]

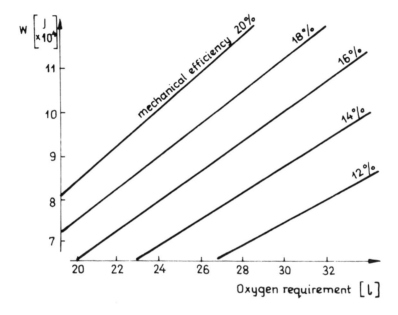

FIGURE 48. The relationship between oxygen requirement, total mechanical work done by rowers, and mechanical efficiency in rowing.[82]

A methodological conclusion appears warranted. It is necessary to define finally and precisely in mechanical terms, the work, power, and efficiency and to use standard, uniform units. This will enable us to avoid confusion and inconsistency in the various work and power definitions.

VI. MODEL EXPERIMENT AND COMPUTER SIMULATION APPROACH TO ROWING IMPROVEMENT

The major developments in computer science technology have also lead to the first practical applications of computers in sport biomechanics. Besides standard computer data processing, graphics, etc., a new scientific area — modeling and computer simulation — promises exciting results as a powerful research tool. Before presenting selected meaningful examples concerning the computer simulation approach to the biomechanics of rowing, we will attempt to clarify the issue with definitions of model, modeling, and computer simulation.

Model — A system of objects (assumptions, events, or situations) U_2 investigated instead of a more complex or more difficult system U_1, but similar enough to U_1

Modeling — The kind of experimental approach where the original system of objects is substituted by its mathematical or material representation (model) and this substitute is investigated in a selective manner. The results of the modeling experiment are then applied to the original object.

Computer simulation — A step in the modeling approach when "experiments" on the validated model are carried out by the use of computers.

The general methodology and typical implementation of the modeling experiment in biomechanics research, can be shown in Figure 49. The modeling experiment has many advantages over the common direct experimental approach. The most important of these can be distinguished as follows:

- the model of an athlete's performance may be investigated in a highly selective manner by isolating various factors
- the model makes it possible to avoid direct investigation of an original object (athlete) when the task is impossible or undesirable from the point of view of safety, economy, etc
- there is the possibility of a wide change in the time scale of an experiment
- a considerable shortening of the time period for sport performance should generally be attained
- the model and simulation procedure may be a useful means of communication between a coach and an athlete.

However, the shortcomings of the modeling experiment must also be stated. Any kind of model can be validated only in a given number of known situations, while the main purpose of the modeling experiment is to predict behavior in some unknown situations.[24]

Most modeling studies in sport are dedicated to an optimization of motion performance in a given sport discipline or exercise. The problem of optimization has usually been solved by use of:

- one of the standard optimization algorithms — in most cases the use of complex, nonlinear algorithms is necessary (Gosh and Boykin,[45] Hatze,[20] Hubbard,[21] and Komor[22])
- interactive input by an experienced operator (coach) with the simulation software (Bauer,[85] Morawski, and Wiklik,[86] Dal Monte, Komor, and Leonardi[32,87]).

The models already developed for rowing can be classified as: prediction-orientated models (Secher and Vaage,[51] Williams[88]); and mechanical models concentrating on rowing performance optimization (Dal Monte, Komor, and Leonardi,[32,87] Pope,[2] Schneider,[50] Senator,[52] and Wellicome[39]).

The first group of models is represented by the interesting study of Secher and Vaage.[51] Their study concerned the prediction of a given race final time by the use of a simple mathematical model based on an analysis of body dimensions as exemplified by body weight. The goal of the study resulted from a peculiarity of the FISA rules; men's events are held separately for lightweights (maximum mass 75.0 kg and average mass 72.5 kg) and for the open class (weight of crew unlimited). They discovered that rowing performance was determined significantly by body dimensions. Based on the theory of the influence of body dimensions on muscular work (Astrand and Rodhal,[89] and McMahon[90]), the model of the global energy balance equation was formulated:

$$t^{1.95}(k_1 w + k_2 w^{2/3} t) n^{0.44} \, \eta_m = k_3 (w + m_B)^{0.56} \, d^{2.95}$$

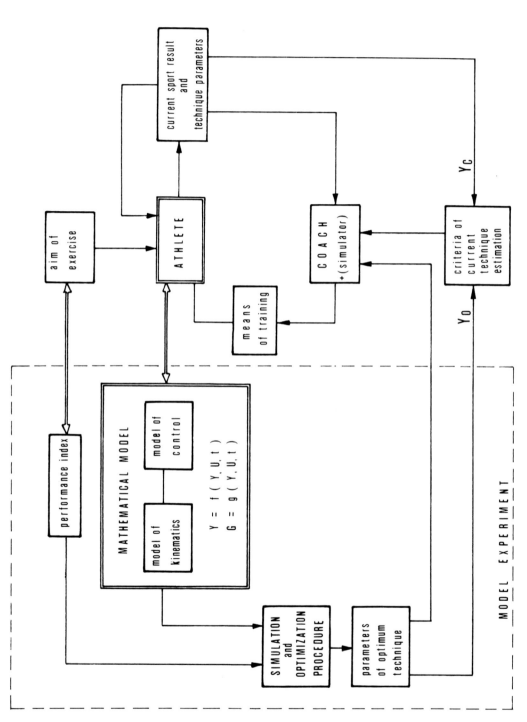

FIGURE 49. A model for experiments in biomechanical research.

where

$$t = \text{duration of event}$$

$$k_1, k_2, k_3 = \text{constants}$$

$$w = \text{body mass}$$

$$n = \text{number of oarsmen}$$

$$\eta_m = \text{mechanical efficiency}$$

$$m_B = \text{boat mass per oarsman}$$

$$d = \text{distance rowed} \tag{28}$$

The constants k_1 and k_2 were calculated from the energy equation of the measured oxygen deficit and total oxygen uptake ($k_1 = 1.2$ J/kg, $k_2 = 91$ J/kg$^{-2/3}$/sec), while k_3 was estimated as 0.2632 N kg$^{-0.56}$ $V_B^{-1.95}$ (single scull). The predictions as a result of solving Equation 28 are presented in Figure 50. The advantage in final time of heavyweighted oarsmen over their lightweighted counterparts, measured against boat mass and the distance rowed, are shown in Figure 51 (a) and (b), respectively. Although the lightweight category is not yet accepted by the International Olympic Committee, such a study seems to indicate that some consideration of the effects of the athletes' weight appears appropriate.

The second category of models is primarily represented by a classical mechanical study of four-oared shell dynamics which was done by Pope[2] (Figure 52). The motion equations of the boat-oars-crew dynamics were defined as follows:

$$(m_1 + m_2)\, \ddot{X} = nF_1 \cos \phi - k_o \dot{X}^2 \text{ (pull phase)}$$

$$(m_1 + m_2)\, \ddot{X} = -k_o \dot{X}^2 \text{ (recovery phase)}$$

where

$$m_1 = \text{mass of the shell,} \quad m_2 = \text{mass of crew,} \quad \text{and} \tag{29}$$

$$n = \text{number of oarsmen}$$

Without going into mathematical detail, the steady-state- and optimum solutions were sought. These considered one cycle and imposed sufficient constraints to ensure periodic movement. The three main factors were analytically defined and based on Equation 29:

— velocity of the boat at the beginning of the stroke

$$V_{Bo} = \frac{\gamma c \lambda}{2a\Delta} \left(\frac{1}{\lambda} - 1 \right)^2 (\phi + \sin \phi \cos \phi)\big|_{\phi_1}^{\phi} \tag{30}$$

— average force delivered by an oarsman during the stroke

$$\bar{F} = \frac{1}{\Delta \tau} \int_o^{\Delta \tau} \frac{c}{b} k_1 \, V_o^2 \cos^2 \phi \left(\frac{1}{\lambda} - 1 \right)^2 dt \tag{31}$$

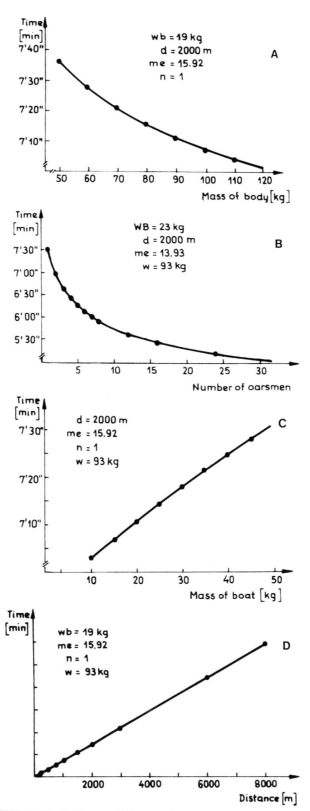

FIGURE 50. Influence of (A) mass of oarsman's body; (B) number of oarsmen; (C) mass of boat per oarsman; and (D) rowing distance on rowing time (Adapted from Secher and Vaage[51]).

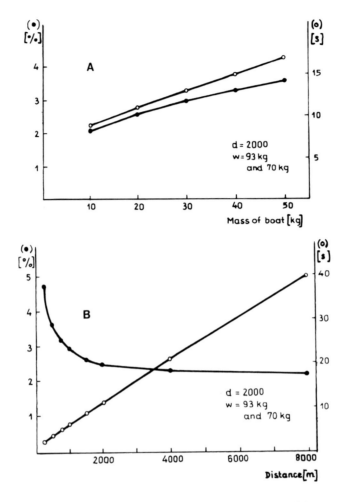

FIGURE 51.   Advantage in final time of heavy oarsmen over lighter oarsmen vs. (A) boat mass; and (B) distance rowed.[51]

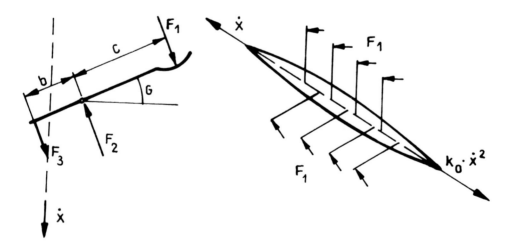

FIGURE 52.   Mechanical model developed by Pope.[2]

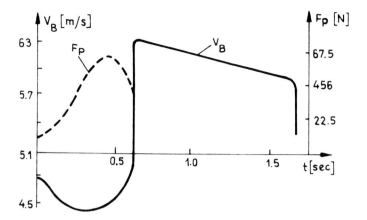

FIGURE 53. Thrust and boat velocity transients: results of simulation by Pope.[2]

— average power exerted by an oarsman during the stroke

$$\overline{P} = k_1 \, V_o^3 \, \frac{1}{\lambda} \left(\frac{1}{\lambda} - 1 \right)^2 \frac{(\phi + \sin \phi \cos \phi)|_{\phi_1}^{\phi}}{\ln \left(\dfrac{1 + \sin \phi_2}{1 - \sin \phi_2} \cdot \dfrac{1 - \sin \phi_1}{1 + \sin \phi_1} \right)}$$

where

$$t_s = \text{time of stroke}$$

$$\tau t_s = \text{part of time representing the pull phase}$$

$$a, \, b, \, c, \, \lambda, \, \gamma, \, \Delta = \text{constants} \tag{32}$$

$$k_1 = \text{coefficient representing total drag}$$

Based on Equation 29 the simulation of one stroke dynamics for a given eight was performed. The thrust at oarlocks and the velocity of boat transients as a solution of Equation 29, are shown in Figure 53.

According to the author,[2] the simulation results were very close to the experimental data. The optimum value of the coefficient defining the pull phase time as a part of the whole cycle time (t_s) was found to be approximately 0.4. Several details of the effect of the sliding masses were also revealed. For example, it was proved that it is ineffective to slide quickly during the pull even though this technique increases the velocity of the shell momentarily. The model also helped in careful analysis of the unorthodox style called "octaped" ineffective. Similar models were also studied by Senator[52] and reasonably exact data were obtained (optimum stroke fraction $\tau = 0.4$, necessary mean power function, etc). Additionally, the results indicated an improvement in overall rowing efficiency by the use of sliding seats, wider blades, and shorter stroke intervals.

While the models previously presented were focused on an intensive mechanical study of rowing dynamics, the final example of a mathematical modeling approach to rowing represents a more practical approach where computer simulation of rowing contributes to technique improvement.

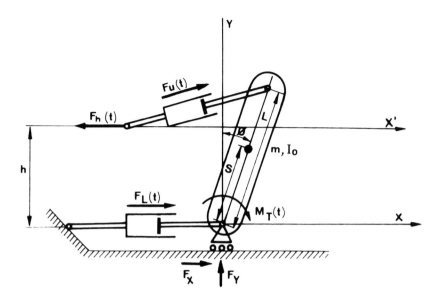

FIGURE 54.   Mechanical model developed by Dal Monte, Komor, and Leonardi.[32]

Based on present experience in the implementation of modeling in the biomechanics of sport, an improved model of rowing technique was proposed. Of greatest importance was the improved simulation methodology which involves a coach directly in the simulation and optimization process (Dal Monte, Komor, and Leonardi[32,87]).

The main goals of that approach were: to identify the factors limiting rowing performance; and finding the best sequence of muscle groups in order to produce the greatest output, that is force impulse applied to the oar. The assumed mechanical model is presented in Figure 54.

The model equations were formulated based on the Lagrange principle:

$$\frac{d}{dt}\left(\frac{\partial T}{\partial \dot{q}}\right) - \frac{\partial T}{\partial q} + \frac{\partial V}{\partial q} = Q$$

where

$$T = \text{kinetic energy of the system}$$

$$V = \text{potential energy of the system}$$

$$Q = \text{external forces}$$

$$q = \text{system variables} \tag{33}$$

and have the following form:

$$(I_o + ms^2)\,\ddot{\phi} - ms \sin \phi\, \ddot{x} = M_t - F_u\, 1 \sin \phi - mgs \cos \phi$$

$$- ms \sin \phi\, \ddot{\phi} + m\ddot{x} - \cos \phi\, \dot{\phi}^2 = F_1 + F_u \tag{34}$$

The main constraints subjected to the model are: geometric (athlete's body structure); and force constraints, maximum forces an athlete is able to exert, in the form (Komor[91]):

$$U_i(t) \leq U_{imax}(q, \dot{q})$$

where

$$U_{imax}(q, \dot{q}) = (a_{1i} q_i^2 + a_{2i} q_i + a_{3i})(1 - \dot{q}_i/q_{imax}) \tag{35}$$

an approximation of maximum muscular torque (force) limits measured under dynamic conditions.

q_{imax} = maximum angular (linear) velocity of selected body segments activated by a given muscular group.

Taking into consideration the system Equation 34, the problem of optimization of rowing motion is two-fold. The optimal initial conditions should be chosen, and optimization of the motion pattern with respect to the control set available to the rower, should be performed. In the example of optimization presented, a simple performance index of maximization (normalized force impulse applied to the oar) was formulated:

$$I_p = \frac{\int_o^{t_s} F_h(t)\, dt}{t_s} \cdot \frac{S_o}{S_s} \rightarrow max$$

where

$$F_h(t) = \text{force applied to the oar handle}$$

$$S_o = \text{simulated oar handle displacement}$$

$$S_s = \text{standard distance to be covered by the oar handle} \tag{36}$$

$$\text{for a given athlete}$$

As was stressed before, model validation should be an essential part of any model experiment. The extended experimental measurements for different athletes during "rowing" on the ergometer were made in order to validate the model and to obtain necessary data for the simulation procedure (anthropometric, dynamometric, and dynamographic). As an example of the comparison of simulated and experimental results, the shapes of force F_h (simulated and real) are shown in Figure 55. Based on a comprehensive analysis of the main kinematic and dynamic parameters from model simulation and real motion, it was proved that the model was very similar to real motion.

In order to perform easy, user-oriented simulation and optimization, a unique software package was developed on a desktop computer which included special programming aids for the user (Figure 56):

- continuous calculation of the performance index and its gradients with respect to selected system parameters such as input conditions, control parameters, etc. (user support subpackage)
- continuous estimation of a temporary solution with regard to a predefined state and control variable transients (simulation results control)
- easy modification of system parameters (input package)

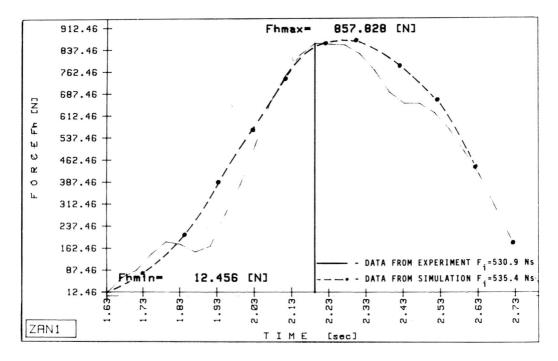

FIGURE 55. Comparison of real and simulated forces applied to the oargrip.

As a typical output the stick-figure graph with preselected kinematic and dynamic parameter graphs, were easily obtained via preprogrammed soft keys (Figure 57). The first simulations were done for "rowing" on a rowing ergometer where the boat motion was neglected. The following aspects of the rowing technique were studied with the interactive optimization approach:

(1) evaluation of the influence of the initial conditions on the performance index. For example, the effects of changing the distance between the oarlocks and feet support (D_s) and initial trunk position, are shown in Figure 58 and Figure 59, while the performance index function with respect to the D_s parameter, is presented in Figure 60.

(2) evaluation of the effects of synchronization of various muscle groups. As an example, the effect of changing the activation time instant of the upper extremities (t_{oa}) is presented in Figure 61 while the performance index sensitivity versus t_{oa} is given in Figure 62.

Based on these studies, the initial optimum position as well as the optimum muscle co-activation was easily found in a few interactive steps, and an improvement of approximately 5% of the performance index was found with respect to a real motion pattern of studied power ($I_{Preal} = 487$, $I_{Popt} = 507$).

Important and interesting results were also obtained when it was assumed that the athlete under investigation was "selectively stronger" by approximately 10%. This meant that at first, the effect of only stronger lower extremities was assumed and examined, later the trunk, and so on. Finally, an improvement of approximately 7.5% of I was found with the necessary changes of force activation. The examples of this "prediction" study are shown in Figure 63.

The approach just presented seems to be particularly useful in biomechanics studies of rowing performance optimization, as an educational tool, and can even be used for direct

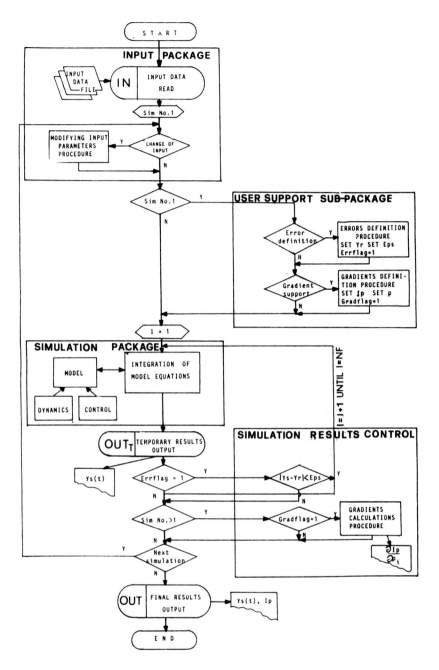

FIGURE 56.   Structure of software package for rowing simulation.

support of a training process. The first attempts have already been done while training top-level Italian oarsmen. It is the fervent hope of the authors that selected presentation of modeling and the computer simulation approach to biomechanical research in rowing, has proved that such an approach is not only an abstract art, but also has many practical and direct applications in rowing research and training.

VII. SOME BIOMECHANICAL ASPECTS OF BREATHING DURING ROWING

A biomechanical study of rowing cannot be considered fully examined without taking

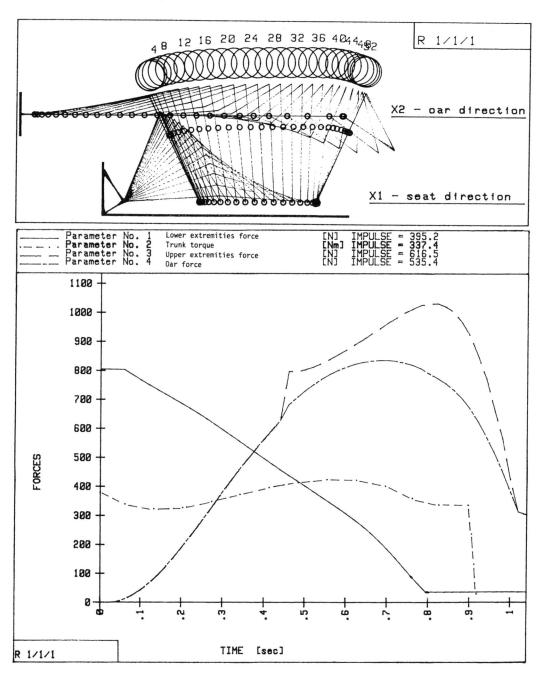

FIGURE 57. Example of simulation output.

into account the mechanics of breathing. The rowers, during their activity, need to perform a very intense hyperventilation. There are a lot of individual differences in the way in which this hyperventilation is performed during rowing. Maximal oxygen consumption brings the respiratory system to its highest level of ventilation.

The biomechanical problem of breathing in rowing, is represented by the interference between the movement of the thorax and the abdomen (through the diaphragm) and the movement of the rower's body parts involved in applying the pulling energy to the oar. The muscles that are considered to be the actuators of the oar movement are situated mainly in the thorax.

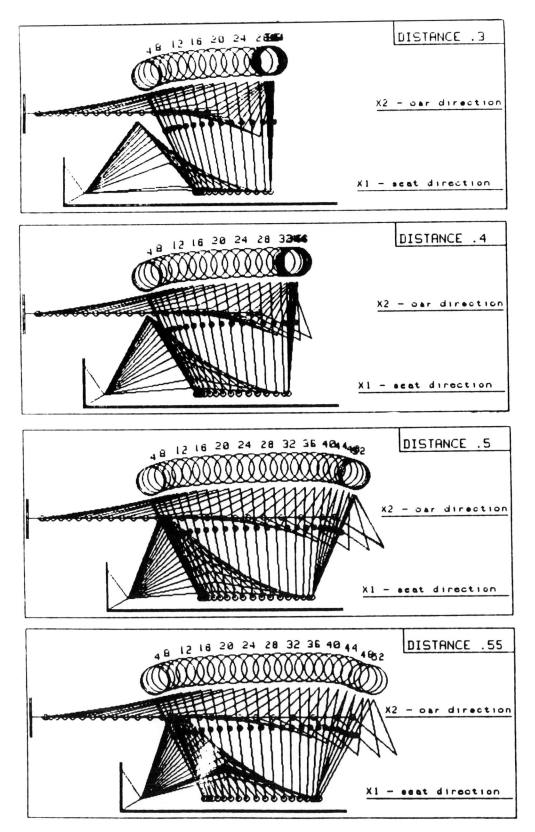

FIGURE 58.   Simulated effect of changing the distance D_S between oarlocks and feet support.

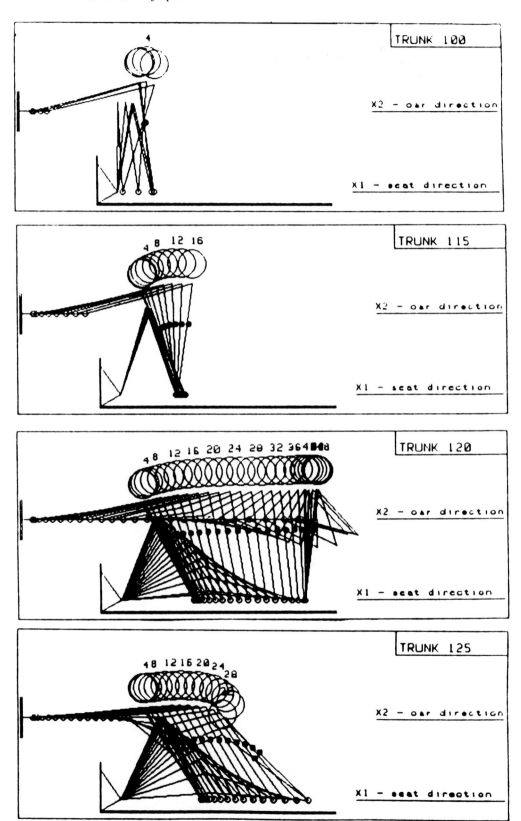

FIGURE 59.   Simulated effect of changing the initial position of the trunk.

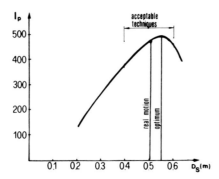

FIGURE 60.   Performance index vs. D_s parameter.

During the rowing activity, the thorax has to perform a double task. The first is to support the upper limbs and the muscles that actuate their movement. The second is to bring about the continuous variation in the diameter of the chest according to the respiratory phases.

These two activities of the thorax unfortunately are not accomplished in a synchronized rhythm. The frequency of the rowing strokes and the respiratory frequency, can be considered compatible only at the lower speed of the boats. When rowing boats move at racing speed this synchronization between the oar strokes and the breathing rhythm, is broken. From a mechanical viewpoint it is very difficult to synchronize the ideal breathing frequency when maximal ventilation is required, i.e., of approximately 50 breaths per min, while the average oar stroke frequency is 36 which represents the mean value during a regatta.

Direct control of the mechanics of breathing and the mechanics of the oars, both in the laboratory and in the boat (with telemetric equipment), has shown that at a low frequency of rowing, the rowers used to breath twice per stroke.[27] This means that at 20 to 22 strokes per min the respiratory frequency is 40 to 44 per min. When the strokes of the oarsman become more frequent, i.e., 32 to 38 strokes per min, the respiratory frequency reaches 65 to 70 breaths per min. This is undesirable for mechanical efficiency. At such a high frequency, the oarsmen rebreath their dead space many times per min, while the tidal volume is significantly reduced in comparison with the ideal distribution of the amplitude of each breath.

Good efficiency in breathing and lower oxygen uptake for the respiratory muscle mass, is represented at the higher ventilation by a tidal volume of approximately 50% of total vital capacity. At such a high frequency of breathing (65 to 70), the tidal volume is no greater than 30% of vital capacity as seen in Figure 64a. However, at lower frequencies there are some significant advantages: the rebreathing of the dead space is not so frequent and the tidal volume is usually higher. Then the index of tidal volume/vital capacity is better and nearer to the optimum theoretical value of 50%, shown in Figure 64b.

Several investigations have been performed in order to analyze optimum breathing during rowing races.[27,30,84] Among other parameters, the influence of fatigue on breathing frequency, as well as its relationship with the ECG, have been widely studied.

Taking into account the selected results of experiments concerning the ''breathing technique'', it is possible to observe that the timing in rowing can be represented by three different fundamental aspects: the ratio of breath:oarstroke can be 2 breaths 1 stroke (Figure 65a) or 1 breath 1 stroke (Figure 65b), or breathing absolutely independently from the rowing rate (Figure 66). The more rational pattern of breathing is the ratio 1:1, but very few athletes are able to perform this way during the total time of the competition.

In the final part of a regatta the pulmonary ventilation is higher than 130:1 with a breathing frequency of 35 to 40 per min. The ventilation in this condition is totally sufficient to accomplish the needs of oxygenation of the blood and to evacuate the carbon dioxide

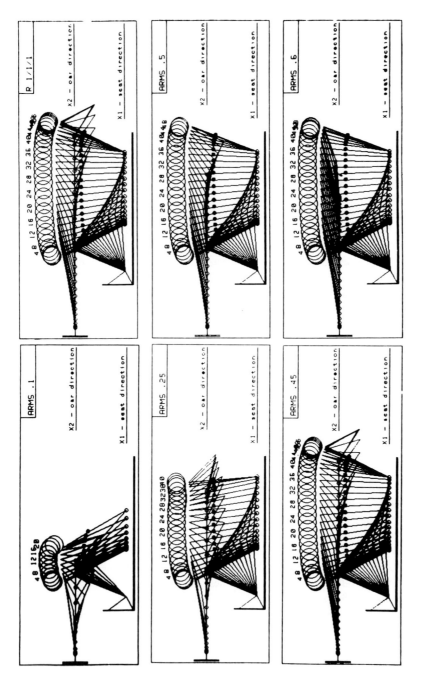

FIGURE 61.   Simulated effect of varying the time instants of upper extremities activation.

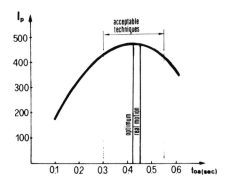

FIGURE 62.   Performance index vs. t_{oa}.

emerging from the working muscles. However, the effect of fatigue produces a breakdown of feedback in the ventilation process, and the athletes are not able to maintain the correct breathing ratio for the whole period of the race (7 minutes). They usually assume a higher frequency of breathing, totally unrelated to the rowing frequency.

Comparison of a synchronized ventilation-rowing stroke at a 1:1 ratio at the beginning of the race, and the effect of poor coordination in the final part of the race, can be seen in Figures 65b and 66 respectively. It is clearly evident that irregular breathing (Figure 66, curve 2) interferes considerably with the ECG (Figure 66, curve 3) and the latter is practically impossible to analyze. Such effects do not appear, while the coordinated ventilation with rowing action exists (Figure 65a). Of course it is not the cardiac activity that is affected by the irregular timing of breathing, but incorrect and unsynchronized activity of the thorax and abdominal muscles. These produce interference in the electric biopotential activity. This effect creates particular diagnostic problems; when evaluation of the cardiac activity is strongly recommended from a medical point of view, a proper reading of the ECG is difficult to obtain. This leads to a strict requirement for improving ECG measurement technique, while the ECG is significantly affected by thorax- and abdomen-muscle activity.

This brief analysis of the biomechanical aspects of breathing during rowing can be concluded by the following remarks:

(1)   the pneumotachographic diagrams show that a higher energy cost in breathing is accomplished when the ratio between strokes and breathing frequencies is different (from 1:1 or at least 1:2).
(2)   the electrical activity of breathing muscles often interferes considerably with the ECG (in the final part of races) and the ECG is altered so that it is not possible to have a correct reading. In order to reduce health hazards resulting from erratic ECG recordings, special equipment, designed especially for rowing, should be developed and used.

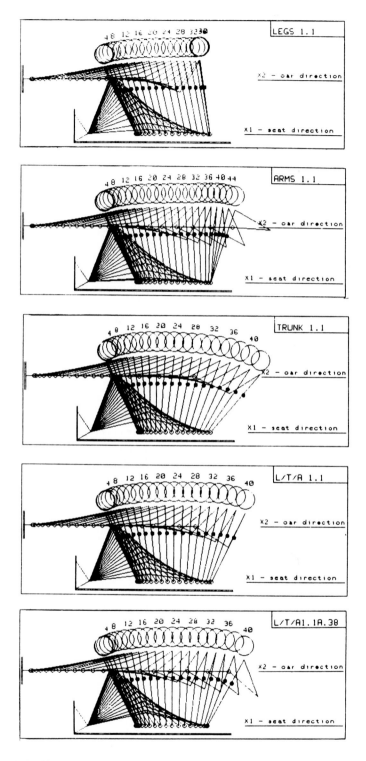

FIGURE 63.   Simulated effect of increasing the strength of selected muscular groups.

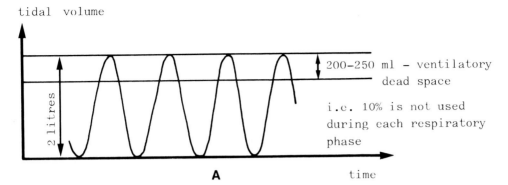

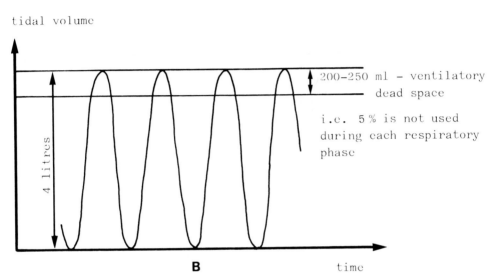

FIGURE 64.   Ventilatory dead space with respect to tidal volume as a result of different breathing: (A) low-efficiency breathing; and (B) high-efficiency breathing (Adapted from Dal Monte[30]).

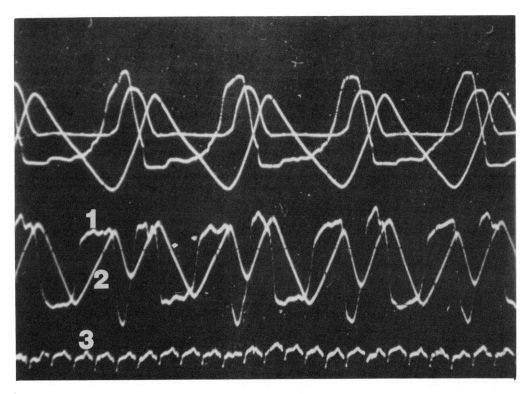

FIGURE 65.   Transients of (1) pneumatachogram; (2) ventilation; and (3) electrocardiogram for 1 to 1 breathing and for 1 to 2 breathing. Upper curves (not marked) represent transients of the force applied to the stretchers, force applied to the oargrip, and angular motion of the oar (Adapted from Dal Monte[27]).

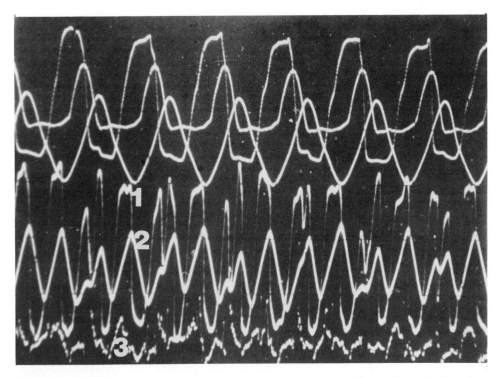

FIGURE 66.   The effect of unsynchronized breathing frequency on the electrocardiogram (the explanation of curves is as in Figure 65) (Adapted from Dal Monte[27]).

REFERENCES

1. **Marchesi, B.**, II. Canottagio per tuti, Gremese Editore, Roma, 1984.
2. **Pope, D. L.**, On the dynamics of men and boats and oars, *Mechanics and Sport, Am. Soc. Mech. Eng.*, 1973, 113.
3. **Williams, J. G. P.**, Rowing: Art or Science? in *Rowing, A Scientific Approach*, Kaye & Ward Ltd., London, 1967, 10.
4. **Endlerg, M., Haber, P., and Hofner, W.**, Wirbelsäulenveränderungen und ihre Mechanopathologie bei Leistungsrudern, *Z. Orthop.*, 118, 91, 1980.
5. **Atkinson, E.**, A rowing indicator, *Natural Science*, 8, 178, 1896.
6. **Atkinson, E.**, Some more rowing experiments, *Natural Science*, 13, 89, 1898.
7. **Lefeuvre and Pailliote**, Étude graphique du coup d'aviron en canoe *Bull. de l'Association Techn. Maritime*, Paris, 1904, 115.
8. **Alexander, F.**, Die vorwärtstreibende Wirkung des Ruderns, *Wassersport*, 41, 1023, 1930.
9. **Edwards, H. R. A.**, The way of a man with a blade, London, 1963.
10. **Herberger, E.**, *Rudern*, Berlin, 1970.
11. **Schroeder, W.**, Rudern Training, Technik, Taktik, Rowolth Taschenbuch Verlag, Reibek bei Hamburg, 1978.
12. **Nolte, V.**, Die Effektivität des Ruderschlages, Bartels & Wernitz, 1985.
13. **Schneider, E.**, Leistungsanalyse bei Rudermannschaften, Limpert Verlag, Bad Homburg, 1980.
14. **Williams, J. G. P.**, Some biomechanical aspects of rowing, in *Rowing, a Scientific Approach*, Kaye & Ward Ltd., London, 1967, 81.
15. **Zatziorski, V. M. and Jakunin, N.**, Biomechanika akademiceskoj grebli - obzor (Biomechanics of rowing - review) *Teor. Prakt. Fiz. Kult.*, 1, 8, 1980.
16. **Hay, J.**, The biomechanics of sport techniques, Prentice-Hall, Englewood Cliffs, N. J., 1973.
17. **Nigg, B. M.**, *Biomechanik*, ETH, Zurich, 1977.
18. **Lisiecki, A.**, Proba oceny wioslarzy centralnego szkolenia na podstawie wybranych parametrow kinematyczno-dynamiczynch mierzonych na basenie (An attempt of top-level oarsmen performance evaluation on the base of selected kinematic and dynamic parameters measurement on the training pool) *Monografie AWF*, Poznan, Poland 61, 37, 1975.
19. **Rulffs, M.**, The problem of technique in rowing, in Proc. *"A Basic-Level Rowing Clinic"*, Princeton University, 1970, 59.
20. **Hatze, H.**, Myocybernetic optimization of sport motion — model, methods for parameter identification, practical implementation, *Rep. Natl. Res. Inst. Math. Sci.*, CSIR Pretoria, S. Arica, 1981.
21. **Hubbard, M.**, Dynamics of pole vault, *J. Biomech.*, 13, 1980.
22. **Komor, A.**, Zastosowanie metod modelowania w sporcie (Application of mathematical modelling in sport sciences) Institute of Sport Publishers, Warsaw, Poland, 1982.
23. **Komor, A.**, Modelli mathematici della technica sportiva, *Rivista di Cultura Sportiva*, 3, 51, 1985.
24. **Vaughan, C.**, Biomechanics of running gait, *CRC Crit. Rev.*, 12, 1, 1977.
25. **Korner, T.**, Einige grundsätzliche Gedanken zur Rudertechnik und ihre internationale Entwicklungstendenz, in *Proc. 7. FISA Trainerkollquium*, 1979, 13.
26. **Morzevikov, N. V. and Sljokov, S. K.**, Techniceskaja podgotovlennost grebcov na adademiceschich sudach (Technique training of oarsmen) *Teor. Prakt. Fiz. Kult.*, 9, 6, 1982.
27. **Dal Monte, A.**, The stroke and the timing of muscular action, in *Proc. 8. FISA Trainerkolloquim*, 36, 65, 1979.
28. **Baird, E. D., and Soroka, W. W.**, Measurement of force-time relations in racing shells, *Am. Soc. Mech. Eng.*, 58, 77, 1951.
29. **Celentano, F., Cortili, G., Di Pampero, P. E., and Cerretelli, P.**, Mechanical aspects of rowing, *J. Appl. Physiol.*, 36, 642, 1974.
30. **Dal Monte, A.**, Quando il laboratore mette la ruote *Canottagio*, 56, 26, 1977.
31. **Dal Monte, A.**, Veloci in barca per avere brabche veloci *Canottacheo*, 56, 10, 1977.
32. **Dal Monte, A., Komor, A., Leonardi, L. M.**, Biomechanical analysis and mathematical modelling of human motion during rowing, *Inst. of Sport Sci.*, Rome, 1985.
33. **Nolte, V., Klauck, J., and Mader, A.**, Vergleich biomechanischer Merkmale der Ruderbewegung auf dem Giessing Ergometer und fahrenden Boot, *Rudersport*, 33:711-714, 1982.
34. **Schneider, E., Morrell, F., and Sidler, N.**, Long-time investigation in rowing by multitelemetry, in *Biotelemetry IV*, Doring-Drück, Braunschweig, W. Germany, 1978, 211.
35. **Yamamoto, S.**, Energy cost of rowing motion (in Japanese), in *Proc. Jpn. Conf. Biomech.*, 1984, 70.
36. **Wyganowska, A.**, Opory hydrodynamiczne w wioslarstwie (Hydrodynamic drag in rowing) *Sport Wyczynowy*, 5, 27, 1969.
37. **Gerdes, R.**, Grossenverhältnisse des Falchwasseinflusses, *Rudersport*, 1965, 19.

38. **Gerdes, R.,** Wissenschaftliche Forschung am Rennboot, *Rudersport,* 7, 1966.
39. **Wellicome, J. F.,** Some hydrodynamic aspects of rowing, in *Rowing, A Scientific Approach,* Kaye & Ward Ltd., London, 1967.
40. **Nolte, V.,** Die Handschift des Ruderers, *Masstechnische Briefe,* 3, 49, 1973.
41. **Dal Monte, A.,** Analysis of physical capacity in sport and methods of functional evaluation, in *Acts. Intl. Symp. Olymp. Solid. the I. O. C.,* VII Asian Games, Tehran, Iran, 1974.
42. **Secher, N. H.,** Isometric rowing strength of experienced and inexperienced oarsmen, *Medic. Sci. in Sports,* 7:280-283, 1975.
43. **Dal Monte, A., Faina, M., Cecioni, N., and Leonardi, L. M.,** Analysis of the inertial forces in rowing by use of force platform, in *Biomechanics IX-B,* Human Kinetics Publishers, Champaign, Ill., 1985, 481.
44. **Dworak, L., Kabsch, A., Lambui, W., and Lisiecki, A.,** Charackterystyka wybranych parametrow dynamicznych u zawdnikow centralnego szkolenia (Characteristics of selected dynamic parameters of top-level oarsmen) *Monografie AWF,* Poznan, Poland 61:29-36, 1975.
45. **Gosh, T. and Boykin, W.,** Dynamics of human kip-up maneuver, *J. Dynam. Syst. Meas. Contr.,* 97, 1975.
46. **Ishiko, T.,** Biomechanics of rowing, *Biomechanics II,* S. Karger, Basel, 1971, 249.
47. **Martindale, W. and Robertson, D.,** Mechanical energy in sculling and in rowing ergometer, *Can. J. Appl. Sport Sci.,* 9, 153, 1984.
48. **Kabsch, A. and Dworak, L.,** Problem of muscle coordination in a rowing cycle in electromyography, in *Abstr. 2nd Sem. ICSPE "Biomechanics",* Eindhoven, The Netherlands, 1969, 52.
49. **Drisko, B.,** Man-powered oscillations, in *Technol. Rev.,* 6:4-5, 1973.
50. **Schneider, E. and Hauser, M.,** Biomechanical analysis of performance in rowing, *Biomechanics VII-B,* University Park Press, Baltimore, Md., 1981, 430.
51. **Secher, N. H. and Vaage, O.,** Rowing performance, a mathematical model based on analysis of body dimensions as exemplified by body weight, *Eur. J. Appl. Physiol.,* 52, 88, 1983.
52. **Senator, M.,** Why sliding seats and short stroke intervals are used for racing shells, *J. Biomech. Eng.,* 103, 151, 1981.
53. **Versinkas, R. S., Zatziorski, V. M., Kajmin, M. A., and Jakunin, N.,** Osobennosti dvizenija systemy sportsmen-lodka v akademiceskoj odinockie s podviznoj ukljucnoj. (Peculiarities of boat-oarsman system motion (single scull) with sliding oarlocks), *Teor. Prakt. Fiz. Kult.,* 1, 10, 1984.
54. **Gutschow, W.,** Mechanik des Getriebes Ruderer/Ruder, *Schiffstechnik,* 3, 128, 1955.
55. **Bernfield, J.,** Effect of stroke rate on the velocity-time curve of a rowing shell, MSc. thesis, State University College, Brockport, N.Y., 1977.
56. **Cameron, A.,** Some mechanical aspects of rowing, in *Rowing, A Scientific Approach,* Kaye & Ward Ltd., London, 1967, 64.
57. **Kabsch, A., Dworak, L., Lambui, W., and Lisiecki, A.,** Characteristics of kinematic and dynamic parameters of the rowing movement in rowing pool and ergometer (in Polish), *Roczniki Naukowe AWF,* Poznan, Poland, 65-73, 1977, 65.
58. **Martin, T. and Bernfield, J.,** Effect of stroke rate on velocity of a rowing shell, *Med. Sci. Sports Exerc.,* 12, 250, 1980.
59. **Usoskin, E.,** Zrozumienie i anliza czynnikow determinujacych technike wiorslarska (Analysis of factors determining the rowing technique), *Sport Syczynowy,* 15, 32, 1977.
60. **Bompa, T. O.,** A biomechanical analysis of the rowing stroke employing two different oar grips, in Poc. XXI World Congr. Sport Med. Brazil, 1978.
61. **Korner, T.,** Zum Kraftverlauf an der Dolle während des Ruderschlages, *Rudersport,* 2, 1979.
62. **Foppl, O.,** Die Windkrafte an Platten und anderen Versuchskörpern nach dem heutigen Stand von Theorie und Versuch, Z. *Vereins Dtsche. Ingen.,* 56, p. 1930, 1912.
63. **Gutsche, F.,** Beitrag zur Hydrodynamik des Ruderbootantriebes, *Schiffstechnik,* 4, 89, 1957.
64. **Gerdes, R.,** Der unbekannte Ruderschlag, *Rudersport,* 9, 1977.
65. **Minienkow, V.,** Eksperimentalnoje opredelenije lopasti vesla ademiceskoj grebli (Experimental method of design of oar blade), *Teor. Prakt. Fiz. Kult.,* 5, 41, 1967.
66. **Gutsche, F.,** Die Suche nach der besten Blattform, *Rudersport,* 29, 684, 1962.
67. **Nolte, V.,** Die Rudertechnik, *Rudersport,* 34, 1, 1982.
68. **Nolte, V.,** Rudertechnik und ihre Analyse — der Arbeitsbereich im Skullboot, *Rudersport,* 20, 468, 1982.
69. **Nolte, V.,** Die Stemmbretteinstellung der Ruderwinkel in der Rucklage, *Rudersport,* 25, 544, 1982.
70. **Marchaj, C.,** Sailing theory and practice, Dodd, Mead & Co., New York, 1964.
71. **Dworak, L.,** Wybrane zagadnienia biodynamiki fazy pociagniecia w cyklu wioslowania (Selected aspects of biodynamics of pull phase in rowing), *Monografie AWF,* Poznan, Poland, 50, 123, 1974.
72. **Hay, J.,** Rowing analysis of the New Zealand Olympic selection tests, *N. Z. J. Health, Phys. Ed. Recr.,* 1, 83, 1968.
73. **Madler , A. and Hollmann, W.,** Zur Bedeutung der Stoffwechselleistungsfähigkeit des Elite Ruderers in Training und Wettkampf, *Beiheft Leistungssport,* 9, 8, 1977.

74. **Strydom, A.,** A scientific approach to the selection and training of oarsmen, *S. Afr. Med. J.,* 1100, 1102, 1967.

75. **Lazareva, A., Zigatov, I., and Morzevikow, V.,** O silovoj charakteristikie rabocej dejatelnosti grebcor w akademiceskich lodkach (Force characteristics analysis of oarsmen), *Teor. Prakt. Fiz. Kult.,* 9, 15, 1968.

76. **Adam, K.,** Die Suche nach der besten Blattform, *Rudersport,* 33, 718, 1961.

77. **Fukunaga, T.,** Biomechanics of rowing motion, *Jpn. J. Sport Sci.,* 3:57-71, 1984.

78. **Tasaki, Y., Saito, S., and Suzuki, M.,** Tsukuba rowing style, *Health Sport Sci.,* Tsukuba University Japan, 2, 69, 1979.

79. **Szapkov, J.,** Analiza cykul wioslarskiego — ruchy robocze (Analysis of rowing cycle — active phase), *BTS Pkol,* Warwaw 1969.

80. **Di Pampero, P., Pinera-Limas, F., and Sassi, G.,** Maximal muscular power (aerobic and anaerobic) in 116 athletes performing at XIX Olympic Games in Mexico, *Ergonomics,* 13, 665, 1970.

81. **Cerretelli, P. and Radovani, P.,** Il massimo consumo di O_2 in ateleti olimpionici di varie specialita, (Maximum oxygen consumption in Olympic athletes from varying disciplines) *(Boll. Soc. Ital. Biol. Sper.,* 36, 1871, 1960.

82. **Asami, T., Adachi, N., and Yamamoto, K.,** Biomechanical analysis of rowing performance in *Biomechanics VII-B,* University Park Press, Baltimore, Md., 442, 1981.

83. **Ueya, K.,** A kinesiological study of rowing motion in view of energy equation, *Jpn. J. Phys. Ed.,* 22, 363, 1978.

84. **Di Pampero, P., Celentano, F., and Cerretelli, P.,** Physiological aspects of rowing, *J. Appl. Physiol.,* 31, 853, 1971.

85. **Bauer, W.,** Mathematical modelling and optimization and their influence on sport movements — possibilities and limitations, in *Biomechanics and Performance in Sport,* Hoffman Verlag, 129-144, 1980, 129.

86. **Morawski, J. and Wiklik, K.,** Application of analog and hybrid simulation in sports, in *Simulation of Control Systems,* Troch, I., Ed., North-Holland, Amsterdam, 1978.

87. **Dal Monte, A., Komor, A., and Leonardi, L. M.,** An application of mathematical modelling and interactive computer simulation to rowing technique improvement, in *Abstr. Sport Biomech. Conf.* Santa Barbara, Calif., 1985.

88. **Williams, L. R. T.,** The psychological model of multiple discriminant function analysis of high-caliber oarsmen, *Med. Sci. Sports,* 9, 174, 1977.

89. **Astrand, P. and Rodhal, K.,** in *Textbook of Physiology,* McGraw-Hill, New York, 1977, 367.

90. **McMahon, T.,** Rowing — a similarity analysis, *Science,* 7, 349, 1971.

91. **Komor, A.,** Identification of force constraint functions of human joints under dynamic conditions, in *Biomechanics IX,* Human Kinetics Publishers, Champaign, Ill., 1985, 115.

92. **Morkovkin, W. and Tarabrin A,** Na veslach (The oars), *Fizkultura i Sport,* Moscow, 1963.

93. **Sestoperov, J.,** Grebnyj sport (Rowing Sport), *Fizkultura i Sport,* Moscow, 1973.

94. **Usoskin, E.,** Zrozumienie i anliza czynnikow determinujacych technike wioslarska (Analysis of factors determining the rowing technique), *Sport Wyczynowy,* 15, 32, 1977.

95. **Aleksander, F.,** Biomechanika (Biomechanics), *Fizkultura i Sport,* Moscow, 1970.

96. **Klavora P,** Rowing strategy: physiological consideration, *Coach. Rev.,* 6, 45, 1978.

Chapter 4

BIOMECHANICS OF SPEED SKATING

G. J. van Ingen Schenau, R. W. De Boer, and G. De Groot

TABLE OF CONTENTS

I. INTRODUCTION

An American reporter once characterized speed skating as watching grass growing. In at least two countries (Norway and Holland), the large attendances at national and international competitions prove that many would disagree with this statement. Nevertheless, we are of the opinion that speed skating has to be practiced before one can understand why this sport has become a national sport in some countries. It is the experience of a proper gliding technique and the possibility of making long trips into a wintry landscape which has made speed skating so popular in countries with a suitable climate and enough lakes and canals with dead water. Another way to highlight the popularity of this sport is to review its remarkable and unique biomechanical background, which is the purpose of this chapter. Since speed skating is still somewhat unknown in many countries, we shall make a few remarks on the development of this sport in the past, and its present significance as a sport and as a subject of scientific research.

A. Skates and Skaters

According to Goodman,[1] speed skating has experienced a wooden, a bone, and an iron age. Archeological discoveries and old Scandinavian and Icelandic legends show that the original roots for speed skating as well as for skiing, have to be dated more than 3,000 years ago.[4,6] Prehistoric men moved on snow and ice on pieces of wood looking for food.[1-7] A separation in the development of skiing and skating occurred with the introduction of skates made of polished bones. With the help of sharpened sticks one could push one's self forward over the ice in a more or less comparable manner to the usage of ski-poles in present cross-country skiing. Although this mode of locomotion on ice has little to do with actual skating, this history of gliding on bones is still present in the Dutch name "schenkel" (shank) for the iron blades in modern skates. The origin of the actual skating technique ("the Dutch roll")[6] which is characterized by a sidewards push-off using sharp whetted iron blades, is often credited to Holland. There is, however, no decisive evidence for such credit. Other possible locations are Scandinavia, Northern Germany, or even Poland. A wood carving from the 15th century, however, shows that skating on skates with iron blades has existed in Holland for at least 600 years (Figure 1). There are few other countries where skating has been such a popular amusement in these past 600 years as Holland. The popularity of skating in the past is closely related to local geographical and climatological conditions. Skating in Holland was able to develop into a national sport thanks to the large amounts of dead water in the western and northern parts of the country. Up to the middle ages, this land consisted mainly of peat-swamps, lakes, and ditches. In severe winters, skating allowed the inhabitants to increase their range of action and to visit friends or family in areas which were normally almost inaccessible to them. In fact, this state of affairs did not change much when the peat regions were brought into cultivation. Due to uncontrolled peat areas, the rising of the sea level, and many inundations in the middle ages, the amount of surface

123

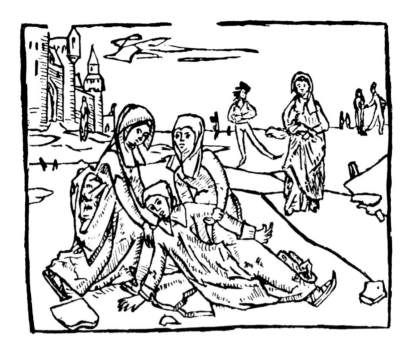

FIGURE 1. The fall of Lidwina of Schiedam in 1395. Lidwina has become the Patron Saint of skaters throughout the world.[5,6]

water increased markedly. Up to the beginning of the present century, the ice allowed the Dutch to visit many friends in one day which would normally have taken them several days. It may be that the possibility of using skates as an effective way to travel a long distance might also explain why skating has become popular in Norway. For skating, one needs a climate in which temperatures are not too low and where there is not too much snow. Moreover, one needs a large amount of surface water. However, it would seem that there is no country which meets all of these requirements. In Scandinavia, the ice in the many lakes is often covered with large amounts of snow. Moreover, it can be extremely cold there, Norway having relatively the mildest temperatures. The same conditions (low temperatures and snow) are often found in Russia and North America. In Holland, Germany, and England the climate is actually too mild. The average period that the Dutch can skate on natural ice is approximately only 10 days per season. In many seasons skating is not possible at all. According to Buisman[9] who described almost all winters in Europe of the past seven centuries, this situation was not much better in the past. Nevertheless, the circumstances for speed skating in Norway as well as in Holland may be relatively the best in Europe. It should be noted that England also has a rich skating history. This holds in particular for an area called the Great Fenns or Moores near London which was geographically similar to Holland.[5,6] Skating on bones was already popular there in 1190.[6] In later centuries, skating on the Fenns became a recreational activity. Old prints also show that in harsh winters, the English could even skate on the Thames[5], with skating and high spirits going hand in hand. Such prints and other paintings prove that speed skating can be regarded as one of the oldest recreational pursuits for the broad public in the northern part of Europe. From the 16th century on, the poor could win prizes in local competitions which were mostly organized by the nobility! During the short periods of ice-cover in Holland there was often a complete fair on the ice with warm drinks, spirits, music, jesters, etc.[3,7]

The first competitions were mostly held over short distances (up to a few hundred meters). Skating events over extremely long distances were reported already in the 17th and 18th

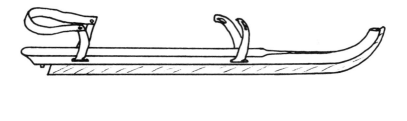

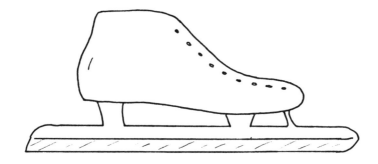

FIGURE 2.   The two major types of skates: the ''wooden'' skate and the ''Norwegian'' skate.

centuries.[3] In 1673, a man visited 12 cities in the western part of Holland in one day. In 1763, the so-called ''Elfstedentocht'' was mentioned for the first time. This trip (200km) along the 11 cities of Friesland has evolved into the most famous long-distance competition in the world. In 1985, 16,176 skaters participated, and due to the good ice and weather conditions, approximately 13,000 completed the race. (In the last, but one race in 1963 only 156 out of the 10,000 participants reached the finish).

In the 19th century, national speed-skating competitions were organized in several countries. The first official World Championships were held in 1891 in Amsterdam and in 1892 the International Speed Skating Association was formed.

During the six to seven centuries since the development of speed skating, the skates have basically not changed. They consisted of a wooden footplate and an edged iron blade. This type of skate is still seen in Holland and is strongly recommended by Dutch coaches for teaching the youngest skaters the basic skating technique. The advantage of these skates for learning purposes is the short distance between foot and ice. The smaller this distance the better the stability of the ankle in the frontal plane. Such skates, however, do not allow a large horizontal component in the push-off (the footplate then touches the ice). This disadvantage in competitive skating was removed by the introduction of the so-called Norwegian skates by Axel Paulsen at the end of the 19th century. Apart from the quality of shoes and blades, these Norwegian skates have not basically changed since then. Both types of skates are presented in Figure 2.

An overview of the European and World Championships over the past 90 years, highlights the tremendous strength of the Norwegians, particularly in the first 60 years of competitive speed skating. Subsequently, possibly as a result of the introduction of artificial ice rinks which made the skaters less dependent on natural ice, the Dutch played an important role. In the last two decades, many nationalties from North America, Europe, and Japan have been seen in international competitions. From a small intimate party of Norwegians, Dutch, and Russians, speed skating has now grown to full maturity.

B. Competitions and Points

The most important international competitions in speed skating are:

1. All round (400 m rink).
   Men: European and World Championships including 500 m, 1,500 m, 5,000 m, and 10,000 m.
   Women: European and World Championships including 500 m, 1,500 m, 3,000 m, and 5,000 m.
2. Sprint (400 m rink).
   World Championships for men and women including 2 × 500 m and 2 × 1,000 m.
3. Olympic Championships for all rounders and sprinters on 500 m, 1,000 m, 1,500 m, 5,000 m and 10,000 m for men and 500 m, 1,000 m, 1,500 m and 3,000 m for women.
4. Short track (110 m rink).
   World Championships including 500 m, 1,000 m, 1,500 m, 3,000 m, and 5,000 m.

In several countries, open long-distance competitions are organized on natural ice. Apart from the Elfstedentocht which can only be skated sporadically, alternatives have been held in Finland, Canada, and Poland. In Norway, the 200 km tour on the Mjosa near Lillehammar, is well known.

On a national level, the marathon competitions in Holland should be mentioned, finally. This is a race over 100 and 35 laps for men and women, respectively. Each season 25 to 30 competitions are organized. It is reasonable to expect that marathon speed skating will become a new offspring in international speed skating in the not too distant future.

C. Scientific Research on Speed Skating

The fact that for a long time speed skating has been a part of the cultural heritage of a few countries only, is more or less reflected by the number and origin of scientific papers on this subject. In particular, the biomechanical aspects of speed skating have been investigated by only a few groups of scientists. This makes it difficult for the present authors to write a critical review on this subject. Naturally, therefore, this chapter will contain some egocentrical aspects and some self-criticism.

Considering all the literature on speed skating, the main studies appear to have been performed in East and West Germany,[8,10-22] the Soviet Union,[23-31] North America,[32-40] Scandinavia,[41-44] and Holland.[45-60]

II. MECHANICAL TOOLS AND DEFINITIONS

The mechanics of speed skating have much in common with the mechanics of other endurance sports. Many models used later in this chapter are essentially the same as the models which are, or could be, used in cycling, rowing, swimming and, to a lesser extent, running. These more general models are discussed first.

A. General Models

The mechanical tools used in modeling movements in sports can be roughly subdivided into two groups:

1. Multi-segment models
2. Models using the whole body as a free-body diagram

In both applications Newtonian and Lagrangian equations of motion are used to calculate unknown variables (force, moment, power, etc).

1. Multi-segment Models

In studying muscle function and coordination of muscles or predicting optimal push-off strategies, the use of multi-segment models is self evident. As indicated by Miller,[61] segment models are, however, hampered by the well-known indeterminacy problem. Because of antagonistic actions of muscles and ligaments, for example, one always has an insufficient number of equations to solve for a large number of unknown variables. Moreover, Williams and Cavanagh[62] showed that it is difficult to relate energy utilization to mechanical work with the help of such models. Many criteria are used to solve the problems connected with the use of multi-segment models, all of them being open to dispute. Nevertheless, in the present state-of-the-art, one has to apply such models for the goals indicated. This yields models which are to be used in predicting optimal work output during push-off in speed skating. It has already been shown that segment models can provide at least a qualitative impression of muscular function and coordination if they are combined with the calculation of muscle contraction velocities and measurement of the activation of the muscles involved.[63-65] This application has also been used to study muscle coordination in speed skating.[66]

2. Free-body Diagrams of the Whole Body

For many purposes, the indeterminacy alluded to above can be avoided by taking the whole body as a free-body diagram. Particularly in swimming, rowing, cycle racing, and speed skating, speed (and thus performance) is directly related to the external power used to overcome friction. Moreover, at constant speed the propulsive force averaged over one or more strokes has to be equal to the mean frictional force. Based on Newtonian mechanics the following equations can be formulated:

Force and force-time integral — The starting point is Newton's second law:

$$\sum F = ma \tag{1}$$

where F means force and m and a are respectively the mass and the acceleration of subject(s) and equipment (cycle, boat, skates). Integration of this equation yields:

$$\int_o^T \sum F \, dt = m\Delta v \tag{2}$$

with T the time-interval of the integration and Δv the change of velocity during interval T. With F_p the resultant propulsive force and F_f the sum of frictional forces this equation can be expanded to:

$$\int_o^T F_p \, dt - \int_o^T F_f \, dt = m\Delta v \tag{3}$$

At constant speed, Δv is approximately zero and thus the mean propulsive force has to be equal to the mean frictional force:

$$\frac{1}{T} \int_o^T F_p \, dt = \frac{1}{T} \int_o^T F_f \, dt \tag{4}$$

This equation is a valuable tool in calculating mean propulsive forces at known frictional forces or vice versa.

Although these forces are often studied by themselves, it is also essential to know them in order to calculate the mean power output of the athlete(s). With respect to the mean friction force, one should keep in mind that friction in fluids and gases is more or less dependent on the square of the speed.[50,67-70] In sports like rowing and swimming, where the speed v can vary considerably,[69] one cannot simply take the mean speed to calculate the friction. For speed skating, Delnoy et al.[58] showed by measurement as well as by simulation that speed fluctuations can be neglected ($<1\%$). In contrast to speed skating, rowing, and cycle racing, where either the propulsive forces[71,72,80] or the frictional forces[50,73,67,74,75] can be measured, the study of these forces in swimming, is hampered by the fact that both forces are difficult to measure. The mean propulsive force calculated by Schleihauf[76] appears to be two to three times smaller than the value reported for the so-called active drag.[77-79] Since active drag is two to three times larger than passive drag on a towed swimmer,[79,81] it is assumed that a moving body causes much more friction than a passive body.[77-79] This was not found for a moving skater in windtunnel experiments.[50] Moreover, Hollander et al.[82] developed a system to measure the propulsive forces of moving swimmers directly, and found values of the same magnitude as reported by Schleihauf[76] and the values reported for passive drag.[79,81] So the indirect active drag measurements introduced by Di Prampero et al.[77] and by Clarijs[79] seem to be open to question.[82]

Power and energy — This chapter on speed skating will emphasize the significance of power-balance models. Basically, such models are simple equations incorporating power delivered by the athlete(s) and power losses. One point should not be overlooked when applying energy-flow equations; in contrast to the applications of Equations 1 to 4, one has to take into account the movement of the points of application of the propelling force. Apart from running and cross-country skiing where the push-off takes place against more or less fixed points on the earth, most endurance sports show a push-off force with a moving point of application with respect to the earth. In swimming and even in rowing, there is always some displacement of hands or blades in a backward direction for the simple reason that one cannot derive a propulsive force from the water without some "slip" with respect to the water.[76,83,84] In skating and cycling the point of application of the push-off force is displaced in a forward direction. Most publications on endurance sports do not take into account the consequences of this phenomenon, and particularly in swimming this can lead to large errors.

It holds for all endurance sports (and many other activities) that the impulse expressed in Equation 2 is derived at the expense of a change in the momentum of the mass against which the push-off takes place according to:

$$\int_o^T F_p \, dt = -m_u \Delta v_u \tag{5}$$

where m_u and Δv_u are the mass and the change of velocity of the mass against which the push takes place. In terms of momentum, there is little difference between the different endurance sports. If, however, the energy expenditure is taken into account, large differences exist.

In each time-interval T an amount of energy $E = 1/2 \, m_u \, \Delta v_u^2$ flows to m_u. As long as m_u represents the entire earth, this amount of energy is completely negligible. If, however,

m_u represents the parts of water which are accelerated as a result of the push-off against the water,[70,83,84] there is a considerable flow of energy to the water which is not used to overcome friction. If this flow of energy to m_u is called P_k and the power losses to friction P_f, this phenomenon can be expressed by the propelling efficiency e_p.[70,85]

$$e_p = \frac{P_f}{P_f + P_k} \qquad (6)$$

In human swimming, this propelling efficiency is not specifically investigated, but it can be estimated that approximately half the total external power P_o ($= P_k + P_f$) flows to the water as a result of this push-off mechanism.[47,83] This means that the actual mechanical efficiency in swimming is much larger than the reported values[77,78,86] derived by calculations of energy consumption and P_f alone.

Since the energy flow P_k can also be expressed as $P_k = \bar{F}_p \cdot \bar{u}$ with $\bar{u}$ being the velocity of the point of application of $\bar{F}_p$, a general power equation for endurance sports can be formulated as follows:

$$P_o + \bar{F}_p \cdot \bar{u} - P_f = m\bar{v} \cdot \bar{a} \qquad (7)$$

$\bar{a}$ being the acceleration of the athlete(s) and boat, cycle etc. (For up- or downhill cycling, of course, a term has to be added to this equation as well as to Equations 3 and 4). The term $\bar{F}_p \cdot \bar{u}$ taken positive since the direction of $\bar{F}_p$ and $\bar{u}$ will be such that the scalar product of the vectors will be negative. As long as one is not pushed forwards by an external-power-delivering system (not allowed in most endurance sports) one can imagine beforehand that a general expression can be formulated for all types of locomotion:

$$\bar{F}_p \cdot \bar{u} \leq 0 \qquad (8)$$

At first sight, this is not the case in cycling and skating. In cycling, it seems obvious that this term represents a positive flow of power from the earth to the cyclist since both $\bar{F}_p$ and $\bar{u}$ are directed forwards. Although $\bar{u}$ seems to be equal to the velocity of the point of contact between the earth and the tire (which is equal to the velocity of the cyclist), this is an optical illusion. The velocity of the part of the tire which is in contact with the ground is zero and consequently $\bar{u} = 0$ too. In fact a wheel can be seen as a structure with a large number of rotating legs, every leg pushing off against a fixed point in the road. Thus $e_p = 1$ in cycling. The situation in speed skating, however, cannot be compared with such a stepwise displace-ment of the point of application of the push-off force. In proper skating technique it is essential that during the push-off phase, the push-off skate continues to glide in a forward direction.[26,48] So the push-off takes place while the point of application of $\bar{F}_p$ is continuously displaced ($\bar{u} \neq 0$). Nevertheless, $\bar{F}_p \cdot \bar{u} = 0$ in speed skating, too. Speed skating is possible thanks to the special properties of ice. Under high pressure, ice becomes water. Since the gliding surface of the blades of skates is small, the pressure under the skate is high (up to 20×10^6 N/m²). The result of this pressure is that there is always a film of water between skate and ice as long as the ice temperature is not too low. In the fore-aft direction, this film of water allows the skate to glide over the ice with very little friction. Since the skate sinks slightly in the ice (the volume of water is smaller than the volume of ice), it is possible to thrust against the ice with the edge of the blade in a direction at right angles to the gliding direction. With skates properly wetted and as long as the ice temperature is not too low, one is able to push-off in that direction at full effort without any side-slip. In fore-aft direction no push-off is possible. Since the skate is gliding forwards, it is essentially impossible to push-off in a backwards direction. In the forward direction, the push-off force cannot exceed

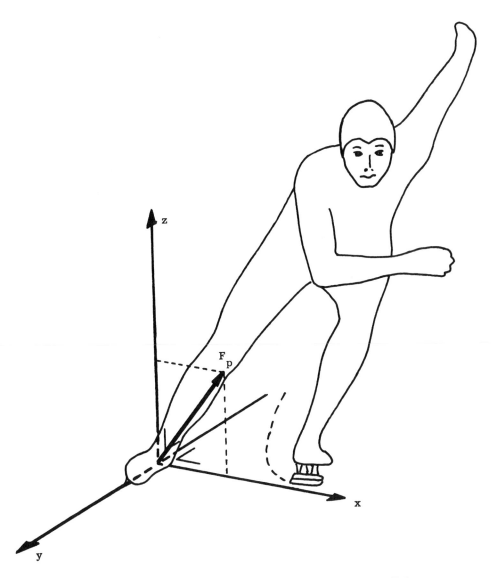

FIGURE 3. In the proper gliding technique, the skate continues to glide during push-off. As a consequence the push-off force F_p lies in a plane (xz) at right angles to the gliding direction (y) of the skate.

the friction force which is less than 1% of the actual push-off force. Moreover, it is not likely that skaters will try to push-off in that direction. It can thus be concluded that the propulsive force $\overline{F}_p$, which is the reaction force from the ice on the skate, lies in a plane perpendicular to the gliding direction of the skate. This (xz) plane is visualized in Figure 3.

Since $\overline{F}_p$ is obviously perpendicular to $\overline{u}$, there is no loss or gain ($\overline{F}_p \cdot \overline{u} = 0$) in speed skating as a result of push-off. From an energy expenditure point of view, the push-off can be compared with a push-off against a fixed point on the earth ($e_p = 1$). For speed skating the power balance is thus reduced to:

$$P_o - P_f = m\,\overline{v} \cdot \overline{a} \qquad (9)$$

It should be noted that in this Equation, external power is defined as the power which is available to overcome friction or to increase speed. Internal mechanical power losses as a result of, for example, antagonistic actions of muscles or unnecessary movements of the trunk or arms, are thus not reflected by P_o. Although such a definition is customary in this and other sports as well as in bicycle ergometry,[42] it should be noted that P_o does not represent the total mechanical output of the involved muscles. To achieve a more complete impression of the total output, one might use a segment model. In the next paragraph, however, it will be argued that such models contain too many uncertainties to solve this problem. Therefore, Equation 9 is chosen as one of the basic tools for the remaining part of this chapter. For the sake of completeness, it should be pointed out that it can be convenient to integrate Equation 9 over a time-interval T (stroke, start):

$$\int_o^T (P_o - P_f) \, dt = \Delta \, 1/2mv^2 \tag{10}$$

With this Equation, it can be calculated, for example, that skaters show a mean power output during the start (first 100 m) of a 500 m race which exceeds 1000 W.

B. Flow of Energy

External power P_o in endurance sports is the result of aerobic and anaerobic power liberated in the involved muscles. The quotient of external power and the mechanical equivalent of metabolic power $\dot{E}$ is defined as mechanical efficiency e_m[42]:

$$e_m = \frac{P_o}{\dot{E}} \tag{11}$$

It should be noted that in this definition of e_m, P_o means the useful external power. Thus, the effectiveness of the use of the mechanical power for external work, does not affect e_m. This means that mechanical or technical parameters do not only influence the relationship between P_o and the speed, but they do also affect e_m. In all endurance sports, P_o is equal to the product of the amount of work per stroke (or cycle) A and the stroke (or cycle) frequency f:

$$P_o = A \cdot f \tag{12}$$

In the production of external power, both factors seem to be important and will be discussed later in this chapter.

Since $\dot{E}$ is derived from oxidation of fat and glycogen, it is possible to represent an endurance sportsman as a system where several variables determine the flow of energy. This representation is shown in Figure 4. The diagram clearly demonstrates that a discussion of mechanical aspects can hardly be isolated from other factors. Of course many of the factors that determine external power and speed, will be interrelated. The representation depicted in Figure 4 is the main approach used in the remaining part of this chapter.

It is understood that this approach, which implicitly or explicitly is used in many other studies[62,67,70,74,75] is just one of many other possible approaches. Particularly in sports like running where most mechanical power is lost internally, this approach is not useful at all. It should be noted, however, that the segment models used in running lead to many uncertainties too[62] which in part are due to disputable assumptions concerning external power, the role of storage and reutilization of elastic energy and the magnitude of mechanical efficiency[62,87,91] Recently, Ward-Smith[88,89] has presented an interesting model for running where all these uncertainties seem to have been by–passed. The aerobic and anaerobic energy

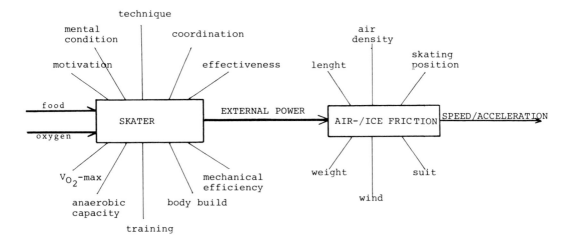

FIGURE 4. The flow of energy during skating.

production are directly related to frictional losses, the change in kinetic energy, and a large residual term Hv where H is a constant and v the speed of the runner:

$$\dot{E} = Hv + P_f + m v a \tag{13}$$

Despite fair agreement between model predictions and reality, this approach does not seem to be a useful alternative for the models presented above.[88] The weak point in Ward-Smith's approach concerns the large term Hv. The statement that all internal losses are simply proportional to running speed, and independent of external factors (wind, slope), does not hold. If, for example, the data of Davies[90] (who measured energy consumption during running in different wind velocities) are substituted in Ward-Smith's model, it appears that this assumption concerning Hv, can be rejected. This will please many physiologists, since the statement concerning Hv means that Ward-Smith assumes an "apparent efficiency" (also called work efficiency) to be equal to 1.0. This would be a nice thermodynamic and physiological problem. It is concluded that in sports like speed skating, where most mechanical energy is used to overcome frictional losses[58,101] the approach presented above appears to be obvious, despite its uncertainties concerning the relationship between effectiveness and mechanical efficiency.

Although models can be regarded as very appropriate tools in studying human movement, there are of course other possible approaches. One can measure kinematic variables, forces etc., without the use of mechanical models. Such descriptive studies can be very meaningful, not only for training purposes, but also to achieve insight into mechanical, physiological, anatomical, or even psychological backgrounds of certain phenomena. Therefore, some attention is paid to these types of studies that have been undertaken.

C. Kinematic Analysis

One of the kinematic variables which is always measured in endurance sports, is speed (or time) and speed variations during a race. This measurement provides proper feedback for the athlete during and after the race. An extensive scientific study on the measurements of speed variations, during and between laps in speed skating, was performed by Kuhlov.[10,12] A remarkable observation made from the measurements during sprint championshps, was the fact that skaters achieved their highest speed during the 500 m race prior to the first curve. This is not in agreement with the opinion of skaters and their coaches, who had (and many still have) the feeling that the highest speed is achieved on the second curve. This feeling, however, is likely to originate from the fact that skaters experience difficulties in following the second curve. It will be explained later that this is more likely the result of local fatigue than of a higher speed. For long distances, Kuhlov found that the best skaters showed the lowest increases in lap times.[10] This result was also reported by Michailow[25] and by Ingen Schenau et al.[49]

Although many coaches explicitly train their athletes to skate at equal lap times, one can dispute whether skating at a constant speed is really the most economic strategy. One might also argue that skating at a constant race-speed is rather a demonstration of strength than a chosen strategy.

A few investigators have subdivided the strokes of skaters into different phases.[26,27,37] In particular, the results of Djatschkow[26] can be explained properly from a mechanical point of view, and will be referred to later in the discussion on skating technique.

A last kinematic study which needs to be discussed concerns a Fourier analysis. Orlov et al.[92] analyzed the movements of skates, knees, and the pelvis of skaters in a frontal plane. The results showed an increase of energy content of higher frequencies with increasing speed. These results seem typical for this type of study. In particular, in cyclic movements, speed is controlled mainly by stroke frequency.[54,93-95] Thus, it seems a matter of course that the frequency spectrum of the movements of body landmarks or ground reaction forces,[96-98] shows a shift in energy content towards higher frequencies at increasing speed. One can argue that such analysis provides information mainly about speed in a rather circumstantial way.[99] Though Fourier analysis is necessary to be able to choose proper cut-off frequencies in smoothing and differentiating kinematic data, they scarcely provide useful information concerning the biomechanics of human movement.[100]

III. FRICTION

As is the case in most other endurance sports, speed skating can be seen as a struggle to overcome friction. To be able to understand the typical skating position when discussing technique, one needs to have some insight into the factors influencing air and ice friction. Therefore, these factors are discussed first.

A. Air Friction

Since air friction in speed skating is not essentially different from air friction in other sports it is not necessary to present an extensive discussion of general aerodynamics.[73] In summary, air friction has two components, friction drag and pressure drag. Friction drag is caused by friction in the layers of air along the body and is dependent on, for example, the roughness of the suit. In speed skating, friction drag is relatively small with respect to pressure drag. According to Bernoulli's law, the pressure in front of a skater is higher than the pressure behind the skater as a result of a difference in the relative velocity of the air with respect to the body. This pressure difference is mainly determined by the dynamic pressure $1/2 \, \rho v^2$ where ρ is the density of the air and v velocity of the air with respect to the body.[32] Given a cross-sectional area (the surface within the contour of a frontal picture) A_p, the pressure drag equals $1/2 \, \rho v^2 A_p$. This relationship, however, does not account for the influence of streamlining, and the contribution of friction drag. Therefore, a dimensionless coefficient C_D is added to this equation and is called the drag coefficient. This drag coefficient can only be determined experimentally. Total air-friction force F_w thus equals:

$$F_w = 1/2 \, \rho v^2 A_p C_D = k_1 v^2 \tag{14}$$

It has often been assumed that k_1 can be taken independently of speed in sports like speed skating,[101] cycling,[67] and skiing.[102] Pugh[69] as well as Shanebrook and Jaszczak,[68] however,

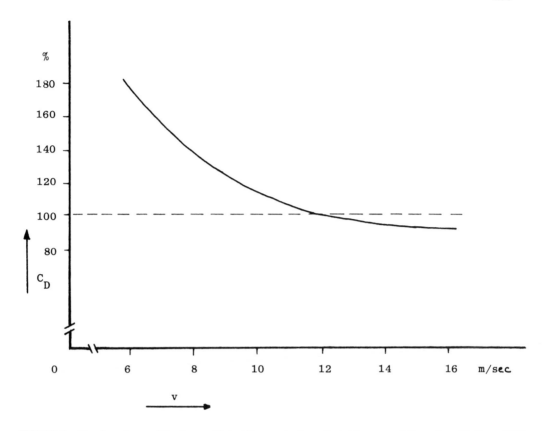

FIGURE 5. The dependency of the drag coefficient C_D on velocity v. C_D is taken as a relative value with $C_D = 100\%$ when v = 12 m/sec.

drew attention to the fact that C_D can decrease when the Reynolds number (R) (which is dependent on v) becomes critical (R > 10^5). Wind-tunnel experiments on speed skaters,[50] indeed, showed a strong dependency of C_D (and thus k_1) on v as seen in Figure 5. In the range of velocities in competitive races (8 to 15 m/sec) it is clear that this dependency has to be taken into account when calculating external work in speed skating. The decrease of C_D at increasing air velocity is explained by a decreased wake behind the body as a result of small turbulences in the boundary layer.[103] Since those turbulences can be reinforced by small disturbances on the suit, one can speculate that suits might be developed in the future which are faster than the present so-called "skin suit" or "fast" suit. Wind-tunnel experiments[50] showed that the skin suit is 2 to 3% faster than the old-fashioned woollen suits at velocities of 10 to 14 m/sec. At velocities below 6 to 7 m/sec, however, the rough woollen suit is faster than the smooth skin suit. The woollen suit obviously reinforces the turbulences in the boundary layer at lower Reynolds numbers. So younger skaters or recreational skaters will be faster in the old-fashioned woollen suit, although the psychological effects of the "fast" suit should not be underestimated.

In the wind-tunnel experiments referred to in the above discussion, a number of other factors were determined[50]:

Skating position — The skating position can be defined with the help of three angles as shown in Figure 6. Trunk position is defined by the angle θ_1 (the line between the middle of the neck and the greater trochanter and the horizontal), the knee angle θ_0 ($= \theta_2 + \theta_3$), and the angle θ_3 defining the position of the lower leg.[48]

Since in particular θ_1 and θ_0 will particularly influence both the cross-sectional area as well as the streamlining, the influence of both angles on drag (k_1), has been investigated

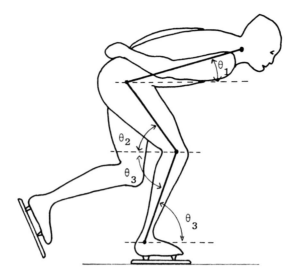

FIGURE 6.   The angles which define the skating position. The
knee angle θ_0 is equal to the sum of θ_2 and θ_3.

separately. The results show a strong influence of position on drag.[50] In particular, the position of the trunk is very sensitive. A vertical deviation of the trunk from the horizontal position by only 20° causes an increase in drag force of more than 20%. Although coaches in speed skating will all stress the importance of skating with a horizontal trunk position, it is remarkable that in cycle racing this factor has been overlooked for a long time. Although much attention is paid to streamlining frames etc., it was only recently that the first bicycle was built which allowed the cyclist (Moser) to keep his trunk more horizontal without changing the angles between his trunk and legs.

Body mass and body length — Since both C_D and A_p will depend on anthropometric measurements, many parameters concerning body-build measured on six different skaters, were correlated with k_1. The best fit appeared to exist with a simple expression $l \cdot m^{1/3}$ including body mass m and body length l. Although this correlation was found by trial and error, it might be a logical result since this expression has the dimensions of a surface (i.e., length squared), if it is assumed that body mass is proportional to body volume.

Active drag — In a few (unpublished) experiments, a skater made skating-like movements on a force plate in a wind tunnel. The mean drag appeared not to exceed the measured passive drag by more than 10%. Since the trunk position could not be accurately defined, it was unclear to what extent this slight increase was due to the movements, or to a larger value of θ_1, that which the skater was asked to adopt before he started to move. Nevertheless, the published data concerning air friction in speed skating might be slightly underestimated, since they are all based on "passive" skaters.[50]

Shielding — For running as well as for cycling, it has been demonstrated that the air friction can be considerably reduced if one is shielded by another runner or cyclist.[73,104] The same appeared to be true for speed skaters during the wind-tunnel experiments. At a distance of 1 m between the skaters this shielding caused a decrease in drag by 23%. Using a model of total frictional losses which will be discussed below, it can be calculated that the speed of a group of five or more skaters can be 5 to 7% higher than the speed of the individual skaters, at the same power output. In allround and sprint speed skating this shielding effect is of course of little significance since both skaters race in separate lanes.

Finally, it should be remarked that the position of the arms will have some influence on drag. From wind-tunnel experiments on skiers,[102,105] it was demonstrated that lateral excursions of the arms can double the drag. To the best knowledge of the present authors, the influence of different positions of the arms in speed skating, has never been published. Particularly on shorter distances, skaters use their arms to support the push-off. It is still an open question as to what extent this support is cancelled out by an increased air-friction force. Recently, Magnussen[43,106] reported about wind-tunnel experiments (unpublished) showing that even the position of the hands on the back is important. Skaters should keep their hands flat on their backs.

From the above it can be concluded that many problems exist concerning air friction and these certainly need further attention. In particular the problem of disturbances of the boundary layer and the influence of moving arms (and legs), deserve closer examination.

B. Ice Friction

There are only a few studies published on the nature of ice friction in speed skating. It is assumed that ice friction can be described by its well-known relationship to surface friction[50,107]:

$$F_{ice} = \mu N \qquad (15)$$

where N equals the normal force (approximately equal to body weight) and μ is the ice-friction coefficient. For properly treated ice rinks, Kobayashi[107] reported friction coefficients between $\mu = 0.003$ (optimal conditions) and $\mu = 0.007$. The lowest friction coefficients were found on natural ice at an ice temperature of $-0.5°C$. Our own (unpublished) experiments with a sledge on skate blades equipped with a sensitive accelerometer, yielded comparable data to those reported by Kobayashi. These data were used in all our previously published studies. From the experiments performed with that sledge, it was found that on artificial ice rinks μ can vary considerably in the timespan of a few races during a competition. In bad weather conditions (high air temperature and high humidity) μ can change by 0.001 or even 0.002 between the periods that the ice is treated as a result of frost. It can be demonstrated that one can really have bad (or good) luck in this sport as a result of variable ice conditions.

It is questionable, of course, to what extent a sledge with blades which are always at right angles to the ice, provides reliable data concerning friction which is exerted mainly on one blade at a time. Furthermore, the blade is often at an angle to the ice (particularly in the curves). It is only recently that we have succeeded in measuring ice friction during actual skating (paper in preparation). The first (and preliminary) results showed that the magnitude of the actual ice friction when averaged over an entire lap might be approximately 50% higher than the values measured with the help of the sledge. However, additional tests will be necessary to test the reliability of the data measured with these new (and complicated) skates. Figure 7 shows a force-time curve of the friction force measured with one of the two special skates.

C. Total Frictional Losses

In the above it was demonstrated how, with the help of wind-tunnel experiments and with the help of a sledge, the magnitude of air- and ice-friction forces can be determined. Although the position of a skater during actual skating is changing continuously, it is assumed that the position of the trunk and the knee angle just before push-off are somewhat representative of the mean position of the entire stroke. These values of θ_1, θ_2, and θ_3 (see Figure 6) were obtained from film analysis during actual races.[48,49,53-58] All films were taken from outside the crossing at right angles to the lane. If the correction for the influence of C_D on speed is called H(v), correction of the basis of actual trunk position $F(\theta_1)$, and correction for knee angle $G(\theta_0)$ then the total friction losses to air friction can be calculated according to[50]:

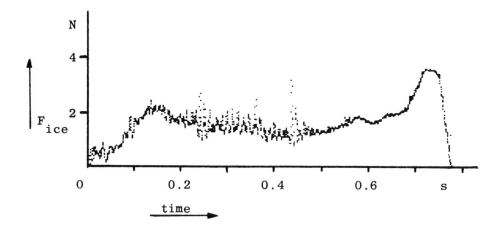

FIGURE 7.   A preliminary result for the measurement of ice friction. This friction force is measured during actual skating. The force-time signals are stored in the memory of a microprocessor system and can be read out in a host computer. The variation in amplitude of the frictional force corresponds with the variation in normal force (see Figure 11).

$$P_f = 0.0205 \ \rho l m^{1/3} \ F(\theta_1)G(\theta_0)H(v)v^2 \tag{16}$$

(See Ingen Schenau[50] for the mathematical expressions for F, G, and H). The density of the air is dependent on the air pressure at sea level ρ_0 and on the altitude h above sea level:

$$\rho = \rho_0 \ e^{-0.000125h} \tag{17}$$

Taking body weight mg as a normal force and assuming a wind velocity v_1, the total friction losses of a skater with a velocity v, a skating position defined by θ_1 and θ_0, body mass m, and body length l can be calculated by:

$$\rho_f = 0.0205 \ l m^{1/3}\rho_0 \ e^{-0.000125} \ F(\theta_1)G(\theta_0)H(v + v_1) \cdot (v + v_1)^2 v + \mu mgv \tag{18}$$

At constant speed, P_f is approximately equal to the external power P_o delivered by the skater according to Equation 9.

A few comments should be made about this Equation which has been used to calculate external power during skating for many male and female skaters:

1.   The relationship between body mass and body length was derived with the help of the data from only six different male skaters. Further experiments will be necessary to investigate if these data are also valid for other populations (males and females).
2.   The influence of body movements is not known exactly (e.g., the movements of the arms are not taken into account).
3.   The model is not corrected for movements in a sideways direction. As a result of the laterally directed push-off, skaters always make sinusoidal trajectories. Recently Delnoy et al.[58] calculated that the use of Equation 18 leads to an underestimation of external power of approximately 2% if these lateral excursions are not taken into account.
4.   As discussed above, the losses of ice friction may be underestimated by as much as 50%. Together with the other points made, this means that the power-output values reported in the publications from our group might contain a systematic underestimation in external power of approximately 10%.

Table 1
MEAN SPEED AND POWER OUTPUT OF ELITE MALE AND
FEMALE SPEED SKATERS AT THREE DISTANCES

	500 m		1500 m		3000 m	
	V(m/sec)	P_f (W)	V(m/sec)	P_f (W)	V(m/sec)	P_f (W)
Males	13.77	454	12.35	349	11.94	310
Females	13.03	373	11.86	303	11.02	261

In Table 1 an (uncorrected) impression is presented concerning the mean power output of elite males and females over three different distances. These power-output values are lower than the power which can be delivered by the same athletes during bicycle ergometer tests[49,52,55,57] and lower than maximal power output during cycling reported for other athletes at the same time-intervals[42] Though it was discussed that the power during skating might be slightly underestimated, this difference will be caused mainly by a large difference in power production during a single cycle. De Groot et al.[57] showed that power production during speed skating lasts only for approximately 10 to 20% of the cycle time, while during cycling, one can deliver power during more than 80% of the total cycle time. Thus, the mean power output during skating is the result of short intensive bursts of power. Peak power during push-off is approximately three times higher than peak power during cycling despite the lower mean power output during cycling.[57] This hypothesis that the lower mean power output is related to technique (and not for example to a large underestimation of internal or external losses), is supported by the corresponding lower-energy-consumption values reported for speed skaters during skating.[30,49] Despite the relatively long, more or less static, gliding phases,[26,48] which also require some metabolic energy, the mechanical efficiency during skating appears to be approximately only 15% lower than the mechanical efficiency during cycling.[49] Thus, it is unlikely that the power-output values presented in Table 1 contain underestimations of more than the 10% discussed above.

IV. MODEL PREDICTIONS

A. Introduction

At constant speed, the mean power output P_o during skating is approximately equal to the power P_f lost to friction. With the equation $P_o = P_f$ it is possible to predict the influence of several variables, such as skating position, fat, altitude, etc., on final times. Although power equations are used in several studies on other endurance sports,[62,67,70,75,74,88,89] such predictions are seldom published. Di Prampero[67] calculated the optimal altitude for cycle racers to establish world records by comparing the decrease in frictional losses (lower air density) with the decrease in aerobic power output as a result of the lower oxygen concentration at high altitude. The optimal altitude appeared to be 3,000 to 3,500 m. Ward-Smith[89] predicted the influence of wind on sprinting times. Power equations, however, make many other predictions possible. For speed skating, such calculations were made to predict the influence of trunk position, knee angle, body composition, ice-friction, wind, and altitude on final times.[50,53] In summary, the procedure for all those calculations was as described below.

First, a standard skater with given mass, length, and skating position was chosen (mean values of elite skaters). In the next step, the power output at a given speed (mean performance level for elite skaters) and under given environmental conditions (P_o, μ) was calculated with the help of Equation 18. Finally, one or more variables were changed and the new speed at the same power output, was calculated. The implicit assumption that the power output remains constant for different conditions, will not of course always be true for a particular skater. For example, a skater who is accustomed to skating with a horizontal trunk position will not be able to achieve the same power output if he is forced to skate with a much more vertical trunk position. However, the model predictions do provide insight into the relative importance of such variables. In other words, they do predict how much power is wasted if one has a nonhorizontal trunk position θ_1. Such data is interesting, apart from the question of the extent to which the involved variable can be changed for a particular skater. In fact, the calculations are a type of partial differentiation of v with respect to a certain variable while holding all other variables constant. Where relevant, the significance of these predictions for training the individual skaters, will be discussed below.

B. Skating Position

Coaches and scientists are well aware of the importance of the skating position with respect to reducing air friction.[26,180] All skaters are instructed to skate with a horizontal trunk position and with a knee angle which, during the gliding phase, is as small as possible. Both positions are, however, difficult to maintain for long periods of time since they require large static forces in the neck, back, hip, and knee extensor muscles. These static loads are regarded as the main causes of local fatigue which is often seen as an important limiting factor for speed skaters to make optimal use of their aerobic and anaerobic capacities during skating.[49,60] An optimal skating position with respect to air friction thus has a limiting effect on the liberation of metabolic energy. With respect to frictional losses, it was calculated that the trunk position in particular, is an extremely important factor. As a rule, one can state that skaters who do not hold their trunk horizontal lose about 0.13 sec per lap for every degree of upward deviation from that optimal position. In a 3000 m race this means that a skater who holds his trunk only 10° towards the vertical will waste approximately 12 sec. For a final time of slightly over 4 min, such a difference can be extremely critical. When viewing old recordings of skaters in the 1950s or 1960s, it is clear that the tremendous improvement in speed-skating performances during the last two decades is due largely to an improvement in the trunk position. Even in the 10,000 m race, the majority of present-day skaters manage to hold their trunk in the optimal or near optimal position. The same recordings show that the current elite skaters have smaller knee angles than the elite skaters in those years, but the difference is not very great. This is understandable since the knee angle in particular has a strong influence on the force of the muscles which have to do external work. This force-level of the hip and knee extensor muscles is, to a large extent, determined by θ_2, the position of the upper leg.[48,54] Coaches of non-elite skaters should realize, however, that skating with a small knee angle is an important prerequisite in speed skating. The model predictions show that, with respect to friction, a reduction in lap time of 0.015 sec was achieved for each degree reduction in knee angle.[60] In the discussion of skating technique it will be shown that skaters should keep the center of gravity line through or just in front of their ankle joint. Due to anatomical limitations particularly in θ_3 (Figure 6), the skater is not entirely free to choose each knee and trunk position without changing the horizontal position of his center of gravity with respect to his ankle joint.[48,50] This might explain why, in particular over short distances, not all elite skaters can be taught to hold their trunk in a horizontal position.

C. Weather Conditions

It is a well-known fact that optimal performances (personal, national, or world records) are often established during weather conditions which are not regarded as "optimal". Even during unstable weather, many good performances are sometimes possible. The opposite is also true. At seemingly optimal conditions (sun, temperature around or just below zero, low humidity, no wind) everyone expects records during national or international competitions, but the times can often be disappointing. Although in particular, the reporters and also the coaches are apt to doubt the expertise of the local ice maker, it is likely that one of the most important factors is often overlooked; the pressure of the air. As shown in Equation 18, the power losses to air friction are dependent on the density of the air. This density is not only dependent on altitude, but also on local air pressure. Since pressure variations between 980 and 1040 millibars at sea level are normal in many countries, these variations can explain the differences in the times. If all other factors remain constant, the model predictions that skaters can skate almost 1 sec per lap faster at 980 millibars than at 1040 millibars,[60] are correct. This is of course a large difference, which explains why an area with very high pressure and beautiful weather is not optimal with respect to personal times in speed skating. Good times may be expected in indoor 400 m rinks with miserable weather conditions outside.

A disadvantage of a low air density at outdoor rinks is of course the wind and high humidity which are mostly the result of low pressure (which in turn causes the relatively low density). Particularly on artificial ice rinks, this high humidity can cause frost on the ice surface. Despite the treatment of the ice (frequently seen during competitions), this frost can strongly influence the final classification.[50] Just after the ice is serviced, the ice-friction coefficient can be much lower than the value found just before the next treatment of the ice. If μ changes from 0.004 to 0.006, the influence on final time is already larger than one point per distance. Thus, one or two seemingly minor changes can completely change the outcome of a championship. It is remarkable that many skaters (of all performance levels) who are quite aware of this problem, do not regard such a lottery as a major handicap. It has been said that this influence of the elements gives a "romantic character" to this sport! In any case, the ice provides these athletes with an elusive excuse for failure.

D. Body Composition
1. Body Build
Two elements concerning body composition have been investigated; the influence of body length and mass, and the influence of fat.[53,60] With respect to body length and mass one can argue that tall and heavy skaters have the disadvantage of higher air- and ice-frictional losses than their smaller and lighter colleagues. On the other hand, taller and heavier skaters will (on the average) be able to produce a larger amount of external power. On the basis of Equation 9 it can be concluded that frictional losses are not proportional to body weight or length. From energy consumption tests it can be seen that this is also true for the liberation of metabolic energy. When expressed per kilogram body weight, tall and heavy subjects experience less friction and have lower energy consumptions than small, light subjects. So one needs regression equations for both aspects; friction and energy liberation (or rather power production) as a function of body composition to answer the question of what body build is ideal for the skater. Since body length and body mass are strongly correlated, one can define a group of standard skaters with body length and weight according to appropriate regression equations. During the last 6 years, the body weight and mass, as well as power output during supermaximal cycling, was measured for several groups of skaters.[49,52,55,57,59] With these data it was possible to construct regression lines between power output on the one hand, and body length or body mass on the other. By comparing a standard small and light skater with a standard tall and heavy skater, it could be concluded that the higher capacity for the taller skater to produce power is completely cancelled out by the increased air and ice friction.[60] Thus, on the basis of this comparison, it would appear that an ideal build for a skater seems not to exist. In the discussion of the technique of skating the curves, however, it should be noted that tall skaters have some advantage over smaller skaters, as a result of a technical peculiarity. Finally, it should be emphasized that the calculations concerning skaters with different body weights and lengths also show that one should not

Table 2
BODY COMPOSITION AND POWER OUTPUT OF
ELITE MALE AND FEMALE SKATERS

	BW (kg)	% Fat	P_c (W)	P_c/BW (W/kg)	P_f (W)	P_f/BW (W/kg)
Males	73.6	9.5	388	5.27	352	4.78
Females	66.3	20.6	340	5.13	304	4.60

Note: The power output P_c during 3 min of supramaximal cycling was measured for 5 males and 5 females. The power output P_f was measured
during 1500 m skating (approximately 2 min) for the same 5 males
and for 10 females (including 4 of the females who also performed the
cycle test.)

use total power output (or energy liberation) in comparing groups of skaters but always
power (or energy liberation) per kilogram of body mass. The same conclusion was drawn
for the runners[111] and cyclists.[112]

2. Fat

In the comparison made above, it was implicitly assumed that both standard skaters have
the same percentage of fat. Looking at the influence of fat, an imaginary standard skater
with given power production, is equipped with a different percentage of fat. By doing this,
the model predicts that skaters can gain 0.15 to 0.20 points at each distance for each kilogram
of lost fat.[53] Such a statement can be misleading. In many sports a knowledge of the influence
of fat has often resulted in uncontrolled diets with a completely opposite effect. It is not,
however, the responsibility of biomechanists to teach coaches that fat can be reduced by
endurance training and normal, intelligent nutrition.[60] An aspect which is interesting from
a scientific point of view, but which is of no use for practical applications, concerns the
differences in fat between males and females. In Table 2 the mean percentage of fat, and
absolute and relative power output during supermaximal cycling and skating of elite male
and female skaters, are summarized from previous studies.[52,53] Although the sample sizes
are small, it is remarkable that, when expressed per kilogram of body weight, the difference
in power output is not significant. With the help of Equation 18, it could be calculated that
the difference in skating performance can almost entirely be explained by the difference in
percentage of fat and a difference in the knee angle.[53] The mean knee angle of the males
($111.6° \pm 6.0°$ was 9% smaller than the knee angle ($121.5° \pm 3.1°$) of the females. If it
is assumed that most of the fat is located proximal to the hip joint, one can even argue that
the difference in performance level is entirely due to the different percentages of the fat
between the groups. Given a certain position θ_2 of the upper leg, the force level in the knee
and hip extensor muscles will be proportional to the body weight proximal to the hip joint.[48]
Assuming a constant (maximal) force level of these muscles, relative to their cross-sectional
area, the difference in fat can explain 50% of the difference in knee angle. Together with
the direct influence of body mass on air- and ice friction, this influence on θ_o and thus on
air friction, explains the difference in performance level between these groups of elite skaters.

If it is assumed that the percentage of fat of the 5 measured females is representative of
the entire group of 10 females analyzed during skating, the results of Table 2 show that
when expressed in power per kilogram of lean body mass, the males are not superior to the
females with respect to power production per kilogram muscle mass. On the basis of both
comparisons (friction and power production) it can be concluded that the difference in
performance level cannot be explained by a difference in work capacity. Comparable results
were reported by Wilmore[110] with respect to leg strength when this strength was taken

relative to body mass. Moreover, Cureton and Sparling[113] showed that by applying excess weights during running, the difference in performance level between male and female distance runners could also be explained by their normal difference in excess weight, i.e., fat. If one compares groups of skaters on the basis of power production, it can be shown in the above that the absolute value is meaningless. An adequate measure is power expressed per kilogram of total body weight. This is not only true for comparing males, but also for comparing males and females. Therefore, Kindermand and Keul[21] seem to make a standard error when they suggest that the difference in performance levels between male and female skaters over short distances is due to the lower muscle force of the females, while at the longer distances the females are handicapped by their lower oxygen-transport capacity. It should be noted that the same authors were co-authors in a previous study (Von Schmid et al.[20]), which showed that oxygen consumption in male and female speed skaters is equal when it is taken relative to body weight. From the above it should not be concluded that female speed skaters might be able to rise to the level of their male colleagues. Without artificial fat-reducing methods there will always remain a difference in excess weight. The differences, however, can be reduced in the future to some extent since both groups seem to be able to lose some fat if their data are compred with American speed skaters[35] or with distance runners.[109]

E. Altitude

It is remarkable that prior to the introduction of indoor rinks, holders of world records in speed skating for males were seldom found among the winners of European or World championships. Most of these records were in the hands of Russian skaters. The majority of the world records (for both males and females) have been established at the famous Medeorink in Alma Ata (U.S.S.R.). With the help of the models used in this chapter, it is possible to prove that this seeming contradiction can be attributed to the decreased air density at the Medeorink which is located 1700 m above sea level. Although there are other skating rinks located at such altitudes (e.g., Davos in Switzerland at 1600 m), there seems to be no other rink with such good climatological conditions (low ice friction) and so many important competitions (mainly among Russian and East German skaters). It might be argued that 1700 m is also a rather optimal altitude for speed skating. Although the air density is reduced by approximately 20%, the reduced oxygen consumption seems not to affect performances at this altitude, at least after some acclimatization. Malhotra and Gupta[114] showed that at 1500 m altitude the maximal aerobic capacity is not significantly different from the values found at sea level. As discussed before[50] such studies show that at altitudes up to 2000 m, one may expect the maximal power output during skating to be almost the same as at sea level. In this respect, it should be noted that speed skaters do not use the maximal capacity of their cardiorespiratory system during maximal skating.[49] This was concluded from the fact that skaters show higher oxygen-consumption values during cycling than during skating.[49,52] Obviously the oxygen consumption during skating is mainly determine by peripheral factors. So it seems correct to assume that skaters can deliver approximately the same power output at sea level and at 1700 m altitude even at the longest distances. Keeping all other conditions constant, the model predicts an advantage for skating at that altitude as summarized in Table 3. As shown before,[50] these predictions are in fair agreement with the actual mean difference of five Russian skaters chosen to test the model predictions (Table 3). The deviation of the predicted gain with the actual differences at 10,000 m is attributed to the known fear (for stiff, painful muscles) skaters have for the 10,000 m race. Most skaters perform the 10,000 m with full effort only at the European and World Championships (held at sea level that season). These predictions, have, of course been made for other altitudes too. As a rule of thumb one might conclude that up to moderate altitudes a skater can gain at least 0.1 points at each distance for every 100 m of increased altitude.[50,60]

Table 3
**THE PREDICTED GAIN IN SPEED FOR SKATING AT AN ALTITUDE
OF 1700 m AND THE ACTUAL MEAN DIFFERENCE OF FIVE
RUSSIAN SKATERS BETWEEN THEIR BEST PERFORMANCE AT SEA
LEVEL AND AT THE MEDEO RINK IN ALMA-ATA, U.S.S.R., (1700 m)
IN ONE SEASON**

	Distance			
	500 m	1500 m	5000 m	10000 m
Predicted gain[a]	1.95	2.05	2.21	2.27
Actual differences	1.91	1.93	2.15	1.61

[a] Expressed in points.

V. SKATING TECHNIQUES

A. Introduction

Speed skating is markedly different from other types of human locomotion if one judges the typical nature of the push-off.[8,15,26,48,60] The so-called "gliding technique" is difficult to learn because it does contradict the intuitive idea that people have about an effective push-off in two aspects, (a) the sidewards push-off; and (b) the absence of plantar flexion.

If one wants to go in a direction $\bar{s}$ it seems obvious that one should push off in a direction $-\bar{s}$. As explained before, this is not possible in speed skating, since one cannot push backwards with a skate that is gliding forwards. One of the first and most important technical skills which is taught to beginners, but which still has to be stressed in training experienced skaters, is the direction of the push-off perpendicular to the gliding direction of the skate. It was argued by Djatschkow[26] that a push-off against a fixed point in the ice as is seen in the majority of recreational skaters, is not possible at speeds higher than 7 m/sec. At higher speeds, every attempt to push against a fixed position will dramatically increase the ice friction. This limited speed of leg extension is closely related to the second peculiarity of the push-off; the unnatural suppression of plantar flexion.

Speed skaters are not able to perform a plantar flexion during push-off, or to formulate this more precisely; to change the position of the foot and skate in a sagittal plane. If one does not avoid this plantar flexion, the tip of the skate will scrape the ice causing a large increase in ice friction. As can be seen at important competitions, even top skaters cannot entirely inhibit the activation of their plantar flexors, especially during the short distances. At the start, but also during the following full lap of the 500 m race, pieces of ice may flow around from the tip of the skate. The coordinated pattern of the leg extensor muscles, as learned in more natural movements such as running and jumping, is obviously difficult to change. These two peculiarities explain part of the mechanical aspects which are typical for speed skating.

1. Location of the Center of Gravity

From a mechanical point of view, it is easy to understand why skaters should maintain a skating position which is such that the point of application of the reaction force on the skate is located under the ankle joint (Figure 8). For the more or less static gliding phase, this means that the center of gravity is positioned above the ankle joint. Taking the foot and skate as free-body diagrams, one can conclude that in that position, the plantar flexors are not to be activated (apart from correcting disturbances of the skater's balance). Every forward displacement of the center of gravity will cause the activation of the calf muscles in order

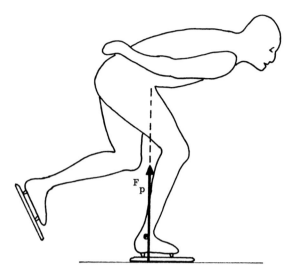

FIGURE 8.   The line of action of the reaction force on the skate should be located through the ankle joint to prevent a strong plantar flexion moment from the calf muscles.

to maintain equilibrium. However, this will cause a plantar flexion as soon as the reaction force on the blade drops at the end of the push-off, and so skaters are taught to "sit" and push-off on the back part of their skates.

2. Trajectory of Center of Gravity

A second notable mechanical result of this push-off is the transverse movement of the center of gravity. When skating along a straight line, the center of gravity describes a trajectory with respect to the ice which can be approximated by a sine wave with an amplitude of less than 0.25 m at high stroke frequencies; up to 0.50 m or more at lower stroke frequencies. These sideward excursions follow directly from the fact that the effective component of the push-off force can only be directed perpendicular to the gliding direction of the skate. This may be explained with the help of Figure 9. Let the skater's velocity prior to push-off be v_1. Since the push-off is directed at right angles to the gliding direction of the push-off skate, the push-off will result in an increase in velocity relative to the push-off skate from zero to v_2. As a first approximation, v_2 is directed at right angles to v_1. Disregarding the small deceleration as a result of frictional forces, the magnitude of v_2 after push-off equals:[54]

$$v_3 = \sqrt{v_1^2 + v_2^2} \qquad (19)$$

Kinetic energy thus increases as:

$$1/2\ mv_3^2 - 1/2\ mv_1^2 = 1/2\ mv_2^2 \qquad (20)$$

This increase in kinetic energy can be regarded as the (useful) amount of work per stroke A.[54] The push-off, however, also causes a change in direction α of the center of gravity which is typical for speed skating only, described by:

$$\alpha = \mathrm{ArcTan}(v_2/v_1) \qquad (21)$$

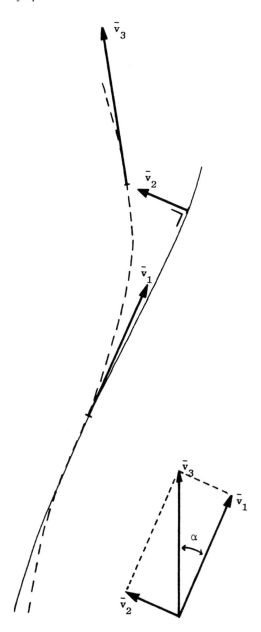

FIGURE 9.   The trajectory of the center of gravity during skating (broken line). The solid line is the trajectory of the right skate. The velocity increment $\bar{v}_2$ is the velocity of the center of gravity with respect to the point of application of the push-off force on the right skate. If $\bar{v}_1$ represents the velocity of the center of gravity just before push-off, $\bar{v}_3 = \bar{v}_1 + \bar{v}_2$ represents the velocity just after push-off. The push-off thus results not only in an increase in kinetic energy but also causes a change of direction.

This change in direction does not only explain the sinusoidal trajectory when skating straight stretches, but will also appear to be a surprising and valuable tool in explaining the mechanics of skating the curves (as described in a later section).

3. The Handicapped Push-Off

A third point which has to be explained in this introduction on skating technique concerns the influence of the absence of plantar flexion on the acceleration of the center of gravity.

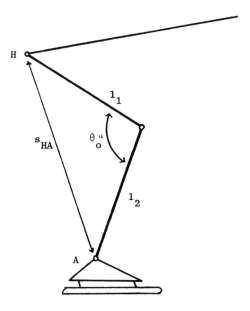

FIGURE 10. The velocity difference V_{HA} ($= ds_{HA}/dt$) between hip and ankle is determined by knee angle and knee angular velocity and is zero by definition at $\theta_0 = 180°$.

It was only recently discovered that speed skaters do not fully extend their knees during push-off.[54,60] This of course was highly surprising since skaters are already handicapped by the constraints concerning trunk position and plantar flexion. In addition to the absence of plantar flexion, skaters do not strongly raise their trunk during push-off to prevent excessive air friction. When compared to jumping, for example, this means that a significant part of the shortening potential of the plantar flexors and hip extensors is not used during the push-off in speed skating. Therefore, it was difficult to understand why even the best skaters in the world appeared to lift the push-off skate from the ice with a knee angle of approximately 160°, instead of performing a full extension of the knee. One reason that this important aspect was not discovered before, might be that almost all skaters complete their knee extension after this lift-off. Moreover, the extension velocity is sufficiently high (approximately 600°/sec) that only selective high-speed film analysis can demonstrate this phenomenon. Since this limited knee extension is not seen in jumping,[64] it seemed obvious to relate this phenomenon to the absence of plantar flexion.[54] With some goniometry it is possible to explain this handicapped knee extension completely.

The aim of every explosive push-off is to accelerate the body center of gravity with respect to the ground. During push-off the center of gravity is accelerated up to a maximal value towards the end of push-off. Lift-off takes place as soon as the larger body segments can no longer be accelerated with respect to the surface against which the push-off takes place. In skating, the velocity of the center of gravity with respect to the blade of the push-off skate is mainly determined by the velocity difference between the hip and ankle joints (Figure 10). This velocity difference is determined by the segment lengths l_1 and l_2 of the upper and lower leg, the knee angle θ_0 and the angular velocity of $d\theta_0/dt$ according to.[54]

$$v_{HA} = \frac{l_1 l_2 \sin \theta_0}{(l_1^2 + l_2^2 - 2l_1 l_2 \cos \theta_0)^{1/2}} \frac{d\theta_0}{dt} \tag{22}$$

Since $\sin \theta_0$ will go to zero at $\theta_0 = 180°$, this velocity reaches its maximal value long before

Table 4
MEAN POWER OUTPUT (P_f), STROKE FREQUENCY (f), AND AMOUNT OF
WORK PER STROKE (A) IN ELITE MALE AND FEMALE SPEED SKATERS
AT DIFFERENT DISTANCES

	500 m			1500 m			3000 m		
	P_f (W/kg)	f (sec^{-1})	A (J/kg)	P_f (W/kg)	f (sec^{-1})	A (J/kg)	P_f (W/kg)	f (sec^{-1})	A (J/kg)
Males	6.20	2.10	2.95	4.80	1.66	2.88	4.15	1.51	2.76
Females	5.65	2.10	2.69	4.60	1.67	2.76	3.95	1.45	2.73

Note: Power output and work per stroke are taken relative to body weight.

$\theta_o = 180°$. Further analysis (publications submitted) showed that v_{HA} − max was reached at $\theta_o = 147°$. If no other segments (trunk and foot) become involved in this transfer of angular velocities of joints into translational velocity of the center of gravity, lift-off should occur at this angle of 147° since the larger segments which have achieved a velocity v_{HA} (trunk with arms and contralateral leg) pull on the smaller segments (lower leg, foot, and skate). The fact that lift-off is visible at $\theta_o = 160°$ might be explained by a slight elevation of the trunk with respect to the horizontal, thus adding a second velocity difference to v_{HA}. In jumping (and most likely in running too), the decrease of v_{HA} is compensated by a fast and powerful plantar flexion reinforced by the biarticular gastrocnemius at the end of push-off.[63-65] It can be concluded that the push-off in speed skating is strongly handicapped when compared with running and jumping. This explains why the push-off has to be performed in a very short time-interval, and why the peak power output often exceeds 2000 W.[57]

B. Work per Stroke and Stroke Frequency
   As in all other cyclic endurance sports, mean power output is equal to the product of work per stroke A and stroke frequency f. In most endurance sports these driving factors can be chosen freely within certain limits. In speed skating practice, stroke length (or number of strokes per lap) is often used as an important mechanical factor. One should realize, however, that stroke length is not an independent variable. It depends on A, f, and friction. One statement concerning stroke length can be useful for training purposes, namely, the longer the stroke at a given speed, the greater must be the amount of work per stroke. In order to train for an overload of the amount of work per stroke at given lap times, this means that the skaters should make longer strokes than they normally do. Without information on speed, stroke length has limited use. One might say that stroke frequency and work per stroke can be directly controlled by the nervous system, and in particular, stroke frequency can be quite easily influenced. It is often suggested that optimal stroke frequency at a certain power output is closely connected to optimal mechanical efficiency.[115-119] However, it is not clear why the ultimate aim of an endurance sportsman (which is the production of an optimal mean power output) should always be achieved at a stroke frequency which coincides with an optimal transfer of aerobic metabolic power into mechanical power. For most endurance sports this relationship between f and e_m is not investigated for supramaximal performances. From a mechanical and psychological point of view, it is interesting that many authors found stroke frequency to be the main factor for the control of speed. This was reported for cross-country skiing,[93] ice hockey,[120] swimming,[94,95] and running.[95] In cycle racing both A and f seem to be increased with speed.[121,71]
   Table 4 shows values for P_f, f, and A for elite male and female speed skaters.[49,54] These data support the results of other endurance sports, i.e., that external power (and thus speed) is determined mainly by stroke frequency. Each skater seems to have a particular amount

of work per stroke available which is more or less independent of the skating distance. This work per stroke will be closely linked to the push-off technique of the individual skater. A constant amount of work per stroke at different power outputs was also reported for a previous group of male speed skaters during the four classical distances (500 m, 1,500 m, 5,000 m and 10,000 m).[48] As discussed before,[50] the magnitude of the values reported in that study contain a systematic underestimation. Nevertheless, based on these studies, one can conclude that stroke frequency in speed skating is mainly used for the control of speed. This, however, does not mean that the best skaters also have the highest stroke frequencies. In elite female skaters there is even a tendency for the opposite; the skaters at the highest performance level have a relatively low mean stroke frequency at one particular distance.[54] On the other hand, it was clear that among males and females, the best skaters show the highest amount of work per stroke, at each distance.[49,54] This means that with respect to these factors, training should be focused mainly on the increase of the amount of work per stroke (push-off technique) and not on an increase in stroke frequency. One could compare work per stroke with the capacity of an engine, while the significance of stroke frequency might be related to the function of the accelerator pedal. As in engines, the performance level is not determined by the accelerator. Finally, it must be remarked that in contrast to skating the straight parts, the stroke frequency in the curves is constrained by other factors, as will be discussed later.

C. Skating Technique on the Straights
A race in all-round and sprint speed skating can be subdivided into three parts:

- the start
- the straights
- the curves

Though large differences in technique exist between these different phases, the majority of the published studies on skating concern the straights.[8,26,48,49,53,54] Haase[15] presented some useful recommendations about the curves, but apart from observations of stroke frequencies[54] and push-off forces,[41,47] no experimental biomechanical studies seem to have been published. Only two studies concerning starting techniques (and these were in ice hockey) have come to the attention of the authors.[122,123]

1. How to Model Work per Stroke
One of our first models published on the technique of speed skating concerned the calculation of the amount of work per stroke on the basis of the knee angle θ_0 prior to push-off.[48] The idea was that the knee-extension range, together with the push-off force, determined to a large extent the external work done. The push-off force was approximated on the basis of the assumption that the center of gravity is displaced only in a horizontal direction.[48] When judging frontal films of speed skating, this assumption seemed reasonable. However, the same study also showed that the amount of work per stroke calculated from frictional losses did not agree with the prediction made on the basis of θ_0. Moreover, the model implicitly predicted push-off forces also. These predicted forces appeared to be lower than the push-off forces which have actually been measured by different authors.[26,41,47] Figure 11 shows a typical example of the push-off forces of the left and right legs measured during skating at a speed of 11.8 m/sec (3000 m level). The peak forces during push-off reach values up to 140% of body weight. According to the model predictions, however, this skater should not show peak forces larger than approximately 125% of body weight. The model predicts that forces lower than body weight cannot be explained if the assumpion of horizontal displacement of the center of gravity is true. As discussed before,[48] skaters

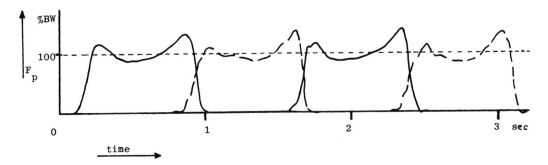

FIGURE 11.   Total push-off force on the straight part measured with skates equipped with strain gauges.[47] Solid line represents the force on the right skate, the broken line the force on the left skate. The forces are expressed in percentage of body weight.

obviously show a passive phase where they rotate around the y-axis (Figure 3). This assumption was validated by a later study concerning the technique of elite female skaters.[54] These arguments, as well as the limited knee extension discussed above, make it clear that θ_0 may be an important prerequisite for producing work during push-off, but that it does not predict the amount of work per stroke. So the model of Ingen Schenau and Bakker[48] has to be rejected. The present idea about the push-off is, in fact, in agreement with the recommendations made by Djatschkow[26] that skaters should make a passive falling movement prior to the explosive push-off.[54] Given the short time-interval in which the push-off takes place, a vertical displacement of only 2 to 3 cm could explain why skaters actually show a much higher amount of work per stroke than was predicted on the basis of θ_0. These latter findings show that the push-off mechanics are much more complicated than what was assumed in the past. Three-dimensional multisegment models will have to be used in the future to investigate whether a new model, which predicts the result of push-off in a direct way, might be valuable. In recent studies, work per stroke has always been calculated indirectly from frictional losses P_f and stroke frequency.[49,53-55] At the end of the next section, we will explain how work per stroke might also be calculated from the horizontal component of the push-off force and the horizontal speed of the body center of gravity relative to the push-off skate. A major problem for such a calculation is the difficulty in measuring the components of the push-off force, separately. In other studies of locomotion, one is able to use force plates which, apart from the start, cannot be used in speed skating.

2. Descriptive Analysis

It has been stated before that the stroke in speed skating can be divided into a gliding phase and a push-off phase. In the gliding phase the skating position of the males is not notably changed. Most elite females appear to show some increase in knee angle during the gliding phase. This results in a larger knee angle prior to push-off than that seen in elite males.[53] At all corresponding distances, the mean value of θ_0 at the onset of push-off is 10 to 12° larger for the females than for males. In Figure 12 a typical example of knee angle and angular velocity of an elite female skater is presented. The beginning of the push-off phase is (arbitrarily) chosen as the point at which the angular velocity continues to increase up to its maximal value. The end of push-off is determined by the time at which it is visible on the film that the skate has been lifted from the ice. It should be noted that the beginning of the stroke is not defined as the beginning of the phase where the skate is placed on the ice which might at first seem logical. According to Djatschkow,[26] the beginning is defined as the time when the contralateral skate is lifted from the ice. It has been assumed by coaches for a long time that weight transfer takes place, at least in part, as soon as the next gliding skate is placed on the ice. However, force measurements have demonstrated that weight

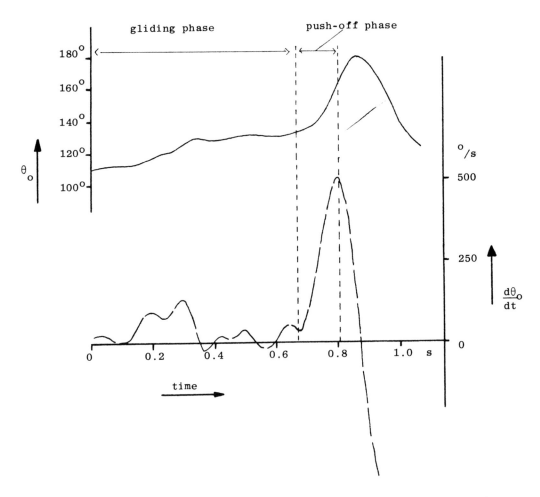

FIGURE 12. Typical example of the knee angle θ_0 and angular velocity ($d\theta_0/dt$) of an elite female speed skater as a function of time.

transfer at this point, which lies approximately at the onset of the passive falling movement prior to push-off, is negligible.[26,41,47] From a mechanical point of view a weight transfer at this point (even in part), would reduce the possibility for a powerful push-off. The placement of the new gliding skate close to the other leg is important so as to be able to accelerate as much mass as possible during push-off.[26] However, it was observed that no weight transfer should take place before the end of the push-off. In this respect, the push-off might be compared to some extent with a jumping-like movement in a horizontal direction.[47] Recently, de Boer et al. (publication in preparation) found a negative correlation (r = 0.64) between the time-span of the push-off phase and performance. This seems to contradict the results of Djatschkow[26] who found a positive correlation (r = 0.98) of performance and the percentage of the push-off time relative to the total stroke time. This apparent contradiction might be explained by a different definition of push-off. Djatschkow defined the beginning of push-off as the point where the trunk begins to rotate externally with respect to the upper leg. However, external rotation takes place prior to the passive falling movement described above. Djatschkow as well as other authors emphasize the importance of this passive movement, which is necessary to position the push-off as horizontal as possible.[8,26,54] Thus, the ratio defined by Djatschkow includes a phase which should be long and a phase which should be short. Moreover, his data were based on competitions held in the late 1960s when it was still common to many skaters to make long strokes (long gliding phases). With respect to the push-off phase as defined in Figure 11, we may conclude that a quick powerful push-off is important in speed skating. In males this is also relfected by a positive correlation (r = 0.60) between peak knee-angular velocity and speed. Surprisingly, such a correlation was not significant (r = 0.10) in a group of elite female speed skaters.[54] This, of course, might be due to the limitation in knee extension during push-off. Maximal extension velocity is reached at approximately the end of push-off (Figure 12). While the maximal value in the velocity difference V_{HA} (Figure 10) is reached approximately 30 msec earlier. Thus, the maximal angular velocity is not a direct measure for the amount of work per stroke. At present, a model is being developed to calculate the actual velocity of the whole body center of gravity from the locations of the segmental centers of gravity.

When considering all the technical parameters measured in a number of studies on this subject (knee and hip angles and angular velocities, stroke frequency, gliding and push-off time, angles of the push-off leg in the frontal plane push-off forces, etc.),[10,26,41,48,49,53,54] the following conclusions can be drawn:

(a) elite skaters can be distinguished from skaters of a lower performance level by their:

- smaller pre-extension knee angle, mainly caused by a more horizontal upper leg position
- considerably greater amount of work per stroke and slightly higher stroke frequency
- higher knee extension velocity
- smaller decrease in lap times (and in A and f) during the course of a race
- brief, but powerful push-off
- more horizontally directed push-off

(b) among groups of elite skaters, the best performers appear to have:

- higher knee extension velocities (males only)
- greater amounts of work per stroke
- more horizontally directed push-off

The last point, the more horizontally directed push-off, seems to be one of the most important technical aspects of speed skating, and needs some further explanation. It was shown before,[54] that using a coordinate system which moves with the push-off skate[48] according to the axis presented in Figure 3, the external work during push-off can be calculated from the energy state $E_T = E_k + E_p$ where E_k equals the kinetic energy and E_p the potential energy of the body center of gravity. Differentiating E_T with respect to time gives the instantaneous external power P of the center of gravity during push-off:[54]

$$P = F_x v_x + F_z v_z \qquad (23)$$

where F_x and F_z are the lateral and vertical components of the push-off force, and v_x and v_z are the velocities of the center of gravity in the corresponding directions. On the other hand, the useful amount of work A per stroke $1/2\ mv_2^2$ as calculated above in Equation 20 is equal to[54]:

$$A = 1/2\ mv_2^2 = \int_0^T F_x v_x\ dt \qquad (24)$$

with T being the push-off time.

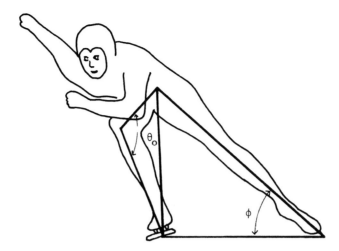

FIGURE 13.   The angle φ between the push-off leg and the ice determines the effectiveness of the push-off.

These Equations show that useful work is determined by the lateral component of the push-off force. The power $F_z v_z$ results in potential energy and vertical velocity which do not contribute to speed. Particularly after a passive falling movement, when some potential energy is converted into useful kinetic energy, F_z can be greater than gravity in order to compensate for the lost potential energy. It is clear that the effect of the push-off is greater if the angle between the push-off force and the ice is smaller. Preventing rotation with respect to the center of gravity means that an effective push-off requires a small angle between the push-off leg and the ice during push-off. This angle φ is indicated in Figure 13. On the basis of this angle a new variable e = ArcCos φ, called ''the effectiveness of push-off'' has been defined.[54] This effectiveness is one of the most important technical aspects to keep in mind when training elite and non-elite skaters.

It should be noted, finally, that one of the very first studies on technique in speed skating, published by Haase[8] in 1953, emphasized the importance of a small φ value at push-off. The same recommendation was given by Djatschkow.[26] It is, therefore, surprising that so many skaters still seem to attempt to push themselves upwards instead of forwards. The reason must be either that those qualitative studies were not convincing enough, or that this effectiveness concerns a technical aspect which is difficult for coaching to influence. Perhaps proper feedback might help to instruct skaters with respect to this angle. This can be done with the help of frontal recordings and also with sagittal recordings of the angle θ_o of the new gliding leg at weight transfer. As shown before, this angle is a proper measure for φ at the end of push-off[8,54] (Figure 13).

D. Biomechanics of Skating the Curves

1. Introduction

The only experimental data published concerning the techniques of skating the curves, have been the measurements of push-off forces,[41,47] and the measurement of stroke frequencies in the curves relative to the stroke frequencies during the straight parts of 10 elite female skaters.[54] This limited number of studies is a source of some disappointment for speed-skating coaches, since most coaches feel that the proper technique in skating curves is much more decisive for competitive skating than the technique of skating the straight parts. Many coaches even state that most of the work should be done on the curves, while the skaters should relax during the straight parts. It is clear that the curves need further attention in the near future. For the present, we will attempt to make some tentative suggestions.

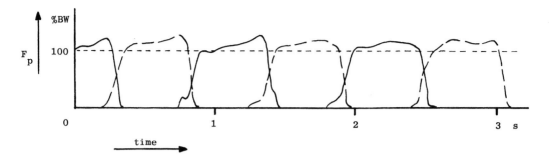

FIGURE 14. Push-off forces while skating round a curve. Note the shorter stroke times when these curves are compared with the curves presented in Figure 11. See Figure 11 for further explanation.

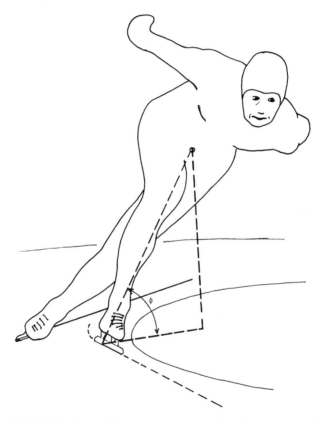

FIGURE 15. The position of the center of gravity while skating round a curve. The angle ϕ should be less than 90° during the entire stroke.

2. Push-Off Force and Stroke Frequency

Figure 14 shows the push-off force in the curve of the same skater (at the same speed) who also produced the force curves presented in Figure 11. The main differences compared with the forces during the straight parts are the shorter stroke time, the lower peak forces at the end of push-off, and the absence of a phase in the middle of the stroke, where the push-off force is less than body weight. This last point is easy to understand since skaters do not rotate from the lateral to the medial side of the skate as they do on the straight part. At weight-transfer, both legs are already placed at an angle to the ice in a way that the center of gravity is on the medial side of the right skate and on the lateral side of the left skate in their period of support. The skater "hangs", as it were, in the curves (Figure 15).

In comparison with the straight part one might say that the first part of the gliding phase is bypassed. This explains the higher stroke frequency in the curves than during the straight parts which is seen in experienced skaters.[54] It is possible that this higher stroke frequency causes lower peak forces at the end of the push-off.

It should be noted that the average level of the push-off forces during skating a curve is not higher than the average force level on the straight parts (cf. Figures 11 and 14). This might be contrary to the intuitive idea most skaters have about the need to oppose a centrifugal force. We will explain in the next paragraph that strokes on the curves are in many respects not essentially different from strokes on the straight parts.

If the stroke frequency on the curve f_c is taken relative to the stroke frequency during the straight parts (f_{sp}), a positive correlation ($r = 0.6$) has been shown with speed for a group of 10 elite female speed skaters.[54] This seems to support the opinion of coaches who state that the best skaters are those who accelerate in the curves. In the next paragraph we will show that this opinion can be completely supported from a mechanical point of view. The only problem, however, is that cause and effect are quite the reverse of what practitioners have assumed; the best skaters are the ones who are forced to maintain a high frequency in the curves as a result of their high speed before they go into the curves.

3. A New Theory

The model discussed below is not based on a critical review of published work. Nevertheless, it is the opinion of the present authors that a chapter on the biomechanics of speed skating would be incomplete if no attention was paid to one of the most important aspects of speed skating (which became clear with the help of a mechanical model recently developed). Since this is an original work, the model is presented in more detail than was done before.

The strokes — As explained before, the effect of the push-off in speed skating is not only an increase of kinetic energy, but also a change in direction of the body center of gravity (Figure 9). This change in direction is used when skating the curves. In a sport such as cycle racing, the required centripetal force for making a curve is delivered by friction between the tire and the road which is directed at right angles to the propulsive force on the bicycle. The cyclist does not have to do work to generate this centripetal force. If speed skaters could make curved strokes according to the radius of the curve of the ice rink, there would be a similarity with cycling. In that case, however, they would not be able to push off. Skaters, therefore, make more or less straight strokes in the curves, particularly when skating at full effort. This means that the only difference with skating the straights is that instead of changing the direction alternately to the right and to the left, the change in direction in the curves is always to the left. This is done both with the right leg and with the left leg. A schematic representation of the trajectory of the center of gravity with respect to the trajectories of the skates is presented in Figure 16. It should be noted that the statement made in the above that the skaters make more or less straight strokes is true to a certain extent for speed skating on 400 m rinks. (Figure skaters and short-track skaters make curved strokes, and so they also generate a centripetal force between the ice and the skate to follow the curve). In speed skating, the centripetal force (necessary to make a curve) is delivered by the same force which does the external work to maintain the speed. This is a unique phenomenon which could explain many of the peculiarities experienced by skaters.

Change in direction and number of strokes — With the help of Figure 9 and Equation 21 we explained before that the change in direction, α, is dependent on the velocity v_1 and the velocity increment v_2 perpendicular to v_1. According to Equation 20, v_2 is the direct result of the amount of work per stroke A, and so the deviation is dependent on the speed v_1 and the amount of work per stroke. For elite skaters, one can calculate from A that v_2 is approximately equal to 2.4 m/sec. Given the same amount of work per stroke, the change

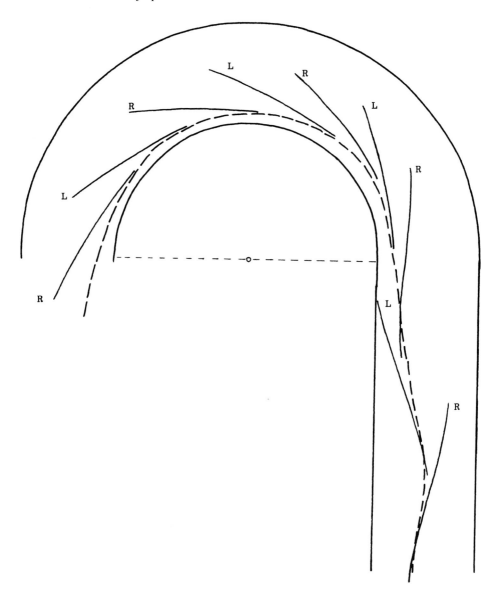

FIGURE 16.   In the curves, the center of gravity (dotted line) describes more or less an arc of a circle which is achieved by pushing the body to the left with the right (R) and left skates (L). This is in contrast to the straight parts where the skater pushes himself alternately to the left and to the right. It should be noted that the actual number of strokes in the curve is considerably higher than the number presented in this figure.

in direction of the center of gravity thus depends on the speed of the skater. This effect is illustrated in Figure 17 with the help of two speeds. At a low speed (5 m/sec) the push-off causes a change in direction of 26°, while the same push-off causes a deviation of only 10.5° at a speed of 13 m/sec (500 m level). The total change in direction which can be made on the curve equals 180°. So the skater with a low speed can make 180/26 = 7 strokes during the entire curve, while the fast skater can make 180/10.5 = 17 strokes if the speed were to remain constant. Given a mean curve length (average of inner and outer lane) of 88 m, the stroke frequency of the first skater has to be 0.4 sec^{-1} and the stroke frequency of the second skater 2.5 sec^{-1}. These stroke frequencies cannot be chosen by the skaters. If they were to increase the stroke frequency they would describe too small a radius. On

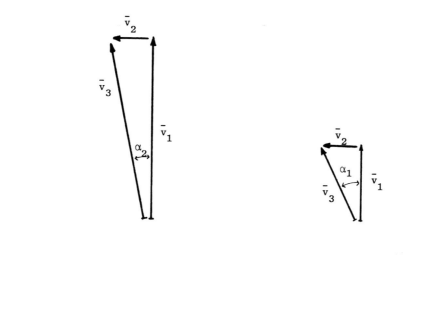

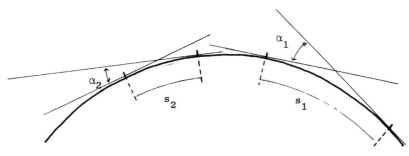

FIGURE 17. The change in direction (α) as the result of the same push-off (resulting in v_2) is strongly dependent on v_1. At a low speed, the change in direction is much larger than at higher speeds. As a consequence the skater can change his direction after a (gliding) distance, s, which is longer for the slower skater (s_1) than for the faster skater (s_2). Together with the difference in speed, this means that the faster skater can maintain a much higher stroke frequency than the slower skater. Note that the tangents indicate the change in direction (these lines should not be confused with strokes).

the other hand at a lower stroke frequency, they would fly out of the curve. This example also shows that at a given work per stroke, the power output $P_o = A \cdot f$ is also determined by the speed of the skater. The slow skater would be forced to produce much less power than he might be able to deliver (in the example only 1.1 W/kg), while the fast skater is forced to deliver an extremely high power output (about 7.8 W/kg). One may thus conclude that the lower the speed of a skater the lower the power output he is allowed to deliver since he has to follow the snow border in the curve. This explains why the best skaters accelerate in the curves and why poor skaters, or skaters who lost speed towards the end of a race as a result of fatigue, have problems maintaining their speed, in particular in the outer lane. On the other hand if a skater cannot deliver the required amount of power at high speeds (for example in the second curve during the 500 m race) he will not be able to follow the snow border of his lane and will describe a larger radius, or he can even be forced to brake. Many other practical problems can be explained by these principles. First, however, a more complete model will be introduced.

A geometrical model of skating curves — Since v_1 is often much larger than v_2 one can, when expressed in radians, approximate α by:

$$\alpha = \text{ArcTan}(v_2/v_1) \approx v_2/v_1 \tag{25}$$

If n equals the number of strokes per curve, then $\alpha n = \pi$ or:

$$n \, v_2/v_1 = \pi \tag{26}$$

Let T be the stroke time ($= 1/f$) and τ the time needed to skate a curve of length πR with R being the radius of the curve. Then $nT = \tau$ and $v_1 T = \pi R$, and we approximate v_1 as the mean speed in the curve. These equations lead to:

$$n = \frac{\pi R f}{v_1} \tag{27}$$

Substituting Equation 26 into Equation 27 yields:

$$v_2 f = \frac{v_1^2}{R} \tag{28}$$

This equation might also be deduced from a first approximation of the mean centripetal acceleration a_c on the center of gravity with $a_c = v_2/T = v_2 f = v_1^2/R$. According to Equations 12 and 20, the external power delivered under these conditions is:

$$P_o = A \cdot f = 1/2 \, v_2^2 f \tag{29}$$

if P_o is expressed in W/kg body weight. Substituting Equation 29 into Equation 28 yields:

$$P_o = \frac{v_1^4}{2fR^2} \tag{30}$$

Since not all variables on the right hand side are independent variables, the significance of this Equation is not easy to understand. It tells us that a skater with a speed v_1 and a certain amount of work per stroke A (resulting in a certain v_2) who is skating a curve with a radius R, is forced to choose a stroke frequency according to Equation 28 and to deliver an amount of external power according to equation 30. Before this model is applied to more practical problems, a few remarks should first be made on its scientific significance.

Validation of the model — Considering the assumptions made in developing the model, the following remarks should be made. First, the assumption that $\alpha = v_2/v_1$ leads to an over estimation of α. This means that f and P will be slightly underestimated (less than 3% at the speeds of interest). Second, the assumption that v_1 equals the mean speed also leads to an underestimation of f and P_o. This error is approximately 6% at a speed of 11 m/sec. Third, in practice, the strokes of many skaters do not exactly describe a straight line. Most skaters are instructed to follow the slight curvature with the curve. Although this can hardly be seen in competitions, one should realize that every stroke less than the n strokes used in the deduction of the model means an overestimation of 8% or more for f and P. Based on these considerations, not much can be said about the validity of the model.

On the basis of experimental data concerning frictional losses, speed, stroke frequency, and amount of work measured previously,[54] one can test if the order of magnitude of P_o (Equation 30) is in agreement with the frictional losses calculated on the basis of the model

Table 5
POWER P₀ PREDICTED ON THE BASIS OF A GEOMETRICAL MODEL OF THE CURVES AND POWER Pf CALCULATED FROM PREDICTED FRICTIONAL LOSSES

	Stroke frequency $f_c(\text{sec}^{-1})$	Speed (m/sec)	P_o (W/kg)	P_f (W/kg)	P_o' (W/kg)
500 m	2.28	12.55	6.94	5.39	6.41
1500 m	1.84	11.37	5.79	4.33	5.01
3000 m	1.66	10.97	5.56	4.08	4.75
5000 m	1.53	10.20	4.51	3.57	3.80

Note: P_o' is an estimation of the power delivered during a full lap (see text). The calculation of P_o is based on the mean values for stroke frequency and speed. Radius (R) is taken as the mean radius of the snow borders of the inner and outer lanes.

derived from wind-tunnel experiments and ice friction measurements (P_f, Equation 18). At the world championships for women in 1983, the frequencies on the curves and on the straight parts were measured separately.[54] Taking the mean values of all the women (n = 10) and averaging the frequencies (f_c) and radii of the inner and outer lane (R = 28.0 m), this comparison was performed for all four race distances of those championships. The results are presented in Table 5. The higher values of P_o were to be expected since these elite skaters would all have been able to accelerate in the curve and relax to some extent during the straight parts, while P_f was a mean value for the entire lap. When comparing the mean stroke frequencies (f_c) in the curves (Table 5) with the mean stroke frequencies (f_s) on the straight sections, (which were 1.97 sec^{-1}, 1.40 sec^{-1}, 1.23 sec^{-1}, and 1.10 sec^{-1} for the four distances, respectively), such a difference in power output is likely. If the stroke frequencies are taken as a measure of power output (thus assuming a constant value for A), an estimation for the mean power output P_o' for the entire lap might be obtained from P_o, f_c, f_s, the length of the curve (88 m), and the straight part (112 m) according to:

$$P_o' = \frac{P_o f_s}{f_c} \cdot \frac{112}{200} + P_o \cdot \frac{88}{200} \qquad (31)$$

these estimations for the mean power output are added to Table 5 as well.

The mean difference between P_f and P_o' is 13%, which is the same order of magnitude as the possible under estimation of P_f discussed before. Together with the strong relationship between P_o' and P_f over the different races (r = 0.995), this agreement is striking. It should be emphasized in this respect that P_o' and P_f are calculated with models and variables which are completely independent of each other. The calculation of P_o' is performed with the help of a geometrical model without any information concerning friction. P_f on the other hand is calculated with a model based on wind-tunnel experiments and ice-friction measurements. Therefore, it is concluded that this agreement is surprising in its support for the validity of the assumptions made in both types of model. Further experiments are performed to test the model presented in Equations 28 and 30 for individual skaters at each lap, separately, with actual velocities measured in the curves.

4. Applications

Generally speaking, the presentation of results of biomechanical studies does not always cause much interest among practitioners. The majority of these results support ideas which are already present among coaches and athletes. Every coach in speed skating knows that skaters should, for example, keep their trunk horizontal, sit deep, not carry too much fat, etc.

The extra dimension a scientist can provide is often limited to support or reject ideas of practitioners with quantitative data. Though the practical significance of such hard data is often underestimated by coaches, it is understandable that many coaches have the feeling that scientists are behind the times. Models not only help to explain or understand reality but can often also be used to make predictions for actual problems. Both aspects (explanations of known facts and predictions of possible solutions for practical problems) appear to be possible with the model discussed in the above. Let us examine a few examples:

1. Poor skaters or skaters who are tired at the end of a race have problems maintaining their speed in the curves. As explained before these skaters are forced to deliver an amount of power which is often much lower than they would physically be able to deliver
2. Elite skaters have problems following the direction of snow border, in particular if they skate the inner lane of the second curve during the 500 m race
3. Although practitioners know that skaters would accelerate in the curves, attempts which have been made to increase the stroke frequency in the curves (e.g., the Norwegian skaters at the end of the 1970s, do not appear to have led to better results
4. A poor skater who can just follow a good skater at submaximal speed during the straight parts often loses contact in the curves
5. A sudden frontal gust of wind prior to the curve (in particular the outer curve) is often fatal. The decrease in speed cannot be compensated for before the next straight part. During the entire curve the skater is forced to deliver submaximal power.
6. Tall skaters often have more problems following the curve at high speeds than small skaters (note the Japanese sprinters). On the other hand, small skaters have, on the average, more problems increasing their speed in the curves at lower speeds (long distance) than tall skaters.

Many of these problems can be explained by the relationship between speed and power output, especially if one realizes the relative influence of work per stroke and stroke frequency. The explanation of the meaning of Equations 28 and 30 was based on a skater with a certain amount of work per stroke. However, skaters differ in the amount of work per stroke. In the discussion of the technique with respect to the straights, we concluded that good skaters differ from poor skaters mainly in the amount of work per stroke. Imagine two skaters with different amounts of work per stroke skating at the same speed before they go into the curve. The skater with the larger A and thus the larger v_2 (proportional to $\sqrt{A}$) is constrained to skate the curve with a lower stroke frequency than the skater with the lower amount of work per stroke (Equation 28). According to Equation 30, the first skater is allowed to deliver a higher power output than the second skater. This explains why good skaters can skate curves better than poor skaters even at submaximal speeds. This also explains the differences between tall and small skaters since tall skaters will tend to show a higher v_2 than small skaters (note that v_2 is an absolute measure, not related to body composition).

From a mathematical point of view this difference in the influence of A and f on curve technique is the direct result of the fact that f is present in Equation 18 to the first power, while A is represented by v_2 which is proportional to $\sqrt{A}$.

Skaters who try to increase their stroke frequency in the curves can achieve this only at the expense of the amount of work per push-off. So an artificial raising of stroke frequency will result in the opposite effect (lower power output) than the skater expected. Such a shift

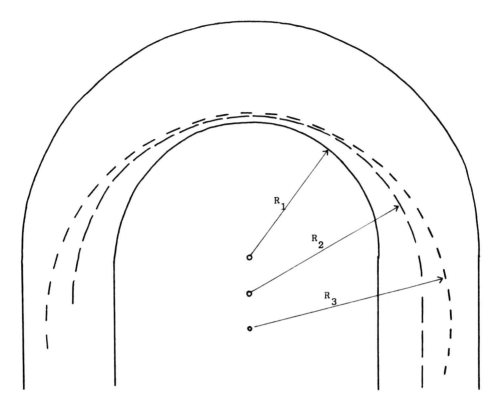

FIGURE 18. If skaters experience difficulties in following the snow border at high speeds (e.g., in a 500 m race), they can increase the radius (R) to some extent.

between f and A can be useful in preventing the problems seen in skaters with a very high speed (point 2).

From the above it can be concluded that by far the most important skill of a speed skater is to deliver a large amount of work per stroke. This was concluded for skating the straight parts and appears also to be the main conclusion for skating the curves. So in training and coaching beginners as well as experienced skaters, one should always pay considerable attention to the optimization of the push-off technique (small knee angle and horizontally directed push-off). An improvement in the amount of work per stroke is the main solution for solving the problems indicated. Apart from such a shift in relative contribution A and f, a few more suggestions can be made. This concerns solutions which, in part, appear to be already in practice:

1. Skaters can manipulate the radius of the curve. As illustrated in Figure 18, the radius can be increased in case of difficulty to follow the snow border at very high speeds. By increasing the radius, the necessity for a higher power output is decreased

2. The relationships derived with the geometrical model are based on straight strokes (Figure 19a). In practice, skaters have the possibility to describe curved trajectories since the blades of the skates would normally have a slight curvature. When a skater has problems following the snow border at high speeds, he or she might make curved strokes as indicated in Figure 19b. On the other hand they might try to make curve strokes as indicated in Figure 19c when their speed is too low. It should be noted that training non-elite skaters to make curved strokes as shown in Figure 19b, which is often seen in practice, seems not to be an appropriate training strategy

3. In particular, when skating the last lap(s) of a race of when the speed has dropped as a result of a head-wind, skaters should try to accelerate prior to the curve.

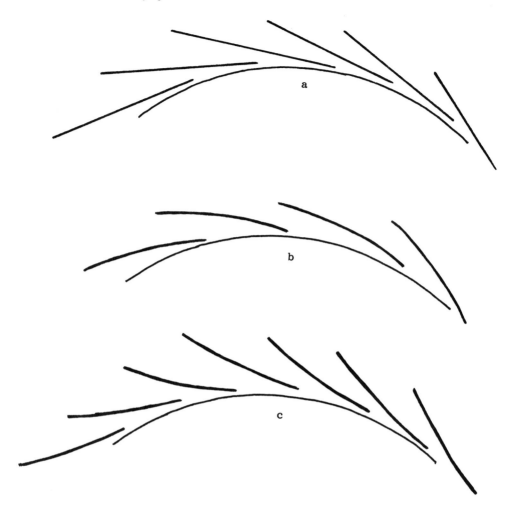

FIGURE 19.   Different curved strokes which might be applied when skating round a curve.

VI. SUMMARIZING REMARKS AND FUTURE DEVELOPMENTS

A. The State-of-the-Art

From the above one might easily draw the conclusion that biomechanical studies confirm the opinion of many coaches that technique is one of the most important and decisive aspects in competitive speed skating. Such a conclusion can be supported by a comparison of the physical condition of speed skaters in the past with the condition of the present elite speed skaters. Enschede[46] measured the maximal oxygen consumption ($\dot{V}_{O_2}$-max) of elite Dutch speed skaters in the 1950s. His results showed that those skaters had approximately the same aerobic power as present day American,[34,36,39,40] Italian,[101] Russian,[30,31] Scandinavian,[44] German,[20] or Dutch[49,55] elite speed skaters. So the tremendous improvement in speed-skating performance in the past two decades seems to be primarily due to an improvement in technique, clothing, and better preparation of the ice. This, however, is inconclusive evidence. A skater cannot be subdivided into a technical, physiological, psychological, or anatomical part. The improvement of technique in terms of, for example, a minimization of frictional losses and an optimization of the amount of work per stroke, is not exclusively a technical or mechanical problem. For example, a proper skating position and effective work output can be the final products of many psychological and physiological factors (see

Figure 4). Even $\dot{V}_{O_2}$-max is not an independent measure of physical condition. It is merely a measure of maximal oxygen consumption for the particular test exercise (normally cycling or running). Many physiological studies show that maximal oxygen consumption is strongly influenced by the type of exercise used, and moreover the training effects of aerobic power are extremely specific.[123-128] Even force development during a contraction appears to show a specific training effect.[129] Though not investigated, one may conclude that based on those studies, it is likely that the specific physical condition of speed skaters has improved markedly over the last two decades. A reason for the larger power output during skating may be found in the intensity of more-specific training methods.[16,17,35] As explained in this chapter, the requirements for speed skating are totally different from those seen, for example, in running, cycling, and jumping. The absence of plantar flexion, the high peak power output during the brief push-off, and the relatively long static gliding phase, requires motor unit levels which are essentially different from many activities which are frequently used as training exercises during off-season in the summer. Recently, de Boer et al.[59] started an extensive study into both biomechanical as well as physiological aspects of most types of exercise frequently used by speed skaters, and compared the results with corresponding variables measured during skating. These training methods concern mainly cycling, running, duck walking, skateboarding, skate jumps, and roller skating.[35,39] The first results showed that the most specific training method appeared to be rollerskating with rollerskates equipped with wheels which are placed one behind the other.[59] Given the specific requirements of speed skating, many other studies of summer and ice training methods and effects will be necessary in the future in order to answer the many questions of coaches. In particular, the problem of overtraining needs further attention. Although all distances in speed skating can be regarded as a supramaximal exercise, such exercise appears to lead easily to overtraining (recall the fear for the 10,000 m race mentioned earlier in this chapter).

Any discussion about the improvement of technique quickly leads to consideration of physiological aspects. The same is true for the psychological factors. Apart from the question of how to train the specific coordination patterns, there are many other problems whch need to be addressed. For example, speed-skating performance appears to be somewhat dependent on arousal level. Often the proper technique is lost at championships which are really important, as a result of too high an arousal level. Another psychological aspect which is closely connected to technique, concerns the application of more-adequate feedback methods to improve the technique. Not only skating position and direction of the push-off, but also speed development during the start, might be appropriate variables to provide as feedback during training sessions.

Considering the results of biomechanical studies as reviewed in this chapter, one might conclude that much is already known about the mechanical background of this sport. A short (and by definition incomplete) overview of a number of questions about unsolved problems proves that the biomechanics of speed skating is still in its infancy. Neglecting the more general and more scientific questions, we still do not know much about:

- the direction and curvature of the strokes with respect to the direction of the (straight) lane. Can the sidewards excursions be decreased?
- the optimal knee angle as a compromise between optimal energy liberation and air friction
- the optimal stroke frequency on the straight parts
- the improvement of the suits and the streamline. Maybe the fastest skates will shown to have the best streamline on the basis of their body build
- the optimal effectiveness. The mechanical optimum ($\phi = 0$)
- how to decrease ice friction. Are there other ice-preparation methods possible? What about the curvature and thickness of the blades under different weather conditions?

- the function of hip extension and external rotation, or at a more general level, how to improve segmental coordination
- the starting techniques. The only thing known about the start is that the opening time of a 500 m race accounts for approximately 80% of the variance of final times
- mobilization of more muscles by the introduction of other techniques
- possible improvements of the skates apart from the blades
- internal losses of mechanical power
- the effect, or even the possibility, of making a counter movement prior to push-off

It is clear that as in other fields, biomechanical scientists do not have to be anxious about finding problems to solve.

B. Future Developments

Many reporters and scientists consider it a pleasant past-time to analyze and forecast past, present, or future world records. These activities have even been elevated to "The study of records."[130] In this last section on speed skating we take the liberty of joining them with some of our predictions concerning future records.

Most analyses of world records appear to be based on world records established in the past and analyzed with the help of curve-fitting techniques. For speed skating, such analyses were performed by McClements and Laverty[33] and by Mognoni et al.[130] In his comment on the study of Mognoni et al., Morton[131] pointed out several methodological flaws in the use of such techniques. It can be argued that this type of analysis can never account for sudden future improvements on the basis of the introduction of new techniques, equipment (suit, skates), etc. Though McClements and Laverty[33] published their prediction for the year 2000 only 9 years ago, most of their predicted records have already been surpassed! For this reason we will try another line of approach.

High performance in speed skating is the simple result of a high power output on the one hand and low friction on the other hand according to Equation 18. Let us assume, therefore, that by the year 2087 the following improvements will have been realized:

- external power: the present problems concerning the limited number of muscles involved and the short duration push-off have all been solved. With their new technique and new skates, skaters in 2087 will be able to liberate the same amount of energy which is measured in distance runners today in 1988. This means that their external power would be increased by approximately 20%.[42] Taking a 1500 m record time of 1 min 55.4 sec at sea level as a starting point, such an increase of external power should result in a new record time of 1 min 47.9 sec.
- frictional losses: many surprising discoveries concerning suit, position, and streamlining have been realized by our aerodynamical engineers. The drag coefficient of skaters has been reduced from $C_D = 0.85$ in 1987 to $C_D = 0.43$ as found in a spherical shape. The ice-friction coefficient, of course, has also been reduced to approximately 50% of its present value (we do not know how, but we do not want to overestimate our forecast). Together with the increased power output, this reduced friction allowed the skaters to set a world record of 1 min 28.0 sec (mean speed: 61 km/hr).

Thus, 1 min 28.0 sec is the ultimate world record which is not to be improved upon. Though . . . why should skaters not exceed the energy consumption of present distance runners and what is more, why should the mechanical efficiency not be improved? It is generally assumed that e_m is approximately 30%, maximally, at the level of muscle output and 25% for external work in complex human movements.[42] On the other hand, Jorfeldt and Wahren[132] found a mechanical efficiency for the legs of only 34%, while Ingen Schenau[87] argued that these low efficiencies might be the result of an unnecessary waste of cross-bridges at the onset of a contraction. And what about the cross-sectional area A_p? The reader will agree that one should limit such speculation, and restrict oneself to more serious problems and go skating!

REFERENCES

1. **Goodman, N. and Goodman, A.**, *Handbook for Fenskating*, Sampson, Low, Marston, Searle and Rivington, London, 1882.
2. **Goodfellow, A. R.**, *Wonderful World of Skates*, Seventeen centuries of skating; Mountainburg, Arkansas, 1972.
3. **van Buttinga Wichers, J.**, *Schaatsenrijden*, Kremer Publishers, Den Haag, The Netherlands 1888.
4. **Schoyen, C. F. B.** *N. S. F. Festskrift i anledning av 25 Aarsjubilat 1893-1918*, 1920.
5. **Goodfellow, A. R.**, *The Skating Scene: The Factbook of Skating*, A. and T. Goodfellow, Tucson, Arizona, 1981.
6. **Bird, D. L.**, Our skating heritage. A centenary history of the National Skating Association, 1879-1979, NSA, London, 1979.
7. **Bijlsma, H. and Verbeek, K.**, *Niet over een nacht ijs*. K.N.S.B., Amersfoort, The Netherlands, 1982.
8. **Haase, H.**, *Zur Entwicklung des Eisschnellaufes. Unsere Läufer lernen von sowjetischen Freunden. I.* Teil Theorie und Praxis der Körperkultur, Heft 12, 1953, 6.
9. **Buisman, J.**, *Bar en boos. Bos en Keuning*, Baarn, The Netherlands, 1984.
10. **Kuhlow, A.**, Running economy in long distance speed skating, *Biomechanics V-B*, Komi, P. V., Ed., University Park Press, Baltimore, Md., 1975, 291.
11. **Nicol, K.**, Computerized method for determination of ice skating velocity, Biomechanics IV. Nelson, R. C. and Morehouse, C. A., Eds., University Park Press, Baltimore, Md., 1974, 251.
12. **Kuhlow, A.**, Analysis of competitors in world speed skating championship. Biomechanics IV. Nelson, R. C. and Morehouse, C. A., Eds., University Park Press, Baltimore, Md., 1974, 259.
13. **Kuhlow, A.**, Geschwindigkeitsverteilung bei 500 m und 1000 m Eisschnellauf von Männern und Frauen. Informationsheft zum Training No. 14, Deutscher Sportbund, 1973.
14. **Weideman, V. H., Roskamm, H., and Reindell, H.**, Ekg-speicher Untersuchungen beim Intervall- und Dauerlauftraining des Eisschnellaufers. *Sportart und Sportsmedizin*, 4, 142, 1967.
15. **Haase, H.**, Zur Entwicklung des Eisschnellaufes. Unsere Läufer lernen von sowjetischen Freunden. II. Teil. Theorie und Praxis der Körperkultur, Heft 1, 30, 1954.
16. **Haase, H.**, Erganzungs- und Spezialübungen des Eisschnellaufes und Ihre Anwendung. Theorie und Praxis der Körperkultur, Heft 7, 1954, 629.
17. **Schmidt, C.**, Über die Entwicklung und Anwendung geeigneter Trainingsmittel zur weiteren Vervollkommung und Leistungssteigerung im Eisschnellauf, Theorie und Praxis der Körperkultur, Heft 12, 1076, 1959.
18. **Kuhlow, A.**, Analyse der Geschwindigkeitsverteilung 2. I.S.U. Sprinter-weltmeisterschaften Inzell 1971, in *Beitrage zur Biomechanik des Sports*. Ballreich, R. and Kuhlow, A., Eds., Verlag Karl Hofmann, Schorndorf, 1980, 168.
19. **Ballreich, R. and Gabel, H.**, Analyse und Ansteuerung biokinematischer Merkmale von Sprintbewegungen, in *Beitrage zur Biomechanik des Sports*, Ballreich, R. and Kuhlow, A., Eds., Verlag Karl Hofmann, Schorndorf, 1980, 22.
20. **Von Schmid, P., Kindermann, W., Huber, G., and Keul, J.**, Ergospirometrie und sportartspezifische Leistungsfähigkeit von Eisschnellläufern, *Dtsche. Z. Sportmed.*, Heft V, 136, 1979.
21. **Kindermann, W. and Keul, J.**, Anaerobic supply of energy in high-speed skating, *Dtsche. Z. Sportmed.*, Heft V, 142, 147, 1980.
22. **Traub, G.**, Zukunftsweisendes Eisschnelllauf-Training, *Leistungssport*, 2, 26, 31, 1972.
23. **Polovcev, V. G.**, Telemetrischen Untersuchungen junger Eisschnellläufern bei Training mit erhöhter Belastung, *Theorie und Praxis der Körperkultur*, Heft V. 364, 1969.
24. **Polovcev, V. G., and J. A. Paryskin.** Anpassungsreaktion des Herzens bei intensivem Trainung jugendlicher Eisschnellaufer, *Theorie und Praxis der Körperkultur*, 24, 161, 1975.
25. **Michailow, W. W.**, Varianten der Kraftverteilung bei Eisschnellläufern, *Theorie und Praxis der Körperkultur*, Heft 3, 212, 1965.
26. **Djatschkow, W. M.**, Die Steuerung und Optiemierung des Trainingsprozesses, Sportverlag, Berlin, 1977, 27.

27. **Doctorevic, A. M.,** Zur Bestimmung von Kriterien einer rationellen Bewegungstechnik im Eisschnelllauf, *Leistungssport,* Frankfurt, Beiheft: *Information zur Training,* 5, 42, 1975.

28. **Krause, O. P.,** New data on the phasic structure of speed skating, *Theory and Practice of Physical Culture,* 3, 15, 1972.

29. **Ivanov, E. B.,** Morfologitsiskaia karakteristika konkobejtsev, *Konkobejnii Sport,* 50, 52, 1978.

30. **Ivanov, V. C., Vasilkovskii, B. M., and Panov, G. M.,** Material ik izutseniiu spetzialnoi prenirovanosti konkobejtzev, *Konkobejnii Sport,* 36, 39, 1977.

31. **Ivanov, V. C., Orlov, K. A., Vasilkovskii, B. M., and Schnaider, V. H.,** Osobennosti funkzionalnoi adaptatzii v skortstnom bege na konkah, *Konkobejnii Sport,* 33, 37, 1979.

32. **Miller, D. I. and Nelson, R. C.,** *Biomechanics of Sport,* Lea & Febiger, Philadelphia, 1973.

33. **McClements, J. D. and Laverty, W. H. A.,** A mathematical model of speed skating performance improvement for goal setting and program evaluation, *Can. J. Appl. Sport. Sci.,* 4, 116, 122, 1979.

34. **Maksud, M. G., Hamilton, L. H., Coutts, K. D., and Wiley, R. L.,** Pulmonary function measurements of Olympic speed skaters from the U.S., *Med. Sci. Sports,* 3, 66, 1971.

35. **Pollock, M. L., Foster, C., Anholm, J., et al.,** Body composition of Olympic speed skating candidates, *Res. Quart. Exerc. Sport,* 53, 150, 1982.

36. **Maksud, M. G., Hamilton, L. H., and Balke, B.,** Physiological responses of a male Olympic speed skater — Terry McDermott, *Med. Sci. Sports,* 3, 107, 1971.

37. **Mueller, M.,** Kinematics of speed skating, Unpublished Master's thesis, University of Wisconsin, 1972.

38. **Morris, A. F.,** A scientific explanation for Erik Heiden's unique Olympic performance, *J. Sports Med.,* 21, 156, 1981.

39. **Maksud, M. G., Wiley, R. L., Hamilton, L. H., and Lockhart, B.,** Maximal V_{O_2}, ventilation, and heart rate of Olympic speed skating candidates, *J. Appl. Physiol.,* 29, 186, 1970.

40. **Maksud, M. G., Farrel, P., Foster, C., et al.,** Maximal V_{O_2}, ventilation and heart rate of Olympic speed skating candidates, *J. Sports Med.,* 22, 217, 1982.

41. **Lier, A.,** *Fraskyvsstrukturen i hurtiglop pa skoyter,* Norges idrettshogskole, NIH-NORA, Oslo, 1975, 37.

42. **Astrand, P. O. and Rodahl, K.,** *Textbook of Work Physiology,* McGraw-Hill, New York, 1977.

43. **Magnussen, B. F.,** Effektbehov og fremdrift ved hurtiglop pa skoter. Paper at the Opsummerings of utviklingsseminar; Norges Skoyteforbunds, Trondheim, April, 19-21, 1985.

44. **Ekblom, B., Hermansen, L., and Saltin, B.,** Hastighetsakning pa skrisko, Idrottsfysiologi, nr. 5, 1967.

45. **Geyssel, J. S. M.,** Training and testing in marathon speed skating, *J. Sports Med.,* 19, 277, 1979.

46. **Enschede, F. A. J.,** On the training of speed skaters, Unpublished thesis, University of Utrecht, 1960.

47. **van Ingen Schenau, G. J.,** A power balance applied to speed skating, Unpublished thesis, Vrije Universiteit, Amsterdam, 1981.

48. **van Ingen Schenau, G. J. and Bakker, K.,** A biomechanical model of speed skating, *J. Human Movement Studies,* 6, 1, 1980.

49. **van Ingen Schenau, G. J., de Groot, G., and Hollander, A. P.,** Some technical, physiological and anthropometrical aspects or speed skating, *Eur. J. Appl. Physiol.* 50, 343, 1983.

50. **van Ingen Schenau, G. J.,** The influence of air friction in speed skating, *J. Biomech.,* 15, 449, 1982.

51. **De Groot, G., Schreurs, A. W., and van Ingen Schenau, G. J.,** A portable light-weight Douglasbag instrument for use during various types of exercise, *Intl. J. Sports Med.,* 2, 132, 1983.

52. **van Ingen Schenau, G. J. and de Groot, G.,** Difference in oxygen consumption and external power between male and female speed skaters during super maximal cycling, *Eur. J. Appl. Physiol.,* 51, 337, 1983.

53. **van Ingen Schenau, G. J. and de Groot, G.,** On the origin of differences in performance level between elite male and female speed skaters, *Human Movement Sci.,* 2, 151, 1983.

54. **van Ingen Schenau, G. J., de Groot, G., and De Boer, R. W.,** The control of speed in elite female speed skaters, *J. Biomech.,* 18, 91, 1985.

55. **Geysel, J., Bomhoff, G., van Velsen, J., et al.,** Bicycle ergometry and speed skating performance, *Intl. J. Sports Med.,* 5, 241, 1984.

56. **van Ingen Schenau, G. J. and Bakker, K.,** A mathematical model of speed skating, *Biomechanics VII,* Human Kinetics Publishers, Champaign, Ill., 1981, 498.

57. **De Groot, G., de Boer, R. W., and van Ingen Schenau, G. J.,** Power output during cycling and speed skating, in *Biomechanics IX,* Winter, D. A., Norman, R. W., Wells, P., et al., Eds., Human Kinetics Publishers, Champaign, Illinois, 1985, 555.

58. **Delnoy, R., de Groot, G., de Boer, R. W., and van Ingen Schenau, G. J.,** Refinements on the termination of power output during speed skating, *Biomechanics X.,* Johnson, B., Ed., Human Kinetics Publishers, Champaign, Ill., 1987, 691.

59. **de Boer, R. W., de Groot, G., and van Ingen Schenau, G. J.,** Specificity of training in speed skating, *Biomechanics X.,* Johnson, B., Ed., Human Kinetics Publishers, Champaign, Ill., 1987, 685.

60. **Rispens, P. and Lamberts, R.,** Physiological, biomechanical and technical aspects of speed skating, Private Press, Groningen, The Netherlands, 1985.
61. **Miller, D. I.,** Modelling in biomechanics: an overview, *Med. Sci. Sports,* 11, 115, 1979.
62. **Williams, K. R. and Cavanagh, P. R.,** A model for the calculation of mechanical power during distance running, *J. Biomech.,* 16, 115, 1983.
63. **van Ingen Schenau, G. J., Bobbert, M. F., Huijing, P. A., and Woittiez, R. D.,** The instantaneous torque-angular velocity relation in plantar flexion during jumping, *Med. Sci. Sports Exercise,* 17, 422, 1985.
64. **Gregoire, L., Veeger, H. E., Huijing, P. A., and van Ingen Schenau, G. J.,** The role of mono- and bi-articular muscles in explosive movements, *Intl. J. Sports Med.* 5, 301, 1984.
65. **van Soest, A. J., Roebroeck, M. E., Bobbert, M. F., Huijing, P. A., and van Ingen Schenau, G. J.,** A comparison of one-legged and two-legged counter movement jumps, *Med. Sci. Sports Exercise,* 17, 635, 1985.
66. **De Boer, R. W.,** Moments of force power and muscle coordination in speedskating, *Intl. J. Sports Med.,* 8, 371, 1987.
67. **Di Prampero, P. E., Cortili, G., Mognoni, P., and Saibene, F.,** Equation of motion of a cyclist, *J. Appl. Physiol. Respirat. Environ. Exercise Physiol.,* 47, 201, 1979.
68. **Shanebrook, J. R. and Jaszczak, R. D.,** Aerodynamics of the human body, *Biomechanics IV,* University Park Press, Baltimore, Md., 1974, 567.
69. **Nigg, B. M.,** Selected methodology in biomechanics with respect to swimming, in *Biomechanics and Medicine in Swimming,* Hollander, A. P., Huijing, P. A., and de Groot, G., Eds., Human Kinetics Publishers, Champaign, Ill., 1983, 72.
70. **Alexander, R. McN. and Goldspink, G.,** Mechanics and energetics of animal locomotion, Chapman and Hall, London, 1977, 222.
71. **Soden, P. D. and Adeyefa, B. A.,** Forces applied to a bicycle during normal cycling, *J. Biomech.,* 12, 527, 1979.
72. **Celetano, F., Cortili, G., di Prampero, P. E., and Cerretelli, P.,** Mechanical aspects of rowing, *J. Appl. Physiol.,* 36, 642, 1974.
73. **Pugh, L. G. C. E.,** Air resistance in sport, in *Medicine Sport. Vol. 9: Advances in Exercise Physiology,* Jokl, E., Anad, R. L., and Stoboy, H., Eds., S. Karger, Basel, 1976, 149.
74. **Whitt, F. R. and Wilson, D. G.,** Bicycling Science; M.I.T. Press, Cambridge, Mass., 1974.
75. **Faria, I. E. and Cavanagh, P. R.,** The physiology and biomechanics of cycling, J. Wiley & Sons, New York, 1978.
76. **Schleihauf, R. E., Gray, L., and de Rose, J.,** Three-dimensional analysis of handpropulsion in the sprint front crawl stroke, in *Biomechanics and Medicine in Swimming,* Hollander, A. P., Huijing, P. A., and de Groot, G., Eds., Human Kinetics Publishers, Champaign, Ill., 1984, 173.
77. **Di Prampero, P. E., Pendergast, D. R., Wilson, C. W., and Rennie, D. W.,** Energetics of swimming in man, *J. Appl. Physiol.,* 37, 1, 1974.
78. **Holmer, I.,** Propulsive efficiency of breaststroke and freestyle swimming, *Eur. J. Appl. Physiol.,* 33, 95, 1974.
79. **Clarijs, J. P.,** Relationship of human body form to passive and active hydrodynamic drag, *Biomechanics VI-B.* Asmussen, E. and Jorgensen, K., Eds., University Park Press, Baltimore, Md., 1978, 120.
80. **Schneider, E.,** Biomechanische Untersuchungen als Leistungsdiagnose und Fortschrittskontrolle im Rudertrainung, *Leistungssport,* 8, 12, 1978.
81. **Malzahn, K. D. and Stafank, W.,** Zur Effektivität verschiedener Bewegungsvarianten in Brust- und Kraulschwimmen, *Theorie und Praxis der Körperkultur,* 22, 725, 1973.
82. **Hollander, A. P., de Groot, G., and van Ingen Schenau, G. J.,** Active drag in female swimmers, *Biomechanics X.* Johnson, B. Human Kinetics Publishers, Champaign, Ill., in press.
83. **Toussaint, H. M., v.d. Helm, R., Elzerman, F. C. T., et al.,** A power balance applied to swimming, in *Biomechanics and Medicine in Swimming,* Hollander, A. P., Huijing, A. P., and de Groot, G., Eds., Human Kinetics Publishers, Champaign, Ill., 1984, 165.
84. **Alexander, R. McN.,** *Biomechanics,* Chapman and Hall, London, 1975.
85. **Bone, Q.,** Muscular and energetic aspects of fish swimming, *Swimming and Flying in Nature. Vol 2.,* Wu, T. Y. T., Brohaw, C. J., and Brenner, C., Eds., Plenum Press, New York, 1975, 493.
86. **Kemper, H. G. C., Clarijs, J. P., Verschuur, R., and Jiskoot, J.,** Total efficiency and swimming drag in swimming the front crawl, in *Biomechanics and Medicine in Swimming,* Hollander, A. P., Huijing, P. A., and de Groot, G., Eds., Human Kinetics Publishers, Champaign, Ill., 1984, 199.
87. **van Ingen Schenau, G. J.,** An alternative view to the concept of utilisation of elastic energy, *Human Movement Sci.,* 3, 301, 1984.
88. **Ward-Smith, A. J.,** A mathematical theory of running based on the first law of thermodynamics and its application to the performance of world class athletes, *J. Biomech.,* 18, 337, 1985.

89. **Ward-Smith, A. J.,** A mathematical analysis of the influence of adverse and favourable winds on sprinting, *J. Biomech.,* 18, 351, 1985.

90. **Davies, C. T. M.,** Effect of wind assistance and resistance on the forward motion of a runner, *J. Appl. Physiol.,* 48, 702, 1980.

91. **Winter, D. A.,** A new definition of mechanical work done in human movement, *J. Appl. Physiol., Respirat. Environ. Exercise Physiol.,* 46, 79, 1979.

92. **Orlov, V. A., Kuznetsov, V. V., Kosmenko, V. G., and Egorova, T. D.,** Kinematics of movements of skaters' biomechanical elements, in *Biomechanics VII-B.,* Morecki, A., et al., Eds., University Park Press, Baltimore, Md., 1981, 488.

93. **Gagnon, M.,** A kinematic analysis of the alternate stride in cross-country skiing, *Biomechanics VII-B,* Morecki, A., et al., Eds., University Park Press, Baltimore, Md., 1981, 483.

94. **Nelson, R. C. and Pike, N. L.,** Analysis of swimming starts and strokes, in *Swimming Medicine IV,* Eriksson, B., and Furberg, B., Eds., University Park Press, Baltimore, Md., 1978, 347.

95. **Farfel, W. S.,** *Bewegungssteuerung im Sport; Sportverlag Berlin,* 1977.

96. **Schneider, E. and Chao, E. Y.,** Fourier analysis of ground reaction forces in normals and patients with knee joint disease, *J. Biomech.,* 591, 601, 1983.

97. **Alexander, R. McN. and Jayes, A. S.,** Fourier analysis of forces exerted in walking and running, *J. Biomech.,* 13, 383, 1980.

98. **Jacobs, N. A., Skorecki, J., and Charnley, J.,** Analysis of the vertical component of force in normal and pathological gait, *J. Biomech.,* 5, 11, 1972.

99. **Rozendal, R. H., Heerkens, Y. F., van Ingen Schenau, G. J., et al.,** Application of vector diagrams in the evaluation of human gait, *Arch. Phys. Med. Rehab.,* 66, 682, 1985.

100. **Lees, A.,** An optimized film analysis method based on finite difference techniques, *J. Human Movement Studies,* 6, 165, 1980.

101. **Di Prampero, P. E., Cortili, G., Mognoni, P., and Saibene, F.,** Energy cost of speed skating and efficiency of work against air resistance, *J. Appl. Physiol.,* 40, 584, 1976.

102. **Watanabe, K. and Ohtsuki, T.,** Postural changes and aerodynamic forces in alpine skiing, *Ergonomics,* 20, 121, 1977.

103. **Schlichting, H.,** Grenzschickt-theorie, Braun, Karlsruhe, 1965.

104. **Kyle, C. R.,** Reduction of wind resistance and power output of racing cyclists and runners travelling in groups, *Ergonomics,* 22, 387, 1979.

105. **Raine, A. E.,** Aerodynamics of skiing, *Science Journal,* 6, 26, 1970.

106. **Magnussen, B. F.,** Personal communication, 1985.

107. **Kobayashi, T.,** Studies of the properties of ice in speed skating rinks, *Ashrae Journal,* 51, 1973.

108. **Hay, J. G.,** The biomechanics of sports techniques, Prentice-Hall, Englewood Cliffs, N.J., 1978, chap. 7.

109. **Pollock, M. L., Gettman, L. R., Jackson, A., et al.,** Body composition of elite class distance runners, *Ann. N.Y. Acad. Sci.,* 301, 361, 1977.

110. **Wilmore, J. H.,** Alterations in strength, body compositions and anthropometric measurements consequent to a 10-week weight training program, *Med. Sci. Sports,* 6, 133, 1974.

111. **Cureton, K. J., Sparling, P. B., Evans, B. W., et al.,** Effect of experimental alterations in excess weight on aerobic capacity and distance running performance, *Med. Sci. Sports,* 10, 194, 1978.

112. **Adams, W. C.,** Influence of age, sex and body weight on the energy expenditure of bicycle riding, *J. Appl. Physiol.,* 22, 539, 1967.

113. **Cureton, K. J. and Sparling, P. B.,** Distance running performance and metabolic responses to running in men and women with excess weight experimentally equated, *Med. Sci. Sports Exercise,* 12, 288, 1980.

114. **Malhotra, M. S. and Gupta, J. S.,** Work capacity at altitude, *Medicine Sport, Vol. 9, Advances in Exercise Physiology,* in Jokl, E., Anad, R. L., and Stoboy, H., Eds., S. Karger, Basel, 1976, 165.

115. **Boning, D., Gonen, Y., and Maassen, M.,** Relation between work load, pedal frequency and physical fitness, *Intl. J. Sports Med.,* 5, 92, 1984.

116. **Jordan, L. and Merrill, E. G.,** Relative efficiency as a function of pedalling rate for racing cyclists, *J. Physiol.,* 49, 50, 1979.

117. **Petrofsky, J. S., Rochelle, R. R., Rinehart, J. S., et al.,** The assessment of the static component in rhythmic exercise, *Eur. J. Appl. Physiol.,* 34, 56, 1975.

118. **Hogberg, P.,** How do stride length and stride frequency influence the energy output during running? *Arbeitsphysiologie,* 14, 437, 1952.

119. **Seabury, J. J., Adams, W. C., and Ramey, M. R.,** Influence of pedalling rate and power output on energy expenditure during bicycle ergometry, *Ergonomics,* 20, 491, 1977.

120. **Marino, G. W.,** Kinematics of ice skating at different velocities, *Res. Quart.,* 48, 93, 1974.

121. **Pugh, L. G. C. E.,** The relation of oxygen intake and speed in competition cycling and comparative observations on the bicycle ergometer, *J. Physiol.,* 241, 795, 1974.

122. **Roy, B.,** Biomechanical features of different starting positions and skating strides in ice hockey, *Biomechanics VI-B.* Asmussen, E. and Jorgensen, K., Eds., University Park Press, Baltimore, Md., 1978, 137.
123. **Daub, W. B., Green, H. J., Houston, M. E., et al.,** Specificity of physiologic adaptions resulting from ice-hockey training, *Med. Sci. Sports Exerc.,* 15, 290, 1983.
124. **Saltin, B., Nazal, K., Costill, D. L., et al.,** The nature of the training response: peripheral and central adaptions to one-legged exercise, *Acta Physiol. Scand.,* 96, 289, 1976.
125. **McArdle, W. D., Magel, J. R., Delio, D. J., et al.,** Specificity of run training on $V_{O_2\text{-max}}$ and heart rate changes during running and swimming, *Med. Sci. Sports,* 10, 16, 1978.
126. **Lesmes, G. R., Costill, D. L., Coyle, E. F., and Fink, W. J.,** Muscle strength and power changes during maximal isokinetic training, *Med. Sci. Sports,* 10, 266, 1978.
127. **Magel, J. R., Foglia, G. F., McArdle, W. D., Gutin, B., et al.,** Specificity of swim training on maximal oxygen uptake, *J. Appl. Physiol.,* 38, 151, 1975.
128. **Pechar, G. S.,** Specificity of cardiorespiratory adaption to bicycle and treadmill training, *J. Appl. Physiol.,* 36, 753, 1974.
129. **Pipes, T. V.,** Variable resistance versus constant resistance strength training in adult males, *Eur. J. Appl. Physiol.,* 39, 27, 1978.
130. **Magnoni, P. , LaFortuna, C., Russo, G., and Minetti, A.,** An analysis of world records in three types of locomotion, *Eur. J. Appl. Physiol.,* 49, 287, 1982.
131. **Morton, R. H.,** Comment on ''An analysis of world records in three types of locomotion'', *Eur. J. Appl. Physiol.,* 53, 324, 1984.
132. **Jorfeldt, L. and Wahren, J.,** Leg blood flow during exercise in man, *Clin. Sci.,* 459, 473, 1971.

Chapter 5

WEIGHT LIFTING AND TRAINING

John Garhammer

TABLE OF CONTENTS

I. INTRODUCTION

The term weight lifting has a variety of meanings to the general public. To many it relates to bodybuilding, to some it refers to competitive sport, and to others it is a form of exercise. In this chapter, the terms weight lifting and weight training will both refer to the use of free-weight equipment (barbells and dumbbells), weight machines, and other machines or devices that provide resistance to movement for the purpose of exercise and/or the enhancement of recreational and sport performance. Under this definition, bodybuilding is a special case of weight training where emphasis is placed on the development of muscular hypertrophy and definition, body symmetry, and the reduction of body fat. Competitive weightlifting is primarily encompassed by two distinct sports (1) powerlifting, which includes the squat, bench press and deadlift movements; and (2) weightlifting (correctly written as one word) which includes the overhead snatch and clean-and-jerk lifts which are contested in the Olympic Games. The clean-and-press was included in weightlifting for many years, but was eliminated from competition in 1972 due to difficulties in defining and judging proper execution technique.

The popularity of weight training in the U.S. and many other countries, is clearly evidenced by the extensive growth of the "Health Spa" industry and sales of resistive exercise equipment for home use. The increased popularity of, and participation in bodybuilding world-wide is also indicative of the level of interest in benefits derivable from weight training. The sport of weightlifting, though not very popular in the U.S., has enormous world-wide popularity with over 120 member nations in the International Weightlifting Federation. Powerlifting, though not nearly as popular world-wide, has grown rapidly in the U.S. in the past two decades with nearly 10,000 active competitors currently registered.

This chapter is not meant to be an exhaustive review of all literature available related to biomechanical considerations of weight lifting and weight training. Rather, it is an extensive review of much of the large variety of research and literature associated with weight lifting and weight training biomechanics that is available in the English language. An associated area of interest is the branch of occupational biomechanics that deals with work-related lifting tasks. Several sources of available literature on occupational lifting have been published.[1,2] This area is not included in this review, although some pertinent references and considerations are integrated into the discussion when particularly relevant. Likewise, the literature addressing the efficacy of use of different equipment and training programs for the improvement of strength and motor performance (e.g., athletic skills), and for rehabilitation, is not covered in any detail, although some discussion and associated references are given to emphasize statements and conclusions based on biomechancial considerations. For more information on this topic see Stone and O'Bryant[3] and Atha.[4]

The review begins with a discussion of types of equipment that can be used for weight training with regard to biomechanical properties, potential advantages and disadvantages, limitations, and manufacturer's claims. This is followed by an investigation of biomechanical information available on a number of common and popular weight-training exercises. Particular attention is given to variables such as speed and pattern of motion (techniques of exercise execution), load lifted, subject skill level, and the effects of changes in these variables on kinematics and kinetics. Since the three lifts contested in powerlifting are also very common weight training exercises, discussion pertaining to this sport is incorporated within the exercise section. Finally, the biomechanical literature on Olympic-style weight-lifting is reviewed and connections to other forms of strength, power, and performance enhancement training are made.

II. RESISTANCE EXERCISE MACHINES

Machines used for weight training may not actually utilize weights of any kind. For example, air-compression cylinders, hydraulic mechanisms, springs, or elastic cables may provide resistance to movement. Of the vast variety of machines currently available for consumer use, however, those most commonly found in public exercise facilities are truly weight machines, that is, their use involves the lifting of weight-plates as part of a weight "stack". The brand name equipment of Universal® and Nautilus® are discussed first since they are widely known and used and are representative of weight machines in general. Isokinetic machines purported to control movement speed by providing "accommodating" resistance are then evaluated.

A. Universal® Machines

Universal® weight machines were commonly available in the 1960s and the company began to promote highly its advanced "Centurion®" design weight machines in the mid 1970s. Several lengthy brochures based on the work of Gideon Ariel were widely distributed explaining the reasoning behind their "dynamic variable resistance" (DVR) machine design.[5,6] A condensed version of this material appears in a recent Universal® equipment catalog,[7] and a summary of the equipments features and training philosophies has recently been published.[8] The major point these brochures made was that the overload imposed on muscles by standard free-weight equipment was submaximal through much of the range of motion for common exercises like the bench press and squat. By utilizing a moving (rolling) pivot at the attachment point of the bench press, leg press, and overhead press station weight stacks on Centurion® machines, the mechanical advantage of a trainee is decreased through the range of motion of the exercise due to changing lever-arm lengths. This requires an increasing effort force as each exercise movement progresses, and the design parameters supposedly result in the resistance felt by a trainee closely matching his or her natural force production capability curve. Independent laboratory evaluations[9] were provided as proof that resistance did increase considerably from the beginning to the end of the range of motion of the above-mentioned stations.

Unfortunately, the range of motion evaluated was much greater than could be executed by anyone other than the tallest of trainees. The DVR exercise stations were said to be designed to average specifications for leverage changes (details were not provided in the Universal® literature), but methods to adjust these devices in any meaningful way for the variety of user sizes, do not seem to exist. Additional DVR rolling-pivot exercise stations have been marketed since the mid 1970s and some stations now incorporate a variable-radius pulley wheel (cam) to alter the mechanical advantage of the trainee. One recent study[10] pointed out the disadvantage (limited movement range) of the DVR "squat" machine due to lack of adjustability to accommodate smaller-sized subjects.

Details of how free-weight bench presses and squats were performed (subject skill level, percent of one repetition maximum (1 RM), speed of execution) for analysis and comparison to DVR bench press- and leg-press "force" curves, were not given in the promotional brochures.[5,6] Theoretical arguments for DVR presented in these brochures, were confusing and denied the length-tension properties of muscle, ignored the existence of force-velocity constraints on muscle function, and confused basic terms such as velocity vs. acceleration and isokinetic vs. isotonic. Reasonable arguments, based on specificity of exercise, were presented in favor of strength-training exercises for performance enhancement that involve multiple joints and muscle groups and that are performed rapidly to involve accelerations as occur in sport activities. These latter arguments seemed to be directed toward competitive machine companies which emphasize slow, isolated joint exercises (see Nautilus® below) or whose equipment minimizes acceleration (see isokinetic machines below). This emphasis on acceleration and ballistic movement seemed contradictory, since DVR tends to minimize such factors due to increases in resistance through the range of exercise motion.

Experimental evidence that DVR does produce superior training results compared to free-weights, was also provided by Universal®.[11] Reported progress of both "experienced" subject groups in the bench press was unusually large, and had the study continued for 30 rather than 20 weeks some world records may have been approached. The superior progress of the DVR group was especially surprising since all testing was done on the free-weight barbell. Independent comparative studies of different weight-training equipment, as summarized by Stone and O'Bryant,[3] fail to support the superiority of any type of equipment over free-weights for the development of strength and power or for performance enhancement. Some additional comparisons of DVR and free-weight equipment are made in Section III.

Universal®, and weight machines in general, do possess other operational properties which can be advantageous. These include ease of resistance adjustment, reduced injury potential, and for some rehabilitation situations, joint and muscle group isolation and constrained-movement patterns. Starr[12] has pointed out additional positive factors about machines in a comparison with free-weights. Exercises which involve the movement of body segments toward each other, as with barbell curls or dumbbell chest flies, are known to require decreasing muscular effort toward the end of the movement range.[13] Machine designs utilizing pulleys and cams to "redirect" the pull of gravity on weights or which by other means increase the range of resistance experienced by a trainee during certain exercise movements, can certainly be considered advantageous in most situations. It should be pointed out that modified free-weight designs planned for marketing in the near future minimize this undesirable reduced-resistance property.[14] Not all free-weight exercises fall into this category, however; in fact, the most important ones do not as discussed in Section III.

B. Nautilus® Machines

Nautilus® machines also began to be promoted heavily in the 1970s. Their machine designs incorporate variable radius pulley wheels or "cams" which alter the mechanical advantage of the machines by changing the effective lever arm of the weight-stack during movement through the range of the exercise. As with the Universal® moving-pivot design, the cam shape supposedly matches the resistance to the user's maximal force-production capability curve.[15] Two independent evaluations of numerous Nautilus® machines, however, indicated that the required machine force curves do not match average human strength curves.[16,17]

The Nautilus® machine designs emphasize isolated joint exercises with the rotational axis of the active joint being in line with the rotational axis of the machine. Nautilus® training philosophy states that movements should be done slowly.[18] This philosophy appears to be related to their machine design, since inertial effects during rapid movements can cause a reduction in the resistance felt by the trainee. In order to justify the principles of slow, isolated joint strength training, Nautilus® supporters have published articles condemning the specificity of this exercise principle,[19] confusing well-established properties of fast- and slow-twitch muscle fibers,[20] and warning of greatly increased injury potential when overload exercise is done with rapid or explosive movements.[20] This latter point is not satisfactorily supported, since it is well known that bone and connective tissues exhibit viscoelastic properties which enable them to withstand greater maximum loads and absorb greater energy before failure when subjected to rapid vs. slow loading. Also unexplained, is why conditioning athletes with only slow exercise movements rather than a combination of fast and slow should better prepare them to withstand rapid muscle and joint loadings and impacts as frequently occur in most sport activities. No independent research is available to indicate any superiority of Nautilus® strength training over other methods, although some evidence indicates the opposite.[3] Of particular interest is a case study involving monozygotic twins where free-weight training produced better results than Nautilus®.[21]

C. Isokinetic Machines

The term, isokinetic, means constant movement, and is generally interpreted as constant movement per unit time or constant velocity movement. As with Nautilus® machines, many isokinetic machine exercises require that the axis of the joint being trained or tested be in line with the machine lever-arm axis. The lever-arm of this type of isokinetic machine is designed to move with constant rotational velocity so that a properly aligned body segment will also rotate with constant angular velocity. This does not mean that any of the involved muscles shorten with constant velocity as demonstrated mathematically by Hinson et al.[22]

Isokinetic exercise has been discussed and studied extensively since the 1960s.[23,24] Devices used to provide isokinetic movement for testing and exercise may involve different means of operation, such as those based on friction, hydraulic, or electromechanical mechanisms. The hydraulic isokinetic machines have the speed of movement controlled by a dial setting that adjusts the size of an orifice through which a fluid (usually light-weight oil) is forced as the machine lever-arm is turned by an externally applied force. Since the fluid is incompressible and flows through the orifice at a rate dependent on its radius, the machine lever-arm moves at a constant angular velocity provided the fluid pressure created by the externally applied force is above a minimal level. Applied-force variations merely alter the fluid pressure which is felt as resistance to movement by the subject. Thus, the machine is said to accommodate the subject's effort by providing more or less resistance while maintaining constant movement speed. For higher speed settings on these machines the subject's initial effort creates a large angular acceleration, since the weight of the lever-arm and fluid flowing through a larger orifice provides little resistance to movement. As rotational speed reaches that corresponding to the dial setting, resistance is suddenly experienced and an equilibrium is reached with constant movement speed occurring. Thus, in reality, exercise on this type (and other types) of accommodating resistance machine is not fully isokinetic. The actual sequence of events that often occurs, for example, is that muscle contraction tension developed in the body acts through its skeletal lever system to create an external force applied at some point on the machine's lever-arm. This applied force creates a torque about the machine's rotational axis, and as its lever-arm initially turns, little resistance is felt and a large angular acceleration occurs until the set rotational speed is reached. At this point, a transition from high acceleration plus low resistance movement, to zero acceleration plus accommodating resistance, is made during which velocity fluctuations occur while a steady-state fluid-flow through the orifice of the machine is established. The higher the speed setting on the machine the more extensive these undesirable effects will be.[25,26] Less than half the range of motion, for example, may be traversed at constant speed when the angular velocity is greater than 1.75 rad/sec (100°/sec).[26] These undesirable effects do not seem to occur or are very minimal at low applied-force levels and slow speeds as may typically occur in rehabilitation situations.[24]

Some studies indicate greater electromyography (EMG) activity from involved muscles when working "isokinetically" at slow speeds compared to fast speeds of movement.[27] This may be partially due to the lack of resistance early in the movement at fast speed settings as discussed above. Others[4] indicate greater EMG activity from involved muscles when similar exercise exertions are made using isokinetic vs. free-weight ("isotonic"., see discussion of this erroneous term below) and isometric equipment. The first case may be the result of neuromuscular effort required to balance and control multidimensional free-weight movement tendencies, while the second case may involve neural inhibition as proposed by Perrine and Edgerton[28] to explain the force decrement in muscle tension capabilities observed at very slow and zero movement velocities.[24] Some studies comparing strength gains in leg extension/flexion after weight machine vs. isokinetic training, have found greater gains from isokinetics.[29] In general, however, studies have not supported the superiority of isokinetic exercise over other methods of resistance training in producing strength and performance improvements. More details related to these considerations have previously been summarized by Stone and O'Bryant[3] and Atha.[4] Some comparisons of exercises performed with free-weights vs. isokinetic or with other equipment, will be presented in the next section.

Isokinetic machines have definitely added a new dimension to muscle training and testing. Despite the limitations pointed out above (which may be decreased by future improvements in equipment) the ability to accurately measure the torque created by muscle contraction through nearly a full range of motion at a variety of selectable speeds for segment rotation, is unquestionably of substantial value. For rehabilitation, patient records with this detail can help make exercise programs more specific and recovery more rapid. For research in muscle physiology and mechanics, the above parameters are very useful and permit easy calculation of other variables such as power (torque × angular velocity). For general training and sport enhancement, the applications are less clear, although use in teaching the concept of rapid explosive contraction for higher speed movement requirements may be very appropriate.

III. WEIGHT-TRAINING EXERCISES

The above section presented information on how a variety of strength-training machines operate and what their limitations are, relative to manufacturer claims and experimental evidence. A large percentage of people participating in weight training utilize free-weight equipment (barbells and/or dumbbells) for all or some of their exercises. The advantages of free-weight use over machine use are numerous, but one of the most significant is the need to balance the weight and one's body, and to control three-dimensional movement tendencies during the execution of exercises. These needs relate well to the requirements of daily work tasks and recreational and sport activities. O'Shea was one of the first individuals to recognize the undesirability of excessive "guided (resistance) apparatus" exercises and to warn of "hindered development of neuromuscular coordination and the antagonistic and assistance muscles."[30] These and many other considerations favorable to free-weight use have been discussed in detail elsewhere relative to general and sports conditioning[3,12,31,32] and rehabilitation.[33,34]

Above all else it must be emphasized that free-weight exercise is in no way isotonic (constant muscle tension) exercise. The load being lifted is constant, but the force applied to it is rarely constant since the lifting action involves movement and acceleration. Newton's second law of motion applied to a free-weight lift shows that the vertical lifting force (F) depends on the weight lifted (W) and its mass (M) and acceleration (A) according to the equation F = W + MA. Due to this fact, many free-weight exercises can be said to accommodate any muscle tension generated and the corresponding lifting force by accelerating at varying rates.[31] Even if the lifting force is briefly constant the muscle tension creating it varies due to leverage changes and the length-tension properties of muscle. Isotonic is a term that should rarely, if ever, be used in connection with weight training and muscle exercise. Isometric exercise is perhaps the only special case where the term isotonic can sometimes be appropriately used. Dynamic, can and should be substituted in almost all exercise literature for the term isotonic.

The following paragraphs discuss biomechanical information about several common weight-training exercises and in some cases contrast their performance on different types of equipment.

A. The Squat

The squat exercise, sometimes called the deep knee bend, has a long history of controversy as briefly reviewed by Rasch and Allman,[35] who point out that published criticism of the lift appeared as early as 1946. Klein's papers[36] are probably the most quoted and debated of those warning of possible dangers associated with squatting. Todd[37] recently provided a detailed history of the use of this lift and insights into the "Klein" controversy. The potential problem debated was that full squats may cause stretching of medial and lateral ligaments at the knee joint, resulting in decreased stability of the knee. It is important to note that the above-quoted literature indicates that only "full" squats (fullest possible range of motion/

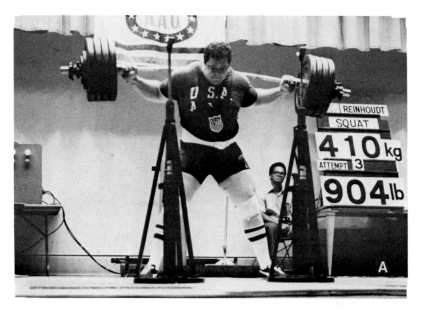

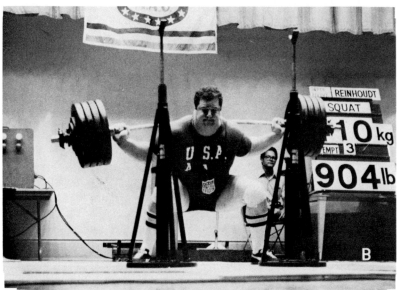

FIGURE 1. The squat exercise as performed in competition. (A) The start and finish position. (B) The bottom or minimum low position (thighs parallel) accepted during the squat exercise in competition. (Photo by B. Klemens.)

maximum knee flexion) were criticized and even Klein himself recommended half squats, which were defined as knee bends to the point of the thighs being parallel to the floor or slightly below (cf. Figure 1). The vast majority of competitive and exercise squats done today are to this depth, as is commonly recommended.[38-40] A recently published ''roundtable'' discussion[40] involving noted researchers and strength and conditioning coaches clearly shows the support for, and perceived importance of, incorporating squatting exercises into strength-training programs.

Considerable biomechanical research on the squat has been published in the past decade. McLaughlin and co-workers[41] have determined the squat kinematics of competitive pow-

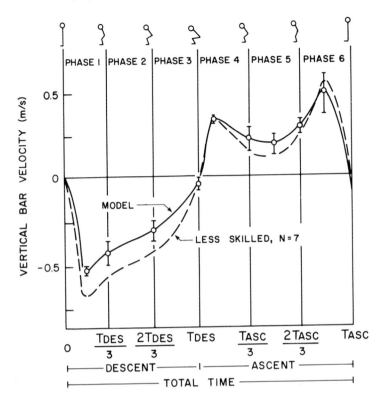

FIGURE 2.   "Model" velocity profile during the squat as performed in competition by elite powerlifters (N = 17) as compared to less-skilled (but still national caliber) powerlifters. TDES is average descent time, TASC is average ascent time, and TOTAL TIME is approximately 4 sec. *Note:* Other research indicates that novices exhibit greater velocity extremes and fluctuations during execution of the squat exercise than shown here. (From Mc-Laughlin, T. M., Dillman, C. J., and Lardner, T. J., *Med. Sci. Sports,* 9, 128, 1977. With permission.)

erlifters from a variety of bodyweight divisions and formulated a model of highly skilled performance based on the pattern of vertical barbell velocity. Contrasting two skill levels showed that the higher skill group (based on world ranking in the squat) (1) descended at a lower rate, and thus approached the lowest (bottom) position more slowly, with less of a "bounce" effect; (2) maintained a more vertical torso position during the entire lift; and (3) maintained a higher vertical bar velocity through the "sticking point" region. This region was characterized by a first minimum (the "sticking point") in vertical bar velocity during ascent, indicating that force applied to the barbell drops below its weight for a short period of time. It was noted that this first minimum of ascent velocity occurred at approximately a 30° thigh angle above the horizontal for all subjects despite a variety of torso and shank angles (cf. Figure 2). Research is needed to investigate the multisegment leverages and single and dual joint muscle interactions that are responsible for this observation.

The average magnitude of both the maximum vertical ascent and descent velocity in the above model was approximately 0.5 m/sec. with the ascent maximum value occurring after the "sticking point". Less-skilled subjects had a slightly greater magnitude for both values. A similar kinematic investigation by Malone[42] involving subjects of considerably lower overall skill level than those analyzed to develop the McLaughlin model, showed much less consistency between and among the two skill-level groups formed. The main similar finding in both studies was the double peak in average ascent bar-velocity curves. In the Malone study, maximum ascent velocity for both groups also occurred after the "sticking point", but was found to average approximately 0.7 m/sec. 40% above that of the McLaughlin model. Other comparisons between these two studies are of questionable value due to the large differences in subject skill levels.

More extensive work has been done involving kinetic as opposed to kinematic analyses of the squat. Plagenhoef[43] used a static three-segment rigid link model to show how segment orientation can affect the dominant muscle torques required for equilibrium at the hip, knee, and ankle joints. Evaluation of one position with excessive forward torso lean resulted in a net flexor torque at the knee, opposite to that expected.

Dynamic three-segment rigid link models have been used to evaluate hip, knee, and ankle forces and torques that are generated while squatting with heavy overloads. Ariel[44] found that the shearing force component at the knee and the net (extensor) knee torque were less for an experienced lifter using 2900 N than for a less-experienced lifter using a lighter weight. A "bounce" action at the lowest position in the squat of this latter subject resulted in a sharp increase in these parameters. Maximum knee torque values for typical subjects were listed at approximately 245 N·m. It was pointed out that forward knee movement during the squat was associated with the development of large shearing forces which could increase injury potential, and that one subject was able to reduce undesirable force components during the squat training period (presumably due to improved lifting technique).

McLaughlin and co-workers performed a similar three-segment dynamic analysis on competitors at the 1974 U.S. National Powerlifting Championships.[45] They found that some highly skilled lifters had lower maximal (extensor) torques at the hip joint than lesser-skilled lifters who were of lighter bodyweight and were squatting with a lighter barbell. This was attributed to greater forward torso lean and the resulting longer lever-arm of the barbell relative to the hip in the less - skilled group. The highly skilled lifters also exhibited larger extensor knee torques than the less skilled, possibly indicating greater reliance on thigh extensor rather than hip extensor musculature. The maximum hip and knee torques calculated were 705 and 500 N·m, respectively. Many peak knee torques were in the range of 100 to 300 N·m which agrees with typical values found by Ariel[44] as stated above. Also in agreement with Ariel was the finding that peak knee torques typically occurred at the lowest position (maximal knee flexion) of the squat. McLaughlin noted, however, that knee torque decreased during early ascent and was relatively low at the "sticking point" position introduced in his previously discussed kinematics paper.[41] Hip torques were generally near maximum at this point.

The above findings can be related to anatomical considerations. Greater forward torso lean requires greater hip extensor torque for equilibrium. The hamstring muscle group would likely contribute to creating this torque and in so doing would generate a flexor torque at the knee, thus reducing the effect of the knee extensors (quadriceps). Rigid-link modeling equations provide "net" force- and torque values at the link joints, so less extensor or even flexor dominance at the knee would be expected and was found for subjects with greater torso lean. Plagenhoef,[43] as discussed previously, showed that excessive forward torso lean results in the calculation of a flexor-dominant torque at the knee for a static squat position. McLaughlin[45] showed that acceleration factors during the heavy squats analyzed were small and that their elimination reduced dynamically calculated joint forces and torques by only approximately 10%. Thus, Plagenhoef's static calculations do provide insights applicable to at least heavy (slow) squats. The above consideration of the dual hamstring effect may indicate that forward torso lean does not necessarily reduce quadriceps activity, but may somewhat negate its effect by producing an opposing flexion torque. It should also be noted that larger magnitude hip extensor torques relative to knee extensor torques do not indicate that hip extensors play a more important role or are more involved than knee extensors in the execution of the lift. Any given net knee extensor torque value could represent maximal tension capability of the associated muscles acting through a given lever arm. A larger hip extensor torque at the same instant could result from submaximal tension of the associated muscles (whose maximal tension may be much greater than that of the knee extensors) acting through a more favorable leverage system. The effect of antagonistic muscle torques in the calculation of net joint torques, must be remembered.

A detailed model of the leg and primary muscles active during squatting movements has been developed by Dahlkvist and co-workers.[46] The model was individualized for six subjects, half of whom performed "fast" squats, while the other half performed "slow" and "fast" ascents from the deep-squat position. No load was used other than bodyweight and details of body segment angles and timing during the squat movements, were not given. However, the model, coupled with EMG data (which was used to determine if a given muscle should be considered a tension producer at any given instant in the activity), did result in estimates of various muscle tensions and joint-force components. Maximal and average quadricep and hamstring muscle forces were found to be greater during "fast" movements compared to slow, but the opposite was generally found for the gastrocnemius. Quadricep muscle tensions ranged from 3.6 to 8.6 times bodyweight depending on the subject and type of squat movement. Corresponding hamstring and gastrocnemius ranges were 0.8 to 2.46 and 0.7 to 1.8, respectively. Average joint-forces normal to the tibial surface ranged from 4.7 to 5.6 times bodyweight, while tangential values were 2.9 to 3.5. Joint-torques, and parameters needed to calculate them, were not given, so that such values from the previously discussed papers could not be compared. It is interesting to note that no reference was made in the paper by Dahlkvist et al. to any published work analyzing the squat as performed for exercise or in competition even though a number were available years in advance of its publication. The detailed model and methods used could provide considerably greater insight into the demands placed on body components (e.g., bones, ligaments, and muscles) if applied to such squats, and may illuminate factors related to the "sticking point" phenomenon. Hopefully, someone will soon accept this challenge.

Cappozzo et al.[47] have determined spinal compressive loads at the L3-L4 joint for two male and two female athletes while performing half squats with a barbell loaded in the range of 0.8 to 1.6 times bodyweight. Methods used are similar to those commonly found in analyses of occupational lifting tasks.[1,2] Fourier analysis of vertical ground-reaction forces and barbell and body segment vertical accelerations, showed that 95% of the signal power fell below 8 Hz. Such information is valuable in determining sampling and cut-off frequencies for data acquisition and smoothing. L3-L4 compressive forces were found to be 6 to 10 times bodyweight and modeled erector spinal forces were found to range from 30 to 50% of published maximal isometric levels for workers. Peak forces occurred at or very near the point of maximum knee flexion (approximately 80°). The spinal compressive forces were increased with forward torso lean and with faster squat-execution times. A shim was placed under the heels of the subjects during the squats, probably to aid in balance. One trial without the shim resulted in the subject leaning further forward. This indicates the importance of joint flexibility in maintaining a more upright torso position and reducing spinal compression and shear forces. Though not discussed, data presented indicated a shift of balance toward the heels during early descent and a shift toward the toes later in descent and during early ascent. The heel shim may have influenced this balance pattern. Balance on the feet during squats with heavy overload has not been, but should be, thoroughly investigated.

The muscle forces required to perform any given weight-training exercise have always been assumed to increase as the weight lifted increased. Hay et al.[48] examined this assumption using dynamic rigid-link modeling techniques with the squat exercise. They found that hip, knee, and ankle torques were linear functions of external load only if the kinematics of the squat were held constant. In practice, when subjects performed squats with increasing loads, the actual torque curves differed from the theoretical curves due to variation in movement kinematics. These differences were generally not large in magnitude, and a similar effect should be expected in the corresponding muscle tensions. Thus, to gain a proportional increase in the tension demands placed on each muscle involved in a multijoint exercise, consistent technique is required.

An extension of the above research included use of a Universal® DVR squat machine.[10] A larger difference in experimental vs. theoretical knee-joint-torque curves was found as load increased on the machine than when using a barbell.[48] A major cause of the torque changes was cited as being an increased torso lean as the machine load increased. This factor has been discussed above as a cause of increased hip/torso extensor muscle tension and spinal compression. Another possible cause (not discussed by the authors) is the fact that machine squats fix the position of both the feet and the shoulders and force the body segments to shift between them during the squat. This movement constraint may result in undesirable and variable segment movement patterns, since the body cannot easily shift balance.[50] Since the squat machine shoulder pads are in a fixed position relative to the ground a subject may unknowingly place his or her feet at slightly different locations under the apparatus for different trials, adding variability to the loading and likely causing movement pattern variability. This problem does not occur with a barbell where balance on the feet can be freely and consistently adjusted to the most comfortable and advantageous leverage position. Also, the DVR machine increases resistance through the range of motion and the pattern of increase may depend on the number and location of plates being lifted as well as subject size. Thus, although the authors suggest that certain types of machines may reduce variability in exercise kinematics, the squat machine seems to have increased torso inclination variability as a function of load more so than occurs with a barbell. (See also the discussion in Reference 50.)

The effects of speed of squat execution on joint-torques, were also investigated.[10] DVR machine and barbell squats were performed with 1-, 2-, and 3-sec ascents, but consistent 2-sec descents. The trend was toward higher joint-torques for faster ascents, as also noted in other studies.[46,47] Since the force-velocity property of skeletal muscle dictates that maximum tension production capability decreases with increasing speed of contraction, the faster squats are likely to require a higher percentage of maximal tension and provide a greater training stimulus. Caution must be exercized, however, since faster squats not only require greater muscle tension, but also increase the likelihood of incorrect technique and injury potential. Speed variation should only be considered for the ascent phase of the squat, never for the descent which should always be done in a slow and controlled manner. It has been shown that squats performed in competition[45] and at reasonable speeds[10] have such low accelerations that these accelerations can be ignored for all or most of the range of motion in dynamic calculations, with the effect being only approximately a 10% reduction in force- and torque values. True "speed" squats, such as jump squats, can (and should only) be done with relatively light weights.

A final topic covered by the same group of researchers involved the concept of joint-shear at the knee during squatting.[49,50] After defining several methods that could be used to calculate joint-shear, it was shown that shear-force components vary during the squat, are maximal at the lowest position of the squat (thighs near parallel), and are larger when the squat is performed fast (1 sec/phase) vs. slow (2 sec/phase).[49] Similar results were found when DVR machine squats were compared to barbell squats.[50] However, greater force levels were found with the machine due to the fact that the resistances used (percentages of 4 RM) were larger on the machine. This was probably related to the fact that no balance was required to use the machine,[10] range of motion was generally smaller on the machine due to lack of adjustability for different sized subjects,[10] and the DVR machine increases resistance through the range of motion. The greater force levels found with machine squats could produce a greater muscular training effect as well as increase injury risk.[50] However, with the free barbell, squat balance and neuromuscular coordination, can be better developed.

In an unpublished study involving only one subject, Malone[51] made several interesting comparisons. He found that fatigue did affect the kinematics of the first two as opposed to the last two repetitions of an eight-repetition set of squats with 90% of 1 RM. Velocities were generally less, particularly in the "sticking point" region, for the later repetitions. Initial acceleration during the ascent was similar in each case and a hypothesis was postulated that elastic energy provided a major contribution to contractile tension during this phase of the lift. Kinematics of the seventh repetition of the training set were later compared to those of a 1-RM squat performed in competition, and no differences were found. Finally, the 1-RM kinematics were compared to those of an isolated squat ascent (barbell lifted from supports) with maximum possible weight. The large initial ascent velocity and acceleration that existed during the 1-RM squat were not found for the isolated ascent and only a very small velocity decrease took place in the "sticking point" region for the latter movement compared to the former. These observations were taken as support for the hypothesis that elastic energy recovery is an important factor in the initial ascent from the low-squat position. Leverage factors were credited with being more important toward the end of the ascent. Malone's reasoning in the above comparison seems to follow that given in studies of vertical jumps with and without counter movement.[52] It is certainly plausible that elastic energy does play an important part in squatting due to the eccentric contractions and muscle stretch that occur during descent and its termination, and the rapid concentric contraction immediately following that permits ascent.[53]

Based on the above research, several summarizing statements are appropriate:

1. There is no objective scientific evidence that the squat exercise to the "thighs parallel" position will damage the knee joint. The possible harmful effects of the full squat on the knee joint are controversial. Any "bouncing" action to help initiate ascent from the full squat position will subject the knee joint to much higher mechanical stress.
2. Squats should be performed with a slow, controlled rate of descent to the "thighs parallel" position followed by an immediate initiation of the ascent if stored elastic energy is to be recovered and aid in the ascent.
3. The torso should remain as close to vertical as possible, relative to the anthropometry and flexibility of the trainee, during the entire lift.
4. The movement of the knees forward during descent should be minimized; maximal forward movement should place the knees no more than slightly in front of the toes.
5. Every effort should be made to maintain stable form (pattern of motion) during every repetition in order to load the muscles in a consistent manner.

NOTE: The depth of a squat is frequently judged in a subjective manner. Such judgements cause controversy in competitive situations and may have important consequences in rehabilitation. With the ever-decreasing price of computers and the increasing availability of electro-optical devices to monitor movement in real time, such subjectivity can, should, and hopefully soon will be eliminated. A hard-wired forerunner of potential future wireless squat depth monitors has already been developed.[54]

B. The Bench Press
The bench press is perhaps the most widely used weight-training exercise in the world (cf. Figure 3). It is the second of the competitive powerlifts and is described in varying detail in almost all weight-training books[3,12,30,39] and in specific articles.[55] Yet, until the last few years, little or no biomechanical analyses of this lift had been published, as evident in a review article written in 1979 by Hatfield and McLaughlin.[56] Part of the reason for this is likely to be the need for three-dimensional considerations and the complex interrelated nature of shoulder and shoulder-girdle movements that occur in the bench press. This fact has also limited modeling of the "shoulder complex" in occupational biomechanics.[57]

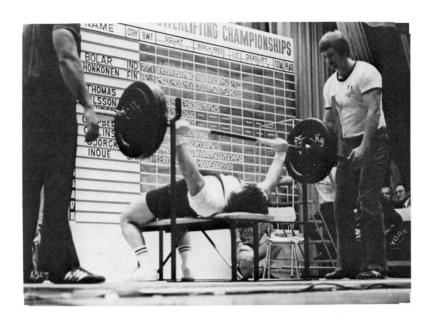

FIGURE 3. The bench press exercise as performed in competition. Shown is the start and finish position. The barbell is lowered to the chest and then raised to the finish position. (Photo by B. Klemens.)

Madsen and McLaughlin[58] have provided some groundwork for future study of the bench press in a paper largely describing and contrasting two-dimensional kinematics of the lift as performed by elite competitive lifters and novice lifters. An extension of this paper provided data for elite heavyweight powerlifters,[59] and McLaughlin has expanded discussion of this research and suggested possible applications in book form.[60] Key differences found between elite and novice groups included a slower rate of lowering the barbell, a movement pattern which kept the bar closer to the shoulder (sagittal plane view), and a more consistent level of force application to the bar for the elite lifters. Some longitudinal data indicate that elite lifters modify technique over time toward the above characteristics.[60] The elite group also followed different bar paths when raising vs. lowering the bar, while the novices followed very similar paths (cf. Figures 4 and 5). Graphs of upward bar velocity showed a minimum between two peaks for almost all subjects, but this minimum was more pronounced for the novices, very similar to what was found for upward velocity in competitive squats[41,45] (Figure 6). Thus, this mimimum velocity point was again labeled the "sticking point". The argument presented previously for elastic-energy recovery being associated with the existence of the sticking region during ascent from a squat,[51] should not apply for the bench press, since the rules of competition require a complete stop at the chest prior to raising the bar (also see McLaughlin[60]. This period of static hold should eliminate or severely reduce elastic-energy recovery.[53] An alternative cause of initial upward-thrust enhancement could, however, be associated with a voluntarily generated intraabdominal/intrathoracic pressure surge and/or recoil of the rib cage due to appropriate muscle contractions.

Differences found between novices and heavy bodyweight elite (HB E) lifters were generally the same as those found relative to lighter bodyweight elite (LB E) lifters. One exception was that HB E lifters generated nearly twice the shoulder joint torque (force on bar × sagittal plane lever-arm) as LB E lifters, although they only handled approximately 30% more weight. The LB E lifters generated approximately the same shoulder-joint torque as novices even though they handled 79% more weight. Body size corrections predicted less than 50% increases in torque for the HB E vs. LB E subjects. Some possible reasons for this discrepancy were presented based on handgrip spacing, bar path geometry, and bar

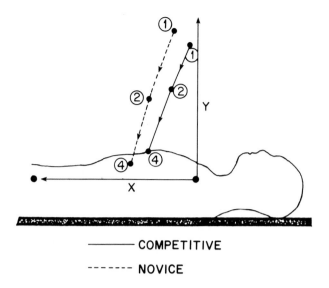

COMPETITIVE

—————— NOVICE

FIGURE 4.   Comparison of paths followed while lowering the bar in the bench press. (1) start, (2) maximum velocity of descent, (4) chest contact. Also see Figure 6. (From Madsen, N. and McLaughlin, T., *Med. Sci. Sports Exercise*, 16, 376, 1984. With permission.)

acceleration differences. Three-dimensional analyses are clearly needed to gain more insight relative to these types of questions.

In a comparison of free-weight and isokinetic bench presses Lander et al.[26] also found that a sticking point (region) existed. In their protocol, subjects were not required to stop the free bar at the chest so that elastic energy utilization was likely. The mean force-time curves for both types of bench presses were very similar, except at the beginning and end of the movement when the isokinetic device provided no resistance (cf. Figure 7). Areas under the curves, which are related to work done, appeared very nearly equal. The isokinetic device used did not provide constant velocity of rotation through the entire range of motion and the isokinetic range decreased as speed increased. The authors felt that both types of equipment accommodated maximal lifting efforts, the isokinetic device via resistance changes, and the free-weights via acceleration changes. The differences found were attributed to a lack of eccentric loading and baseline force with isokinetic equipment and the need for balancing forces with the free barbell. Ability in the free-bar bench press was shown to be related to the ratio of first to second force peak in the isokinetic bench press. Better free-weight bench pressers had lower ratios (0.81), as they did for the same force-peak ratios determined with the free bar (1.25). Other factors subjectively related to ability in the bench press included handgrip spacing, and arm-forearm and arm-torso angles. Mean maximal-force values for the six subjects whose best bench presses ranged from 1333 to 1822 N (1.27 to 2.16 times bodyweight) were approximately 2000 N for the free bar and 1900 N for the isokinetic device. These values compare reasonably with those for HB E, LB E, and novice lifters whose values were 2621, 2004, and 1349 N for mean lifts of 2349, 1814, and 995 N (1.92, 2.36, and 1.32 times bodyweight), respectively.[59]

Minimal data from three-dimensional (3-D) analyses of the bench press have been found. Two published abstracts[61,62] and short sections in McLaughlin's book[60] report the use of EMG with 3-D analyses to study the effects of variables such as handgrip spacing and load. One study[62] indicated that peak shoulder torques were higher for wide grips (97 N·m) than for narrower grips (70 N·m) and were higher when lifts were performed at higher speeds of movement. Load values were not given in the abstract so it was not possible to speculate

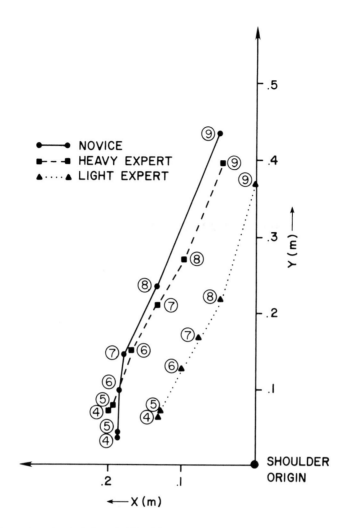

FIGURE 5. Comparison of paths followed while raising the bar in the bench press. (4) chest position, (5) maximum upward acceleration, (6) maximum upward velocity, (7) minimum upward acceleration, (8) minimum upward velocity, (9) finish. (From McLaughlin, T. M. and Madsen, N. H., *Natl. Strength Cond. Assoc. J.*, 6, 44, 1984. With permission.)

on why these values were so much lower than those estimated with 2-D analyses of novice (255 N·m), LB E (261 N·m), and HB E (501 N·m) lifters.[58,59]

C. The Deadlift

The deadlift is the third of three lifts contested in power lifting and it, or one of its several variations, is commonly used in exercise programs (cf. Figure 8). Despite its frequent use, it has received almost no attention from biomechanists. Various lifting postures which have some relationship to the deadlift as performed for exercise and in competition, have been studied relative to occupational applications,[1,2,63] but will not be discussed here. Techniques for performance of the deadlift are presented in most books on weight training,[3,12,30,39] and have been covered in specific articles.[64]

The only pertinent data found were recently published by Brown and Abani.[65] They analyzed teenage powerlifters from film taken during a competition, and compared kinematic and kinetic parameters between "skilled" and "unskilled" subjects who represented almost all bodyweight classes, and successfully deadlifted between 140 and 272 kg. The unskilled

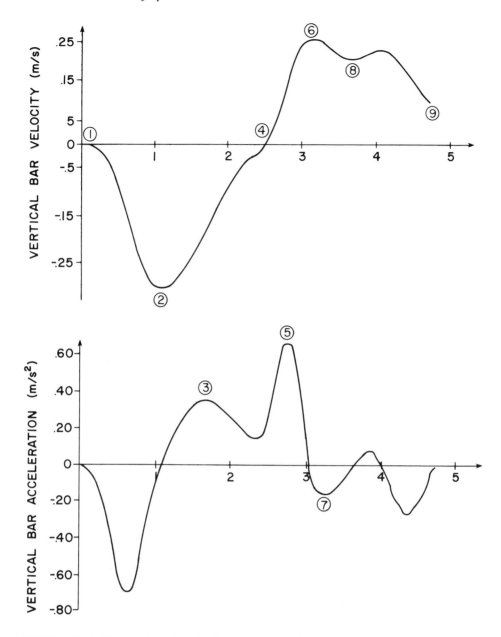

FIGURE 6.   Typical bar velocity and acceleration patterns for the bench press performed by a competitive lifter. Numbered points defined in Figures 4 and 5. Madsen, N. and McLaughlin, T., *Med. Sci. Sports Exercise,* 16, 376, 1984. With permission.)

group had a greater range of motion for the thigh and shank and more forward torso lean during the lift. None of the skilled lifters generated a vertical bar acceleration greater than 0.41 m/sec during a lift, while several unskilled lifters had values more than twice as great. Typical durations from lift-off until completion of a lift were approximately 2 sec. Torques required at the hip, knee, and ankle were greatest at the start of the lift and were larger for the skilled lifters (means of 436, 44, and 190 N·m, respectively). Inertial effects were small in comparison to barbell mass and its lever-arm distance to the joints for torque calculations of both groups. The results of this study indicate that skilled deadlifters maintain a more upright posture during the lift, keep the bar as close to the body as possible so as to minimize

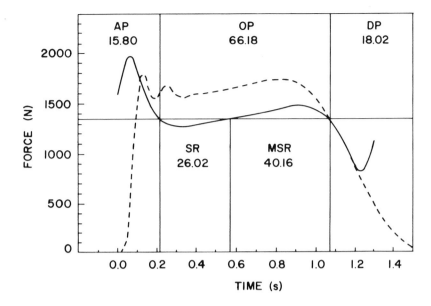

FIGURE 7.   Mean applied force vs. time patterns for free weight (solid line ——, heavy weight condition) and "isokinetic" (dashed line - - slow speed condition) bench presses. Marked phases (AP, acceleration; OP, oscillation; DP, deceleration) and regions (SR, sticking; MSR, max strength) are percentages of the duration of the free-weight activity. (From Lander, J. E., Bates, B. T., Sawhill, J. A., and Hamill, J., *Med. Sci. Sports Exercise,* 17, 344, 1985. With permission.)

lever-arm distances, and apply a more consistant vertical force to the bar so as to minimize acceleration and inertial forces. These characteristics are similar to those noted previously for skilled squatters.[41,45]

D. Power Output

The mechanical power output produced by the body during execution of the above three weightlifting exercises, which are contested in the sport of powerlifting, has been calculated. Values are presented in Table 1 along with typical values for the two Olympic lifts. Power output is lowest for the bench press and greatest for the snatch and the clean. This is to be expected since the bench press involves the smallest muscle mass, while the Olympic lifts involve essentially the whole body and must be executed rapidly (also see Section IV). Another interesting consideration is the order of world-record weights lifted by heavy bodyweight athletes in these five lifts (essentially identical trends also exist for lighter bodyweight athletes). Using approximate values, the order is squat (1000 lb, 4450 N), deadlift (900 lb, 4050 N), bench press (700 lb, 3150 N), clean (600 lb, 2700 N), and snatch (465 lb, 2092 N). Excluding the bench press, the trend is higher power output for lower load lifted. Time of force application during the actual lifting phase of these movements also shows a trend with the Olympic lifts requiring 0.6 to 0.9 sec[66,67] and the power lifts approximately 2 sec.[45,58,59,65] Since the range of motion is greatest in the former and least in the latter lifts, it is evident from the definition of power (force × displacement/time) why the power output order is as listed in Table 1. Also note that vertical accelerations commonly occurring in the snatch and clean exceed 6 and 5 m/sec^2, respectively,[68,69] and result from applied forces far in excess of the static load value (F = W + MA, as discussed previously). On the contrary, accelerations measured for the competitive power lifts are near 1 m/sec^2 or less,[45,58,59,65] resulting in minimal inertial effects. With the exception of the bench press, the above lifts can be considered to involve the major muscle groups and segments (shank, thigh, and torso) of the body. The force-velocity relationship has been well supported for

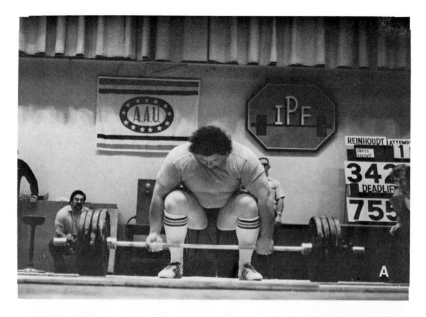

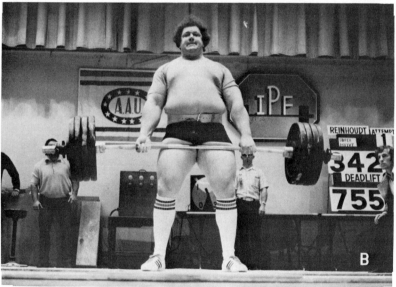

FIGURE 8.   The deadlift exercise as performed in competition. (A) Just prior to the start of "lift-off", (B) finish of the deadlift (Photo by B. Klemens.)

in vivo single-joint human-muscle function,[28] and data supporting the extension of such a relationship for multijoint activities, are also available.[70-73] The above observations tend to lend further support to such a relationship.

Since power output capability is an important factor in most athletic performances, the above data provide some insights useful in developing a power vs. strength training program. The so-called "power lifts" actually are more strength dependent than the Olympic lifts, which are highly power dependent. Also, data provided in Table 1 and elsewhere[73-75] clearly indicate that power generated increases as an athlete executes any of the above lifts with less than a 1-RM load. Bench-press data [74] show an increase from 100 to 60% of a 2-RM load with a large jump between 85 and 80%. Data for the other four lifts cover smaller load

Table 1
POWER OUTPUT DURING EXECUTION OF
SELECTED LIFTS

Lift	Subject	Power (W)	Ref.
Bench Press	Novice (60%—2 RM)	481	74
	Novice (85%—2 RM)	366	74
	Novice (100%—2 RM)	247	74
	Light novice	243	58
	Light elite	267	58
	Heavy elite	415	59
Deadlift	(Similar to squat values)		75
Squat	Heavy elite (93%)	1259	75
	Heavy elite	900	75
Snatch	Light elite (95%)	2821	73
	Light elite	2675	73
Clean	Heavy elite (92%)	3877	73
	Heavy elite	3413	73

Note: All values are for 1 RM unless listed otherwise. Values are for a specific elite athlete for each lift except bench presses which are group averages. All values, except bench presses, include horizontal work and work performed to elevate the body's CG.

ranges as occur in competitions when athletes are "peaked" for maximal performance and are allowed only three attempts at each lift.[73,75] Ueya and Ueya[76] have presented data showing a decrease in power output in the clean-and-jerk after substantial load decreases from maximum. Danoff [77] has shown peak power production to occur at submaximal loads during maximal efforts at elbow flexion. Current data are insufficient to determine the best percentage of 1 RM to train with in any given lift for any specific goal, but since variation in training stimuli is valuable,[3,39,78] it would seem reasonable to emphasize lifts in 70 to 90% of the 1-RM range for a balance of strength and power development. Higher intensities are highly stressful to the body and result in lower power output, while lower intensities will reduce the overload and stimulus for strength gains.

E. Assistance Exercises

The squat, deadlift, snatch, and clean lifts discussed above can be called primary or "core" exercises, since their execution requires a very large percentage of the body's muscle mass to be active. The bench press, behind-neck press, bent-over-row, and leg press are common weight-training exercises which involve several, but fewer, muscle groups and joints in movement patterns that relate well (kinesiologically) to many everyday activities. Still other overload exercises isolate muscles and single joints and can be called assistance exercises, since they generally contribute to specialized needs, such as forearm strength for a tennis player or rehabilitation of an injury. As examples of this type of exercise, arm curls, leg extensions and curls, and sit-ups, will be discussed.

1. Arm Curls

Arm curls are extremely popular among male trainees due to the enhanced size and shape of flexor muscles in the upper arm that results from their use. Hay et al.[13] have biomechanically analyzed two common methods of arm curls performed with the upper arms resting on an inclined support ("preacher bench"). A barbell and a Universal® DVR (see Section II. A) curl machine were the equipment used for three speed and three load conditions. Details of the equations of motion used in the analyses were provided. The loads used (40, 60, and 80% of 4 RM) were found to affect the magnitudes of elbow torque required during the curls, but not the shape of the torque curves. Differences in physical size of the three subjects also had little effect on the shape of the torque curves (values given below are for the middle-sized subject, 1.83 m tall, 841 N bodyweight).

Movement speed (1-, 2-, or 3-sec concentric and 2-sec eccentric phases) and equipment type, had considerable effect on the elbow-torque curves. Barbell curls required an elbow-extensor torque in the region of maximal elbow flexion (60 to 120 N·m) and required the greatest flexor torque (100 to 140 N·m) in the region of maximal elbow extension. The fastest speed of execution required greater torques at the extremes of movement range, but similar torques compared with slow and medium speeds in the mid-range of motion. DVR machine curls resulted in an almost constant elbow-flexor torque (80 N·m) for slow and medium execution speeds, but oscillating values (0 to 100 N·m) for the fast speed. Extensor torque did not develop with the DVR machine. Since skeletal muscle can produce lower maximal forces at higher contraction rates, it was argued that the fast curling speed provided greater overload (absolute and relative to maximal capability). This is true, but injury potential is also increased with speed, especially at the extremes of motion when elbow-torque values were greatest. This is especially true with "preacher bench" curls since the upper arms are in a fixed position. A standing barbell curl may be safer for fast curling speeds since the torso and upper arms can move to absorb kinetic energy at the extremes of motion. Such "body swing", however, is often used to initiate the curl motion and thus reduces flexor muscle range of involvement.

Comparison of the two types of equipment at any given speed was difficult and no definitive choice of one over the other could be made. The barbell required greater torque in the region near full extension, while the DVR machine maintained a flexor torque in the region of full flexion when the barbell created the need for an extensor torque. As stated in Section I.A, a modified free-weight design may soon be marketed which minimizes the shift toward elbow extensor torque in the range of full flexion during a barbell curl.[14]

2. Leg Extensions and Curls

Leg extensions and curls can be performed with a variety of equipment. These exercises work the knee extensors (quadriceps) and flexors (hamstrings) respectively. Probably the oldest equipment used for these exercises is some form of weighted boot attached to the foot or ankle region. Leg extension and curl machines are now more popular, with the original design being a flat bench with a padded lever arm rotating from one end. Free-weight plates are attached to the lever which is forced to rotate by muscular exertion of the trainee who has his or her knee joint(s) aligned with the lever axis and, applies force to the pad in the ankle region. Countless design modifications now exist, such as leg curl bench surfaces equipped with an inclined and declined section to tilt the pelvis posteriorly and provide the hamstrings with a mechanically more advantageous angle of pull. Some newer machine designs, such as compressed air cylinder and isokinetically controlled machines, permit leg extensions and leg curls to be executed continuously from the same seated position. An important property of the "free-weight" leg extension machines is that they provide almost no resistance at the start of movement, since gravity pulls straight downward on the weight plates which hang directly below the lever-arm pivot. As movement occurs, the lever-arm of the weights relative to the pivot increases and so does the joint-torque required to continue the movement. This pattern of increasing overload may be desirable in some rehabilitation situations. However, such a pattern does not exercise the involved muscles efficiently through much of the range of motion. To reduce this inefficiency, cables and pullies were added by many machine companies so that the resistance was more evenly distributed through the range of motion. A design common to several popular brands of machines provides the greatest resistance at the start of motion and a slowly decreasing resistance as the movement continues. These different loading properties based on machine design can be very important relative to the stresses placed on the muscles and joint structures and the specific strengthening effects obtained. It should be noted that basic mechanical equilibrium considerations show that a large shearing-force component is required at the knee toward completion of a leg extension on these machines. Such considerations are often discussed in books on therapeutic exercise.[79]

3. Abdominal Exercises

Sit-ups and other common exercises used to strengthen the abdominal muscles have been studied in considerable detail. Rasch and Burke[80] have summarized the findings of several EMG studies performed in the 1950s. The first part of the sit-up exercise (spinal flexion) is called a trunk curl and it activates the upper rectus abdominis and to a lesser extent the obliques. If resistance is held in the shoulder area the greatest increase in activity occurs in the obliques and lower rectus. The following phase of the sit-up is a flexion of the hips and involves the abdominals only isometrically. Hip flexor muscle activity increases if the feet are held down, while abdominal activity increases if they are not. It is recommended to keep the knees and hips flexed (hook lying position) when performing sit-ups as opposed to extended (long-lying supine position). This position results in an improvement in the mechanical advantage of hip flexor muscles and a decrease in their length, both of which can reduce the tension generated. This is desirable, since excessive pull of the rectus femoris and the illiacus may tilt the pelvis anteriorly causing accentuated lumbar curvature, which may add to a spinal hyperextension effect (psoas paradox) resulting from the direct pull of the psoas major. These undesirable effects may be minimized by strong abdominals which can resist the anterior tilting of the pelvis. Unfortunately, many people with weak abdominal musculature perform full sit-ups to strengthen this muscle group, but soon develop low back pain. Thus, it is reasonable to suggest bent-knee trunk curls as a productive means of strengthening the abdominal muscles without the risk of aggravating the lowerback complex. Similar concerns exist about other common abdominal exercises, such as leg raises, which are primarily hip flexion exercises. Any torso-twisting motion that is added to a trunk curl or sit-up exercise will increase the activity of the internal and external oblique muscles.

The above recommendations are supported by a recent study of four types of sit-up exercises.[81] All resulted in a "hollowing" under the lumbar spine at the start of movement due to forward (anterior) pelvic tilt. The trunk-curl movement resulted in the greatest abdominal muscle activity during the initial 40 to 50° of torso flexion. From the above information it is strongly suggested that a conscious effort be made at the start of sit-up exercises to keep the abdominal wall flat by contraction of all four abdominal muscles, which will minimize forward pelvic tilt and lumbar hollowing (hyperextension). The importance of intra-abdominal pressure (IAP) to lumbar support during lifting and its relationship to abdominal muscle strength and activity, has been supported in many studies.[82,83] IAP effects must be incorporated into future weight-training exercise models.

IV. OLYMPIC-STYLE WEIGHTLIFTING

The biomechanical literature available on Olympic-style weightlifting is much more extensive than that on other lifting exercises. Three papers written from 1979 to 1980[73,84,85] contain reviews of considerable detail on weightlifting biomechanics (note that publication of Garhammer and Hatfield[84] was delayed 5 years and that it contains numerous typographical errors, since an opportunity for proofreading was unfortunately not provided). An additional, but shorter review was written in 1983.[86] Rather than repeating this information it will be

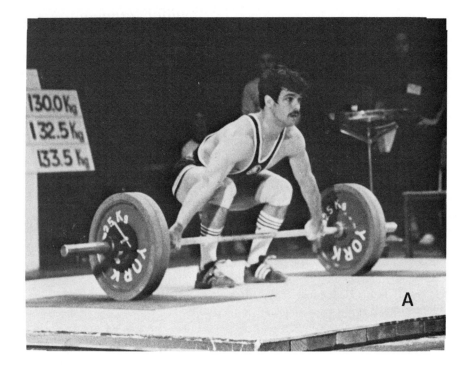

FIGURE 9.   The snatch lift as performed in competition. (A) Start position just prior to "lift-off" or start of the first pull; (B) mid-way through first pull; (C) end of first pull; (D) end of shift, transition or "scoop" phase; (E) top pull position (end of second pull or jump phase); (F) catch or receiving position; and (G) finish. (Photo by B. Klemens. From *Weightlifting USA*. With permission.)

summarized within the current review, which will emphasize other and more recent work, a synthesis of available knowledge in the field, and recommendations for future work.

The two movements now contested in weightlifting are the snatch and the clean-and-jerk lifts (cf. Figures 9 and 10). The snatch requires a barbell to be lifted from the floor to straight arm's length overhead in one continuous motion and is sometimes referred to as the single movement lift. The clean-and-jerk is a double-movement lift where the barbell is first lifted from the floor to the shoulders in one continuous motion and then jerked to straight arm's length overhead using primarily leg and hip thrust. These lifts are done very rapidly with less than 1 sec being used for the propulsion phase of any of the movements. Due to the explosive strength (muscular power) required to perform these lifts they are often used in training by athletes in other sports involving "explosive" actions such as throwing (shot put and hammer) and jumping (volleyball and high jump). Subdivisions of the complete lifts (e.g., high pulls and push jerks) are often described in more detailed weight-training books,[3,39] and are also sometimes used in general strength-training due to the large muscle mass employed and the speed factor.

A. Data on Elite Lifters

An obvious first biomechanics question concerns the kinematics of these lifts as performed by world-champion athletes. Extensive data of this type are available from several sources. The Soviet Union has the largest population of competitive weightlifters and it is not uncommon for eight or nine of the top ten lifters in the world in a given bodyweight division to be from the U.S.S.R. Dr. Yessis has translated countless reports written by Russian weightlifting authorities on analyses of top athletes' training methods and lifting techniques. Many of these contain detailed information about the kinematics (and some kinetics) of one or more lifts performed by specific world champions.[87-97]

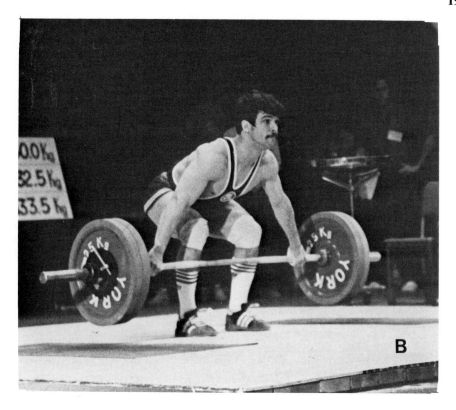

FIGURE 9B.

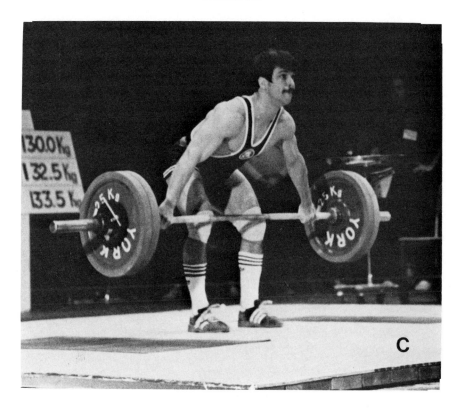

FIGURE 9C.

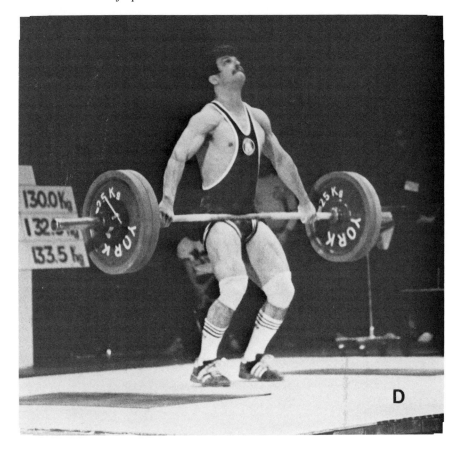

FIGURE 9D.

Recent articles,[87,88] for example, contain the following information on world-record holder U. Zakharevich: height and foot length; sequential photos, and stick-figure representations of key positions during the execution of a world-record snatch (192.5 kg), including joint angles and torso inclination; detailed figures and data tables describing horizontal and vertical bar position (trajectory), and velocity during the third attempt at a world-record lift, a lighter first attempt lift (188 kg), and a missed second attempt at the world record, and durations to a hundredth of a second for all key phases of the lift from prior to lift-off until bar fixation overhead. Discussion includes a comparison of these parameters for the above three lifts.

An additional source of such information is a published collection of approximately 30 individual analyses of world-champion lifters performed by the Soviet experts Roman and Shakirzyanov.[98] *U.S.S.R. Weightlifting Yearbooks,* which generally contain biomechanical data as well as detailed training and technique information, have also been translated and are readily available.[99] Translations from Russian on biomechanical considerations of other specific lifting topics, have been published.[100-105]

Individual authors from other countries have also analyzed world champions and world-record lifts.[67,73,106-113] The parameters studied by these researchers varied, but included bar trajectory,[67,73,106,108,111,113] bar velocity, [67,73,106,108-112] joint- and body-segment angles, [73,107,112] and work/power output.[67,73,106,108-111]

B. Bar-Trajectory Data

Bar-trajectory data, particularly when coupled with bar-velocity data, are very informative about an athlete's technique in the snatch and clean movements. Detailed discussion of a

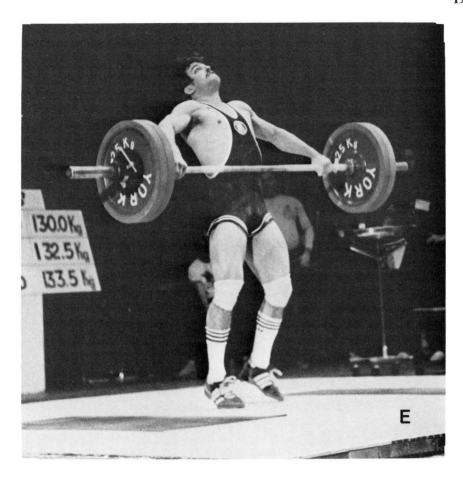

FIGURE 9E.

variety of observed trajectory patterns and a recommended optimal ("rational") pattern, has been given by Vorobyev.[114,115] The optimal pattern consists of initial bar movement after lift-off being toward the lifter (4 to 6 cm) followed by movement away from the lifter, crossing a vertical-reference line passing through the position of the bar prior to lift-off. Movement is then essentially straight upward (during the mid- and final part of the second pull; see below) until the bar hooks back toward the lifter (again crossing the vertical-reference line) and descends as the athlete rapidly moves under the barbell to catch it (see Figure 11).[96,97] Numerous world-record lifts have been found to follow this "rational" pattern (e.g., a clean by Rusev[111] and a snatch by Blagoev,[108] both representing Bulgaria), but many others have not.[87,88] This latter lift followed the most common deviation from the "rational" pattern. The trajectory of Figure 11 is tilted to the right so that the bar-path never crosses the vertical-reference line, and is caught farther back from the initial horizontal position than with the optimal pattern. Such a pattern is most likely caused by premature movement of the shoulders to a position behind the bar during the second pull.[114,115] Although some discussion has been published concerning the effects of relative segment lengths (arm, torso, thigh and shank) on lifting technique[115] much more work is needed, particularly employing mathematical optimization methods.

C. Film Analysis and Computer Modeling

The biomechanical techniques most commonly used to study weightlifting are film analysis, EMG, and force-plate measurement. In addition to many of the studies cited above

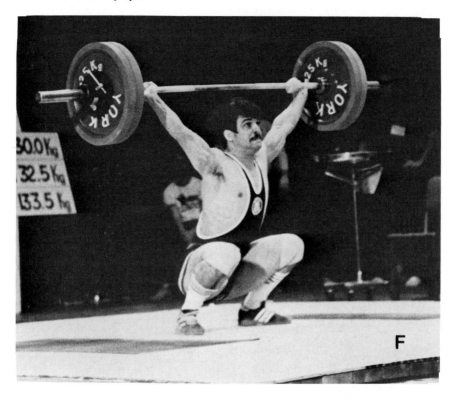

FIGURE 9F.

which employed film-analysis methods, many others have been published which include varying levels of detail and sophistication and subject skill level. Some of these involved comparisons of subjects representing different skill levels and are discussed in Section IV.G. Others simply noted technique characteristics and discussed them relative to mechanical principles and coaching standards.[116-119] Still others utilized rigid-link modeling methods and input data from film analysis to estimate joint-forces and torques. One study[120,121] showed that torque patterns at the knee and hip were distinct for two different lifting styles — the "double knee bend" (DKB, see below) and a style emphasizing hip extension ("frog-leg pull"). By comparing these torque patterns with the corresponding bar-acceleration patterns, it was evident that the former style depended mainly on knee extension to accelerate the barbell during the second pull.

A slight modification of the above modeling technique permitted estimation of the tension in the patellar ligament at rupture during a jerk attempt by a highly skilled lifter. The value was 17.5 times the athlete's bodyweight.[122] In the analysis of Dahlkvist[46] one subject (No. 3) was very similar in size to this injured athlete and was found to have a patellar ligament tension of approximately 3 times bodyweight at 90° of knee flexion (position of injury occurrence) and a maximum of approximately 6 times bodyweight at maximum knee flexion (50°) during a fast squat descent with no load.

The DKB style involves a rebending of the knees after the barbell has been lifted from the floor to just above knee level (first pull). During this second knee bend, the torso rotates to a more vertical position for the final knee extension (second pull), which leads to the top-pull (full extension) position just before the lifter moves under the bar to catch it (cf. Figures 9 and 12). Enoka[123-126] has analyzed the DKB and shown that it permits re-employment of the powerful knee-extensor muscles through their strongest range of motion. Elastic-energy storage and stretch-reflex facilitation of the final knee extension, may also

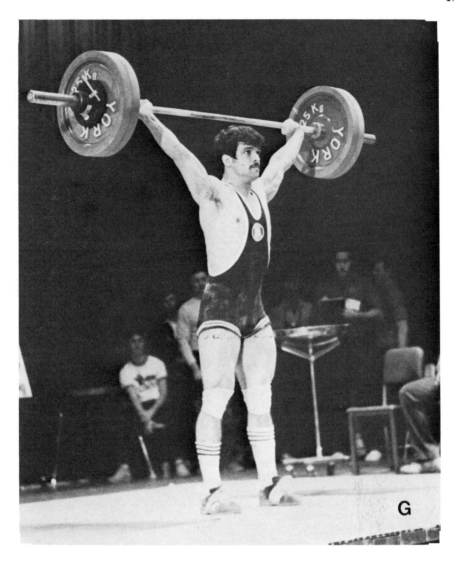

FIGURE 9G.

be very important aspects of the DKB technique. Modeling of the torso, which included consideration of IAP effects, provided evidence that the DKB greatly reduced stress on the lumbar spine.[123,124]

Hall[127] has used rigid-link modeling methods to estimate the net forces and torques acting at the base of the lumbar spine during clean-and-jerk exercises performed at three load and speed conditions. The subjects were not highly skilled due to the low loads lifted (40, 60, 80% of 1 RM, which was less than bodyweight) and IAP effects were not considered. Results, however, were consistent with those found for similar conditions with lifts previously discussed; mechanical stress on the lumbar spine increased with load, speed of movement, and forward torso lean.

D. EMG Studies

Cerquiglini and co-workers[128] used both EMG and phonomyography to study selected muscle activity in weightlifters. Spectral analysis of both signals showed differences between novice and experienced lifters. After a period of training, amplitude and higher frequency

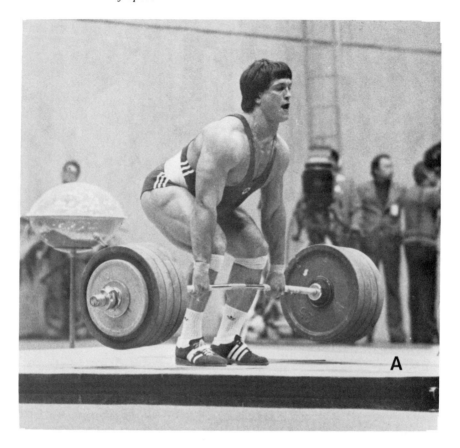

FIGURE 10.   The clean-and-jerk lift as performed in competition. (A) Middle of the first pull after ''lift-off'';
(B) end of first pull; (C) end of shift, transition or ''scoop'' phase — start of second pull; (D) catch or receiving
position for the clean; (E) preparation position for the jerk; (F) lowest point of the dip prior to the upward thrust
to jerk the barbell overhead; (G) catch or receiving position for the split jerk; and (H) finish. Photo by B. Klemens.
From *Weightlifting USA*. With permission.)

content increased for the former group. This may have been related to enhanced recruitment
of fast-twitch motor units, but it was not discussed by the authors. They did, however,
suggest that the acoustic signals could be used for ''feedback'' to aid the lifter in learning
proper technique.

Lehr and Poppen[129] used EMG to compare one skilled lifter with two less-skilled lifters
during execution of the squat and power cleans. Clear differences were found between the
two types of cleans as well as between skill levels. A similar study[130] involved 17 subjects
of varying ability lifting 60, 80, and 95% of 1 RM in the clean-and-jerk. Differences in
muscle activation patterns were again found relative to load and skill levels. In both of these
studies, EMG patterns were clearly related to the major phases of the lifting movements
performed.

Cameron[85] analyzed the clean pull via synchronized EMG and cinematography. Segment
kinematics and electrical activity of four muscles were determined for groups of highly
skilled and less-skilled subjects while cleaning 85% of 1 RM. The former group was found
to follow a movement sequence that resulted in greater extension of the body (higher center
of gravity [CG] position at top pull) and superior leverage for the hip and lumbrosacral
joints relative to the latter group. They also exhibited different electrical-activity patterns in
selected muscles and lower overall EMG activity despite lifting heavier weights. Thus, the
highly skilled group seemed to be more efficient in using their muscle activity and leverages.

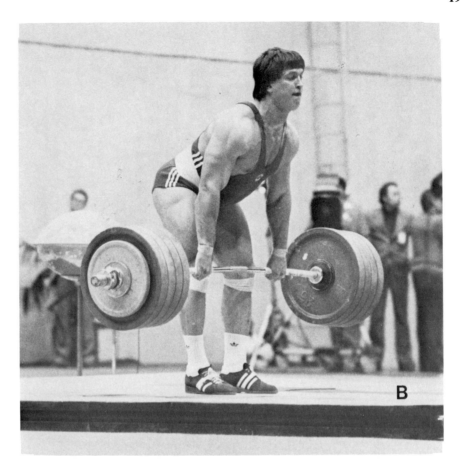

FIGURE 10B.

An interesting hypothesis was made by the author that differences in the movement sequence/pattern betweeen the two groups may have been due to differences in the percentage of bodyweight being lifted. The CG trajectories of the body alone were different, but not those of the combined body-barbell system. Movement sequence/pattern differences may have been a manifestation of attempts by both groups to be more efficient in raising the combined CG of the system. This could be a very enlightening area of study, and Nelson and Burdett[110] have provided some pertinent isolated and combined CG movement data across bodyweight divisions, but did not compare skill levels nor address the above hypothesis.

Connan and co-workers[131] performed a complex analysis of the snatch lift using video, film, EMG (eight muscles), and force-plate records. Three skill-level groups were used and loads lifted ranged from 50 to 95% of 1 RM. Pull height and maximal first-pull velocity decreased with increasing load for all subjects. Variations in EMG patterns decreased for all skill levels as load increased. It was suggested that training resulted in learned muscular patterns needed to lift heavy loads which are not readily adapted to lighter loads. If this is correct it would indicate that excessive training with too light a load could be detrimental to maximal performance. The authors also stated that variations in barbell kinematics and ground-reaction forces resulted more from load changes than from body segment movement/pattern alterations. This could relate to Cameron's hypothesis discussed above. Some additional EMG data are available in other references[143,146] and are discussed in Sections IV.F and IV.G.

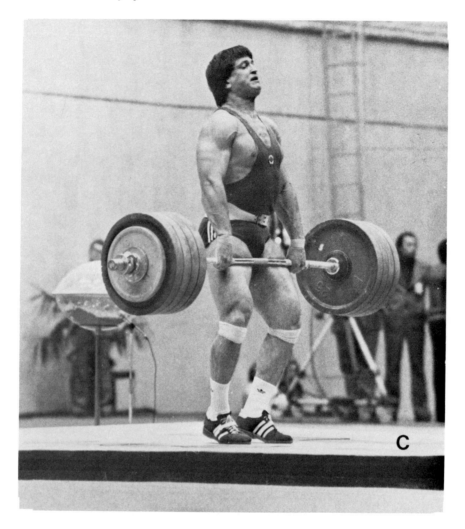

FIGURE 10C.

E. Force-Plate Studies

Payne et al.[132] obtained force-plate data for a number of athletic activities in 1968. These included a power clean-and-press, snatch, and clean-and-jerk for a single experienced lifter. One of the more interesting findings, though not discussed by the authors, was the existence of two vertical ground-reaction force peaks separated by an "unweighting" period during a snatch and power clean pull. This is what is seen with a DKB pull — a technique not commonly taught until the 1970s. Enoka[123-125] has documented and discussed vertical ground-reaction force during the DKB in detail (see also Figure 12).

Garhammer[133] utilized force-plate measurements to study the movement of the center of pressure (CP) on one foot during snatch lifts. For most subjects CP was found to move rapidly from the ball-of-foot/mid-foot area to the heel and back toward the toes during the transition from the first to the second pull. This CP movement was related to use of the DKB pulling method and seemed to be quantitatively related to the extent of horizontal bar movement during the pull. One subject who had difficulty in completing his lifts had a straighter bar trajectory and little movement of the CP from the ball of his foot. Data presented in other studies using a force plate show that extensive anterior-posterior CP shifts take place during snatch and clean pulls,[76,134] but the authors do not discuss this parameter.

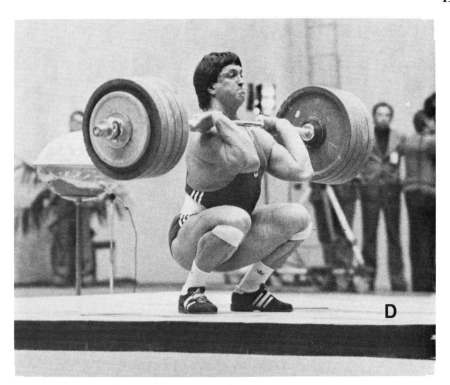

FIGURE 10D.

In an effort to gain more insight into the possible connection between bar trajectory and CP movement, Garhammer carried out additional force-plate work with highly skilled subjects from various bodyweight divisions performing both snatches and cleans.[135,136] Lifts were done with both feet on the plate, and minimal lateral CP movement indicated symmetrical force application.[108] Extensive anterior-posterior CP movement was again found with the pattern being similar to that previously noted.[133] Posterior CP movement during the first pull correlated to movement of the bar toward the lifter both temporally and in magnitude. Anterior CP movement during the transition to, and early part of, the second pull preceded forward bar movement and had some relationship to its magnitude. CP movement pattern consistency was excellent for a given athlete in a given type of lift. It was suggested that coaches consider teaching pulling techique in terms of interrelated horizontal barbell and anterior-posterior CP movement.

Vertical jumps have an "unweighting" phase (countermovement) and thrust phase.[52] This is also true of DKB pulls.[123] The ground-reaction force patterns for these activities have been compared temporally and in magnitude.[137] Similarities were noted, particularly when one subject performed both activities. The maximal force generated was found to decrease as the percentage of maximal effort increased. However, longer force durations at submaximal levels resulted in larger impulses for greater efforts. The use of DKB pulls was recommended for jump training due to the kinetic and temporal similarities found. Similarities of the leg and hip action as used in the DKB pull to leg and hip action in a number of other sport activities, have been pointed out by Miller.[138]

F. Work, Energy, and Power Output

As noted in Section III.D the competitive Olympic lifts are performed rapidly and require a large power output. The power output during a single clean was reported in 1958 as approximately 1940 W (2 hp).[139] The next consideration of work-related parameters in

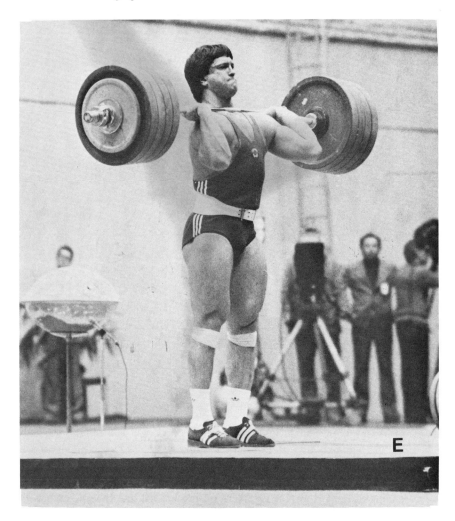

FIGURE 10E.

weightlifting appears to be by Ranta,[140] who developed an objective evaluation scale based on the work-energy principle to compare lifters of different bodyweights. Soon thereafter, Nelson and Burdett[110] published time-, displacement-, work-, and power values obtained from film of world-class lifters performing at an international meet. Power values ranged from approximately 1400 W in the lightest weight class to nearly 3000 W in the heaviest. Their most interesting finding was that average power output in the snatch-and-clean pull was very similar for a given athlete. This observation was supported and extended to other groups of movements by later research.[66,67] The high-skill level and inclusion of work done in lifting the body's CG resulted in these higher values relative to the 1940-W value cited above.

Garhammer[141] modified and extended Ranta's application of work-energy concepts to weightlifting and used the resulting methodology to make precise power-output calculations for five different lifting movements.[66,67] Values obtained were much higher than previously determined and reached approximately 4000 W for complete pulls by heavier lifters and approximately 6000 W for second pulls and jerk thrusts. This calculation technique has been applied to many groups of lifters with similar results.[73,106,108,109,111] When referenced to body weight, power values generally fell in the range of 31 to 37 W/kg for complete pulls by

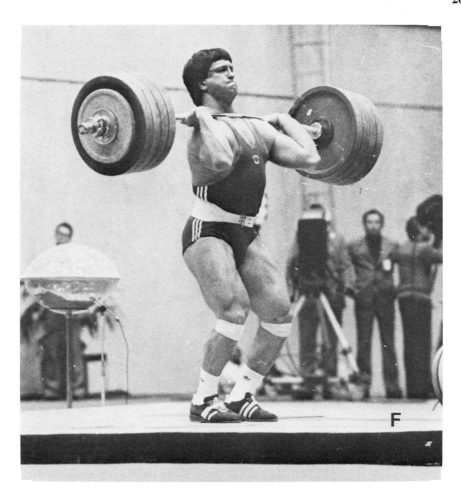

FIGURE 10F.

elite lifters. Second pull- and jerk-thrust values were in the range of 45 to 60 W/kg. These magnitudes are near maximal theoretical values for humans.[73]

Previous discussion (Section III.D) pointed out that power output increases as the load lifted decreases from the 1-RM value. Other studies, though not actually calculating power, have provided data that are indicative of this inverse relationship. Campbell et al.[142] found that maximum bar height and velocity decreased as the load for power cleans increased from 40 to 80% of 1 RM (also see Conan et al.[131] discussed in Section IV.D). Hakkinen et al.[143] found that for both Finnish national level and district-level lifters increasing loads in the snatch-and-clean resulted in lower peak ground-reaction forces (GRF) (in agreement with Garhammer and Gregor[137]), lower barbell velocities, and lower maximal barbell heights.

One paper has analyzed the development pattern of energy in body segments and its transfer between segments and to the barbell during snatch and clean lifts performed by elite athletes.[144] The results provided insights relative to the time-course of dominant muscle group action at the joints and the magnitude and temporal characteristics of energy flow. The method used showed potential as a means of quantifying lifting technique and evaluating rehabilitation exercises and lifting tasks in industry.

G. Comparative Studies

A number of investigators have compared lifters of different skill levels or have compared

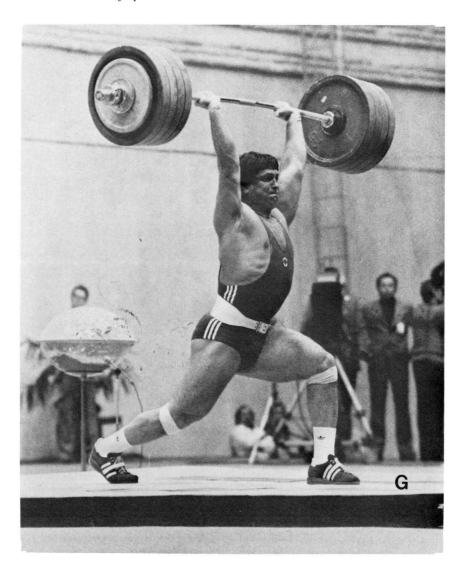

FIGURE 10G.

the kinematics of successful vs. unsuccessful lifts. Comparisons of the former type using EMG, were covered in Section IV. D.[85,129] Kinematics derived from film in various studies showed that some or all of the following characteristics were exhibited by the higher-skilled athletes during the snatch and/or clean[107, 111-113,145,146] (1) faster movement during one or more phases of the lifts (opposite of what was found for higher- vs. lower-skilled powerlifters, see Sections III.A to III.C); (2) greater body extension during the pull; and (3) lower peak bar height relative to body size. In addition, Kauhanen et al.[146] noted greater relative maximal GRFs during each major phase of a lift for the elite vs. district level athletes. They also found correlations between neuromuscular performance parameters (e.g., isometric force level generation times and CG rise in drop jumps) and lifting ability. A report comparing American champions with world champions,[111] showed that the latter group produced higher power outputs, and had greater consistency in power output for similar lifting movements and in the duration of the pull from ''lift-off'' until maximum bar velocity and bar height were attained.

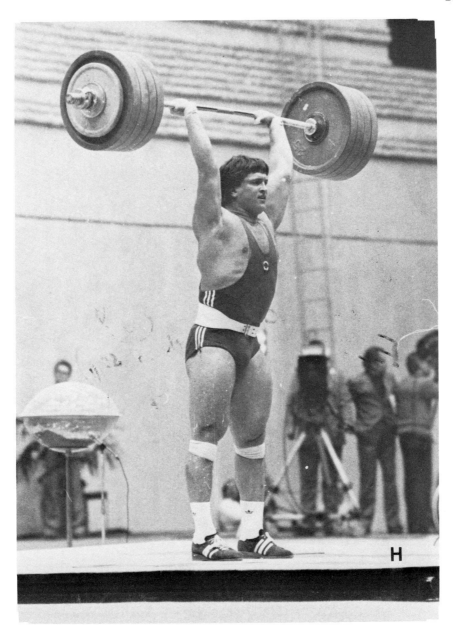

FIGURE 10H.

Grabe[147,148] used a numerical classification analysis method to compare kinematic variables associated with the jerk phase of the clean-and-jerk lift as performed by athletes of differing skill levels. Some reference values were obtained from translations of Russian literature on the jerk characteristics of world champions.[100] Some findings were in agreement with another recent investigation involving the jerk as performed by lifters of different skill levels.[146] Those more highly skilled had a shallower dip and shorter braking phase prior to the jerk thrust, and less horizontal barbell movement. Unsuccessful attempts often had excessive rather than insufficient height.

Successful vs. unsuccessful attempts in the snatch and/or clean were compared in several studies.[112,120,149] Differences between good and missed lifts with equal or slightly different

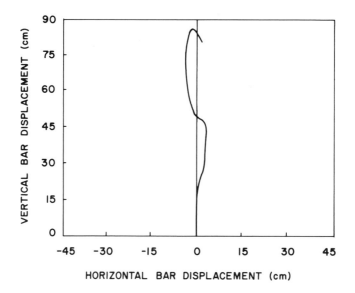

FIGURE 11.   Bar trajectory for a 217.5 kg clean by a 1984 Olympic gold medalist. From Garhammer, J., *Intl. J. Sport Biomech.*, 1, 122, 1985. With permission.)

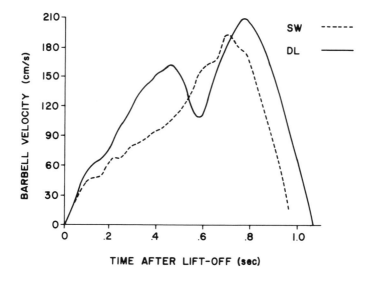

FIGURE 12.   Bar velocity patterns for two snatch lifts at the 1984 Olympic Games (SW—120 kg, DL—172.5 kg). DL used the DKB pulling technique (note the double peak in velocity), while SW used a pulling style more dependent on hip extension — see text for discussion. (From Garhammer, J., *Intl. J. Sport Biomech.*, 1, 122, 1985. With permission.)

weights, were not consistent. Sometimes a missed lift, for example, had a higher maximum vertical velocity than a good lift. Results seem to suggest that timing and duration of the lifting phases may be equally or more important than kinetic variables such as maximum force applied.

A longitudinal comparison of highly skilled lifters has been made by filming them in competitions which occurred 2 years apart.[109] The parameters compared, included peak bar velocities, power outputs, and joint-torque patterns. This method seemed to be sensitive enough to distinguish between performances with regard to the amount of weight lifted. A higher digitizing frequency (50 vs. 25 Hz) would provide greater sensitivity and permit smaller changes in technique to be determined quantitatively.

H. Data Smoothing

Detailed general discussions of data-smoothing techniques have been published with example applications usually related to running and gait.[150] The studies reviewed in this manuscript used a variety of data-smoothing methods including spline functions (SF), digital filters (DF), and "least squares" moving arc (MA) curve fitting. One comparative evaluation of these three methods has been performed.[68] Results indicated excellent agreement between methods when the sampling frequency was 50 Hz. The optimal DF cut-off frequency was approximately 4 Hz for vertical movement and 5 Hz for horizontal movement during a snatch lift. Corresponding values for a clean were 5 and 6 Hz. Grabe and Widule[148] used a DF to smooth barbell- and joint-movement data for jerk lifts. They found these movements were best represented by a third-level harmonic (4 Hz). One analysis of squats[47] found 95% of the signal power for vertical GRFs and barbell- and joint accelerations to lie below 8 Hz. The subjects were not competitive powerlifters, and since they were using squats in sport training they may have moved slightly faster than competitive lifters would while using maximum loads. Optimal SF error estimates were approximately 2.7 mm for both lifts and movement directions.[68] This is in agreement with work by McLaughlin et al.[151] Garhammer has expressed concern about using a MA method with a sampling frequency of 25 Hz, and suggested that 50 Hz or a different smoothing technique could improve accuracy.[73,120,121,144] Due to the ease of use of the MA method, and the minimal differences found between the DF, SF, and MA at a 50-Hz sampling frequency[68], it seems an appropriate and advantageous choice for weightlifting analyses.

V. SUMMARY

Considerable information is obviously available on the biomechanics of weightlifting exercises. Several areas, however, clearly require more detailed analysis. Computer models for lifting movements must be improved. The use of 2-D dynamic rigid-link models to calculate net joint forces and torques, has been employed repeatedly. More detailed joint models must be used to supplement the results of rigid-link analyses[122] or to replace them.[46] Industrial lifting models have advanced more rapidly than exercise models. IAP, for example, is commonly considered in the former, but seldom in the latter. Enoka[123] has used it for lower-back-force calculations in a quasi-static model of the pull for cleans, while Cappozzo et al.[47] have argued that it is not needed for lower-back analysis during squats without providing quantitative data to support their conclusion. Observations such as the "sticking point/region" in the squat[41,45] may be explained if detailed models including dual joint muscles and skeletal geometries, such as in Dahlkvist et al.,[46] are extended to the torso with consideration of IAP.

Force-plate analyses must go beyond vertical GRF patterns. Anterior-posterior- and mediolateral forces as well as balance patterns must be evaluated and interpreted for many additional weightlifting exercises. Force-plate data must also be incorporated into more sophisticated computer models to improve or verify accuracy.

Three-dimensional analysis is needed for many lifting activities, some more than others. Again, occupational models seem to be ahead of exercise models.[2] The bench press appears to be the only lifting exercise where 3-D analysis has even begun.[60-62]

For competitive lifting and many other exercises, combined force-plate- and 3-D film analysis (with or without modeling) would be extremely enlightening. Even combined 2-D film and force-plate data are limited primarily to Olympic lifting studies performed in a laboratory setting (see Sections IV.C and IV.E). The International Olympic Committee and International Weightlifting Federation are taking steps to eliminate this gap in knowledge. One step involved major filming projects at the 1984 Olympic Games.[152] More recently, the 1985 World Weightlifting Championships were held with specially made Kistler force plates used as part of the competitive platform, and with synchronized 35-mm cameras used to record selected lifts. Detailed analyses of these data are planned.[153] Powerlifting needs to move in this direction after preliminary laboratory studies are done. General weight-training exercises should also undergo such detailed study if they are to be more fully understood in terms of stresses placed on the body.

Finally, biomechanists should evaluate new weight (resistance) machines that are placed on the consumer market. Manufacturers often refer to biomechanical principles to justify and support the value of their product. However, it is clear (see Section II.) that advertising claims and objective measures are not in agreement. If biomechanics is to be widely recognized and respected it must serve the common person as well as research interests. Many newer resistance devices add color and "bells and whistles" to exercise, but they may not, for example, accurately control or record movement speed and force level as claimed (to say nothing about providing improved training results). Such limitations must be made known both for fairness to the consumer, who may exercise on the device, and for scientific accuracy in research measurements made using the device. Many of the countless published research papers based on "isokinetic" muscle-function evaluation may now be criticized due to the discovery that movement speed is often not uniform through the range of motion.

ADDENDUM

Since this chapter was completed in early 1986, some of the most recent research in weight lifting biomechanics is not covered. One notable addition includes a 3-D film analysis synchronized with force-plate data made at the 1985 World Weightlifting Championships. (Baumann, W. et al., *Intl. J. Sport Biomech.*, 4(1), 68, 1988).

REFERENCES

1. **Grieve, D. W.,** The dynamics of lifting, *Exercise Sport Sci. Rev.*, 5, 157, 1977.
2. **Chaffin, D. B. and Andersson, G. B. J.,** *Occupational Biomechanics,* John Wiley & Sons, New York, 1984.
3. **Stone, M. H. and O'Bryant, H. S.,** *Weight Training: A Scientific Approach,* Burgess Publishing, Minneapolis, 1987.
4. **Atha, J.,** Strengthening muscle, *Exercise Sport Sci. Rev.*, Miller A. I., Ed., Franklin Institute Press 9, 1, 1981.
5. Understanding the scientific bases behind our . . . *Universal® Centurion®*, 1st ed., Universal® Athletic Sales, Fresno, Calif., 1974.
6. *Universal®'s Amazing New Centurion®*, Universal® Athletic Sales, Fresno, Calif., 1975.
7. Universal®-Physical Conditioning Equipment Catalog, Universal® (subsidary of Kidde, Inc.), Cedar Rapids, Iowa, 1984.
8. **Smith, F.,** Dynamic variable resistance and the Universal® system, *Natl. Strength Cond. Assoc. J.*, 4, 14, 1982.
9. **Pennycook, W. D. and Charley, P. J.,** Evaluation and test results of Universal® variable resistance equipment, Test no. 175190, Truesdail Laboratories, Los Angeles, 1975.
10. **Hay, J. G., Andrews, J. G., Vaughan, C. L., and Ueya, K.,** Load, speed and equipment effects in strength-training exercises, in *Biomechanics VIII-B,* University Park Press, Baltimore, 1983, 939.
11. **Ariel, G. B.,** *The Effects of Dynamic Variable Resistance on Muscular Strength,* Computerized Biomedical Analysis, Inc., Amherst, Mass., 1976.

12. **Starr, B.,** *The Strongest Shall Survive: Strength Training For Football,* Fitness Products, Ltd., Annapolis, Md., 1976, chap. 18.
13. **Hay, J. G., Andrews, J. G., and Vaughan, C. L.,** Effects of lifting rate on elbow torques exerted during arm curl exercises, *Med. Sci. Sports Exercise,* 15, 63, 1983.
14. **Garhammer, J. and Grabiner, M.,** Biomechanical evaluation and comparison of modified design and standard free weight exercise equipment, Technical Report, manuscript in preparation.
15. *Nautilus®: A Concept of Variable Resistance.* Nautilus® Sports/Medical Industries, *Natl. Strength Cond. Assoc. J.,* 3, 48, 1981.
16. **Fleming, L. K.,** Accomodation capabilities of Nautilus® weight machines to human strength curves, *Natl. Strength Cond. Assoc. J.,* 7, 68, 1985; abstract of Master's thesis, University of Alabama, Birmingham, 1984.
17. **Harman, E.,** Resistive torque analysis for 5 Nautilus® exercise machines, *Med. Sci. Sports Exercise,* 15, (Abstr.), 113, 1983.
18. *Nautilus® Instruction Manual,* Nautilus® Sports/Medical Industries, DeLand, Fla., 1980.
19. **Jones, A.,** *Specificity in Strength Training — the Facts and the Fables,* Nautilus® Sports Medical Industries, DeLand, Fla. (Reprinted from Athletic J., May 1977).
20. **Kalas, J. P.,** *Fast-Twitch Slow-Twitch Muscle Fibers: What Is the Truth?,* Nautilus® Sports/Medical Industries, DeLand, Fla. Reprinted from Athletic J. January 1977).
21. **Everson, J.,** Variable resistance vs. isotonic weight training in monozygotic male twins, *Natl. Strength Cond. Assoc. J.,* 5, (Abstr.), 31, 1983.
22. **Hinson, M. N., Smith, W. C., and Funk, S.,** Isokinetics: a clarification, *Res. Q.,* 50, 30, 1979.
23. **Hislop, H. J. and Perrine, J. J.,** The isokinetic concept of exercise, *Phys. Ther.,* 47, 114, 1967.
24. **Noffroid, M. R. et al.,** A study of isokinetic exercise, *Phys. Ther.,* 49, 735, 1969.
25. **Sawhill, J. A.,** Biomechanical Characteristics of Rotational Velocity and Movement Complexity in Isokinetic Performance, Doctoral dissertation, University of Oregon, Eugene, 1981.
26. **Lander, J. E., Bates, B. T., Sawhill, J. A., and Hamill, J.,** A comparison between free-weight and isokinetic bench pressing, *Med. Sci. Sports Exercise,* 17, 344, 1985.
27. **Rosentswieg, J., Hinson, M., and Ridgway, M.,** An electromyographic comparison of an isokinetic bench press performed at three speeds, *Res. Q.,* 46, 471, 1975.
28. **Perrine, J. J. and Edgerton, V. R.,** Muscle force-velocity and power velocity relationships under isokinetic loading, *Med. Sci. Sports,* 10, 159, 1978.
29. **Thistle, H. G. et al.,** Isokinetic contraction: a new concept of resistive exercise, *Arch. Phys. Med. Rehab.,* 48, 279, 1967.
30. **O'Shea, J. P.,** *Scientific Principles and Methods of Strength Fitness,* 1st ed., Addison-Wesley, Reading, Mass., 1969, 62.
31. **Garhammer, J.,** Free weight equipment for the development of athletic strength and power, *Natl. Strength Cond. Assoc. J.,* 3, 24, 1981.
32. **Stone, M. H.,** Considerations in gaining a strength-power training effect, *Natl. Strength Cond. Assoc. J.,* 4, 22, 1982.
33. **O'Donoghue, D. H.,** *Treatment of Injuries to Athletes,* 3rd ed., W. B. Saunders, Philadelphia, 1976, 800.
34. **Nosse, L. J. and Hunter, G. R.,** Free weights: a review supporting their use in training and rehabilitation, *Athletic Training,* Fall, 206, 1985.
35. **Rasch, P. J. and Allman, F. J.,** Controversial exercise, *Am. Correct. Ther. J.,* 26, 95, 1972.
36. **Klein, K.,** The deep squat exercise as utilized in weight training for athletes and its effects on the ligaments of the knee, *J. Assoc. Phys. Ment. Rehab.,* 15, 6, 1961.
37. **Todd, T.,** Karl Klein and the squat, *Natl. Strength Cond. Assoc. J.,* 6, 26, 1984.
38. President's Council on Physical Fitness and Sport. Exercise and the knee joint, *Phys. Fitness Res. Dig.,* 6, 1, 1976.
39. **Garhammer, J.,** *Sports Illustrated Strength Training,* Harper & Row, New York, 1986.
40. The squat and its application to athletic performance. Roundtable discussion, *Natl. Strength Cond. Assoc. J.,* 6, 10, 1984.
41. **McLaughlin, T. M., Dillman, C. J., and Lardner, T. J.,** A kinematic model of performance in the parallel squat by champion powerlifters, *Med. Sci. Sports,* 9, 128, 1977.
42. **Malone, P. E.,** Applicability of the McLaughlin Model of the Parallel Squat to Class II Powerlifters, 1979.
43. **Plagenhoef, S. C.,** *Patterns of Human Motion — A Cinematographic Analysis,* Prentice-Hall, Englewood Cliffs, N.J., 1971, 55.
44. **Ariel, G. B.,** Biomechanical analysis of the knee joint during deep knee bends with heavy load, in *Biomechanics IV,* Nelson, R. C. and Morehouse, C. A., Eds., University Park Press, Baltimore, 1974, 44.
45. **McLaughlin, T. M., Lardner, T. J., and Dillman, C. J.,** Kinetics of the parallel squat, *Res. Q.,* 49, 175, 1978.

46. **Dahlkvist, N. J., Mayo, P., and Seedhom, B. B.,** Forces during squatting and rising from a deep squat, *Eng. Med.,* 11, 69, 1982.

47. **Cappozzo, A., Felici, F., Figura, F., and Gazzani, F.,** Lumbar spine loading during half-squat exercises, *Med. Sci. Sports Exercise,* 17, 613, 1985.

48. **Hay, J. G., Andrews, J. G., and Vaughan, C. L.,** *The Influence of External Load on Joint Torques Exerted in a Squat Exercise,* Proc. Biomech. Symp. Indiana Univ. Oct. 1980, Indiana State Board of Health, 1980, 286.

49. **Andrews, J. G., Hay, J. G., and Vaughan, C. L.,** *The Concept of Joint Shear,* Proc. Biomech. Symp. Indiana Univ. Oct. 1980, Indiana State Board of Health, 1980, 239.

50. **Andrews, J. G., Hay, J. G., and Vaughan, C. L.,** Knee shear forces during a squat exercise using a barbell and a weight machine, in *Biomechanics VIII-B,* University Park Press, Baltimore, 1983, 923.

51. **Malone, P. E.,** An Investigation of the "Sticking Point" Phenomenon in the Parallel Squat, 1980.

52. **Bosco, C. and Komi, P. V.,** Potentiation of mechanical behavior of the human skeletal muscle through prestretching, *Acta Physiol. Scand.,* 106, 467, 1979.

53. **Cavagna, G. A.,** Storage and utilization of elastic energy in skeletal muscle, *Exercise Sport Sci. Rev.,* Hutton, R., Ed., 5, 89, 1977.

54. **Fisher, A. G. and Ramey, J. S.,** Electronic squat monitor, *Res. Q.,* 48, 213, 1977.

55. **Algra, B.,** An in-depth analysis of the bench press, *Natl. Strength Cond. Assoc. J.,* 4, 6, 1982.

56. **Hatfield, F. C. and McLaughlin, T. M.,** Powerlifting, in *Encyclopedia of Physical Education, Fitness, and Sports,* Vol. 4, Cureton, T. K., Ed., AAHPERD, Reston, Va., 1985, 587.

57. **Engin, A. E.,** On the biomechanics of the shoulder complex, *J. Biomech.,* 13, 575, 1980.

58. **Madsen, N. and McLaughlin, T.,** Kinematic factors influencing performance and injury risk in the bench press exercise, *Med. Sci. Sports Exercise,* 16, 376, 1984.

59. **McLaughlin, T. M. and Madsen, N. H.,** Bench press techniques of elite heavyweight powerlifters, *Natl. Strength Cond. Assoc. J.,* 6, 44, 1984.

60. **McLaughlin, T. M.,** Bench Press More Now: Breakthroughs in Biomechanics and Training Methods, 1984, 42.

61. **Madsen, N. and McLaughlin, T.,** Influence of three-dimensional geometry on success in the bench press, *J. Biomech.,* 14 (Abstr.), 493, 1981.

62. **Harman, E. A.,** A 3D biomechanical analysis of the bench press exercise, *Med. Sci. Sports Exercise,* 16, 159, 1984; abstract of Doctoral dissertation, University of Massachusetts, Amherst, 1984.

63. **Troup, J. D. G. et al.,** A comparison of intraabdominal pressure increases, hip torque and lumbar vertebral compression in different lifting techniques, *Hum. Factors,* 25, 517, 1983.

64. **Gotshalk, L.,** Analysis of the deadlift, *Natl. Strength Cond. Assoc. J.,* 6(6), 4, 1985.

65. **Brown, E. W. and Abani, K.,** Kinematics and kinetics of the dead lift in adolescent power lifters, *Med. Sci. Sports Exercise,* 17, 554, 1985.

66. **Garhammer, J.,** Power production by Olympic weightlifters, *Med. Sci. Sports Exercise,* 12, 54, 1980.

67. **Garhammer, J.,** Biomechanical characteristics of the 1978 world weight-lifting champions, in *Biomechanics VII-B,* University Park Press, Baltimore, 1981, 300.

68. **Garhammer, J. and Whiting, W. C.,** A comparison of three data smoothing techniques in the determination of weightlifting kinematics, manuscript submitted.

69. **Garhammer, J.,** unpublished data.

70. **Tsarouchas, E. and Klissouras, V.,** The force-velocity relation of a kinematic chain in man, in *Biomechanics VII-A,* University Park Press, Baltimore, 1981, 145.

71. **Komi, P. V.,** Neuromuscular performance: factors influencing force and speed production, *Scand. J. Sports Sci.,* 1, 2, 1979.

72. **Garhammer, J.,** Force-velocity constraints and elastic energy utilization during multi-segment lifting/jumping activities, *Med. Sci. Sports Exercise,* 13, 96, 1981.

73. **Garhammer, J.,** Evaluation of Human Power Capacity through Olympic Weightlifting Analyses, Ph.D. dissertation, University of California at Los Angeles, 1980; University Microfilms, Ann Arbor, Mich., 1981.

74. **Santa Maria, D. L., Grzybinski, P., and Hatfield, B.,** Power as a function of load for a supine bench press exercise, *Natl. Strength Cond. Assoc. J.,* 6, (Abstr.), 58, 1985.

75. **Garhammer, J. and McLaughlin, T.,** Power output as a function of load variation in Olympic and power lifting, *J. Biomech.,* 13, 198, 1980.

76. **Ueya, K. and Ueya, H.,** Skills of clean and jerk in view of force and power output, in *Science of Human Movement II,* Kyorin Ltd., Tokyo, 1977, 178.

77. **Danoff, J. V.,** Power produced by maximal velocity elbow flexion, *J. Biomech.,* 11, 481, 1978.

78. **Yessis, M.,** The key to strength development: variety, *Natl. Strength Cond. Assoc. J.,* 3, 32, 1981.

79. **Cailliet, R.,** *Knee Pain and Disability,* 2nd ed., F. A. Davis, Philadelphia, 1983, 60.

80. **Rasch, P. J. and Burke, R. K.,** *Kinesiology and Applied Anatomy,* 6th ed., Lea & Febiger, Philadelphia, 1978, 242.

81. **Ricci, B., Marchetti, M., and Figura, F.,** Biomechanics of sit-up exercises, *Med. Sci. Sports Exercise,* 13, 54, 1981.
82. **Grillner, S., Nilsson, J., and Thorstensson, A.,** Intra-abdominal pressure changes during natural movement in man, *Acta Physiol. Scand.,* 103, 275, 1978.
83. **Kumar, S.,** Physiological responses to weightlifting in different planes, *Ergonomics,* 10, 987, 1980.
84. **Garhammer, J. and Hatfield, F. G.,** Weightlifting, in *Encyclopedia of Physical Education, Fitness, and Sports,* Vol. 4, Cureton, T. K., Ed., AAHPERD, Reston, Va., 1985, 594.
85. **Cameron, M.,** A Cinematographic and Electromyographic Analysis of the Clean Pull Used in Olympic Weightlifting, Master's thesis, University of Maryland, College Park, 1980.
86. **Garhammer, J.,** Possible contributions of biomechanics to weightlifting progress, in *1983 American Weightlifting Yearbook,* American Weightlifting Coaches Association, 1983.
87. **Roman, R. A. and Treskov, V. V.,** Snatch technique of world record holder U. Zakharevich, *Sov. Sports Rev.,* 19, 113, 1984.
88. **Roman, R. A. and Treskov, V. V.,** Snatch technique of world record holder U. Zakharevich, *Sov. Sports Rev.,* 19, 199, 1984.
89. **Roman, R. A. and Shakirzyanov, M. S.,** Snatch technique of world record holder, A. Voronin, *Sov. Sports Rev.,* 17, 17, 1982.
90. **Roman, R. A. and Shakirzyanov, M. S.,** Jerk technique analysis of Nedelcha Kolev, *Sov. Sports Rev.,* 16, 114, 1981.
91. **Medvedev, A. S. and Lukashov, A. A.,** Jerk technique of world record holders Alexeev and Bonk, *Sov. Sports Rev.,* 16, 11, 1981.
92. **Roman, R. A. and Shakirzyanov, M. S.,** Jerk technique analysis: David Rigert, *Sov. Sports Rev.,* 15, 127, 1980.
93. **Roman, R. A. and Shakirzyanov, M. S.,** Clean and jerk technique of Valery Shary, *Sov. Sports Rev.,* 15, 22, 1980.
94. **Medvedev, A.,** Snatch technique of Christo Plachkov, *Sov. Sports Rev.,* 14, 56, 1979.
95. **Vorobyev, A. N.,** Jerk technique of Vasily Alexeev's 245.5-kg world record, *Yessis Rev.,* 12, 11, 1977.
96. **Roman, R. A. and Shakirzyanov, M. S.,** Snatch technique of world record holder Pavla Pervushin, Yessis Rev., 10, 10, 1975.
97. **Shakirzyanov, M. S.,** World champion David Rigert — technique essentials, *Yessis Rev.,* 9, 78, 1974.
98. **Roman, R. A. and Shakirzyanov, M. S.,** *The Snatch, The Clean & Jerk,* Charniga, A., transl., Sportivny Press, Livonia, Mich., 1982.
99. *1982/1983 Weightlifting Yearbooks* Charniga, A., transl., Sportivny Press, Livonia, Mich., 1983.
100. **Frolov, V. I. and Levshunov, N. P.,** Phasic structure of the jerk from the chest, *Sov. Sports Rev.,* 17, 120, 1982.
101. **Ilyin, A. P., Livanov, O. I., and Falameev, A. I.,** Duration of the nonsupport phase in the snatch and clean (condensed version), *Sov. Sports Rev.,* 14, 180, 1987.
102. **Frolov, V. I. and Lukashev, A. A.,** Comparative analysis of snatch and clean technique, *Sov. Sports Rev.,* 14, 80, 1979.
103. **Frolov, V. I., Lelikov, S. I., Efimov, N. M., and Vanagas, M. P.,** Snatch technique of top-class weightlifters, *Sov. Sports Rev.,* 14, 24, 1979.
104. **Saksonov, N. N.,** Diagonal foot placement prior to the jerk of the barbell from the chest in the clean and jerk, *Yessis Rev.,* 5, 45, 1970.
105. **Dolenko, F. L.,** Role of functional specialization of the talocrural (ankle) joint in mastering rational weightlifting technique, *Yessis Rev.,* 9, 90, 1974.
106. **Garhammer, J.,** Biomechanical profiles of Olympic weightlifters, *Intl. J. Sport Biomech.,* 1, 122, 1985.
107. **Burdett, R. G.,** Biomechanics of the snatch technique of highly skilled and skilled weightlifters, *Res. Q. Exercise Sport,* 53, 193, 1982.
108. **Garhammer, J.,** The 1982 and 1983 Elite Weightlifting Project Biomechanics Reports, submitted to the Sports Medicine Division, U.S. Olympic Committee, and the U.S. Weightlifting Federation.
109. **Garhammer, J.,** Longitudinal analysis of highly skilled Olympic weightlifters, in *Science in Weightlifting,* Terauds, J., Ed., Academic Publishers, Del Mar, Calif., 1979, 79.
110. **Nelson, R. C. and Burdett, R. G.,** Biomechanical analysis of Olympic weightlifting, in *Biomechanics of Sports and Kinanthropometry,* Landry, F. and Orban, W., Eds., Symposia Specialists, Inc., Miami, Fl., 1978, 169.
111. **Garhammer, J.,** Biomechanical comparison of the U.S. Team with divisional winners at the 1978 World Weightlifting Championships, report to the U.S. National Weightlifting Committee, August 1979.
112. **Ono, M., Kubota, M., and Kato, K.,** The analysis of weightlifting movement at three kinds of events for weight-lifting participants of the Tokyo Olympic Games, *J. Sports Med. Phys. Fitness,* 9, 263, 1969.
113. **Stolberg, D. C.,** Comparison of Techniques of Champion Lifters and Good Lifters, Master's thesis, Michigan State University, East Lansing, 1961.

114. **Vorobyev, A. N.,** The trajectory of lifting weights, *The Strength Athlete (London),* Muirhead, O., (transl.) 175, 5, 1978.

115. **Vorobyev, A. N.,** *A Textbook on Weightlifting,* Brice, W. J., transl., International Weightlifting Federation, Budapest, 1978.

116. **Garhammer, J.,** Cinematographic and mechanical analysis of the snatch lift, *Intl., Olympic Lifter,* 2, 5, 1975.

117. **Whitcomb, B. M.,** A Cinematographic Analysis of the Clean and Jerk Lift Used in Olympic Weightlifting, Masters's thesis, University of Maryland, College Park, 1969.

118. **Boileau, R.,** A Cinematographic Analysis of the Two Hands Snatch as Used in Olympic Weightlifting, Master's thesis, University of Maryland, College Park, 1970.

119. **Webster, D.,** The two-hands snatch, *Strength and Health,* 32, 15, 1964.

120. **Garhammer, J.,** A Dynamic Rigid Link Model Applied to the Olympic Snatch Lift, M.Sc. thesis, University of California at Los Angeles, 1976.

121. **Garhammer, J.,** Biomechanical analysis of selected snatch lifts at the U.S. Senior National Weightlifting Championships, in *Biomechanics of Sports and Kinanthropometry,* Landry, F. and Orban, W., Eds., Symposia Specialists, Inc., Miami, Fla., 1978, 475.

122. **Zerniche, R., Garhammer, J., and Jobe, R. W.,** Human patellar-tendon rupture, *J. Bone J. Surg.,* 59, 179, 1977.

123. **Enoka, R. M.,** The pull in Olympic weightlifting, *Med. Sci. Sports,* 11, 131, 1979.

124. **Enoka, R. M.,** Biomechanical Analysis of the Pull in Olympic Weightlifting, Master's thesis, University of Washington, Seattle, 1976.

125. **Enoka, R. M.,** Ground reaction force during the pull, *Intl. Olympic Lifter,* 5, 32, 1979.

126. **Enoka, R. M.,** The second knee bend in Olympic weightlifting, in *Encyclopedia of Physical Education, Fitness, and Sports,* Vol. 4, Cureton, T. K., Ed., AAHPERD, Reston, Va., 1985, 608.

127. **Hall, S. J.,** Effect of attempted lifting speed on forces and torque exerted on the lumbar spine, *Med Sci. Sports Exercise,* 17, 440, 1985.

128. **Cerquiglini, S., Figura, F., Marchetti, M., and Salleo, A.,** Evaluation of athletic fitness in weight-lifters through biomechanical, bioelectrical and bioacoustical data, in *Medicine and Sport (8), Biomechanics III,* S. Karger, Basel, 1973, 189.

129. **Lehr, R. P. and Poppen, R.,** Electromyographic analysis of Olympic power and squat clean, in *Science in Weightlifting,* Terauds, J., Ed., Academic Publishers, Del Mar, Calif., 1979, 15.

130. **Lecampion, D. and Pottier, M.,** Study of Weightlifting movements by electromyography, *Med. Sci. Sports,* 52, 4, 1978.

131. **Connan, A., Moreaux, A., and Van Hoecke, J.,** Biomechanical analysis of the two-hand snatch, in *Biomechanics VII-B,* University Park Press, Baltimore, 1981, 313.

132. **Payne, A. H., Salter, W. J., and Telford, T.,** Use of a force platform in the study of athletic activities, *Ergonomics,* 11, 123, 1968.

133. **Garhammer, J.,** Force plate analysis of the snatch lift, *Intl. Olympic Lifter,* 3, 22, 1976.

134. **Breniere, Y., Do, M. C., Gatti, L., and Bouisset, S.,** A dynamic analysis of the squat snatch, in *Biomechanics VII-B,* University Park Press, Baltimore, 1981, 293.

135. **Garhammer, J.,** Center of pressure movements during weightlifting, in *Sports Biomechanics,* Proc. 2nd Intl. Symp. of Biomechanics in Sports, Academic Publishers, Del Mar, Calif., 1984, 279.

136. **Garhammer, J.,** Balance on the feet during weightlifting, in *1984 American Weightlifting Yearbook,* American Weightlifting Coaches Association, 1984.

137. **Garhammer, J. and Gregor, R.,** Force plate evaluations of weightlifting and vertical jumping, *Med. Sci. Sports,* 11, (Abstr.) 106, 1979.

138. **Miller, C.,** Rotary action of legs and hips common to many sports, *Natl. Strength Coaches Assoc. J.,* 1, 20, 1979.

139. **Fletcher, J. G., Lewis, H. E., and Wilkie, D. R.,** Photographic methods for estimating external lifting work in man, *Ergonomics,* 2, 114, 1958.

140. **Ranta, M. A.,** A simple mathematical model of weightlifting, in *Biomechanics V-B,* Komi, P. V., Ed., University Park Press, Baltimore, 1976, 337.

141. **Garhammer, J.,** Performance evaluation of Olympic weightlifters, *Med. Sci. Sports,* 11, 284, 1979.

142. **Campbell, D. E., Pond, J. W., and Trenbeath, W. G.,** Cinematographic analysis of varying loads of the power clean, in *Science in Weightlifting,* Terauds, J., Ed., Academic Publishers, Del Mar, Calif., 1978, 3.

143. **Haekkinen, K., Kauhanen, H., and Komi, P. V.,** Biomechanical changes in the Olympic weightlifting technique of the snatch and clean and jerk from submaximal to maximal loads, *Scand. J. Sports Sci.,* 6, 57, 1984.

144. **Garhammer, J.,** Energy flow during Olympic weightlifting, *Med. Sci. Sports Exercise,* 14, 353, 1982.

145. **Hunter, G.,** Velocity, Acceleration and Movement Patterns in the Pulling Phase of an Olympic Lift, Master's thesis, Michigan State University, East Lansing, 1974.

146. **Kauhanen, H., Haekkinen, K., and Komi, P. V.,** A biomechanical analysis for the snatch and clean and jerk techniques of Finnish elite and district level weightlifters, *Scand. J. Sports Sci.* 6, 47, 1984.

147. **Grabe, S. A.,** Kinematics of the jerk from the chest: cluster analysis of Olympic style lifters, in *Biomechanics in Sports II,* Terauds, J., and Barham, J. N., Eds. Academic Publishers, Del Mar, Calif., 1985, 316.

148. **Grabe, S. A. and Widule, C. J.,** Success and failure in the jerk from the chest in competitive weightlifters: comparisons of the classification levels, *Res. Q. Exercise Sport,* (in press).

149. **Ueya, K., Ueya, H., and Sekiguchi, O.,** Mechanical study on snatch technique, in *Science in Weightlifting,* Terauds, J., Eds., Academic Publishers, Del Mar, Calif., 1979, 23.

150. **Wood, G. A.,** Data smoothing and differentiation procedures in biomechanics, in *Exercise Sport Science Review,* Vol. 10, Terjung, R. L., Ed., The Franklin Institute Press, 1982, 308.

151. **McLaughlin, T. M., Dillman, C. J., and Lardner, T. J.,** Biomechemical analysis with cubic spline functions, *Res. Q.* 48, 569, 1977.

152. **de Merode, A., Gregor, R. J., and Komi, P. V.,** Foreword/Introduction, *Intl. J. Sport Biomech.,* 1, 94, 1985.

153. **Baumann, W.,** Biomechanical research into weightlifting, *World Weightlifting (IWF, Budapest),* No. 4, 36, 1985.

Chapter 6

THE THROWING EVENTS IN TRACK AND FIELD

Mont Hubbard

TABLE OF CONTENTS

I. INTRODUCTION

The purpose of this paper is to review and to present a coherent view of the scientific literature concerning the mechanics and biomechanics of the throwing events in track- and field athletics. Many hundreds of papers have been written on these subjects. Because each event is essentially composed of the *mechanical* motion of a competitor and an implement, a majority of the literature can be said to concern mechanics or biomechanics to a greater or lesser degree. Moreover, these papers span the entire spectrum of scientific content, from those which might be classified mainly as anecdotal commentary to those reporting rigorous scientific experiments and/or formal mathematical models and analysis.

It is thus necessary to limit, at the outset, the scope of the literature covered. We have specifically excluded from consideration material from the "softer" end of the science spectrum (whatever its subject), purely qualitative discussions of technique, and all material whose main subject is training, coaching, or psychology. Thus, we attempt to assess the state-of-the-art of the quantitative understanding of the mechanics and biomechanics of these events.

II. THE THROWS — GENERAL CONSIDERATIONS

All motions of the body and of the various implements used in the field events are, of course, ultimately governed by the laws of mechanics. In spite of this apparent unity, the jumps and throws differ rather qualitatively. In the jumps (high jump, long jump, triple jump, and pole vault) the motion of the body itself is of interest and the performer acts continuously throughout the motion to optimize the performance (height or distance) with muscular inputs. Thus, in any complete model of a jump both the three-dimensional motion of a multisegment model of the body and the dynamics of the various muscle groups must be accounted for — a prodigious task to say the least. An additional complication is that nearly impulsive (large magnitudes over relatively short times) forces may act at certain times which can play a large role in the eventual outcome of the jump.

The four throwing events (shot, hammer, discus, and javelin), however, consist of two phases. In the first (launch) phase which ends at release, the thrower imparts release conditions to the implement with time varying muscular inputs. In this phase the same complexity of analysis is needed as in the jumps. The second (flight) phase consists of the airborne trajectory of the implement, during which more clearly defined gravity and aerodynamic forces act. It is the interplay of these two forces and especially their relative magnitudes which determine the character of the flight trajectory of each implement and which distinguish each of the throws.

At the end of the flight phase the performance (range) is measured. Thus, the throws can be characterized as "initial condition" problems (where initial here means at release), since the differential equations which describe the flight are of the form

$$\frac{d\bar{x}}{dt} = f(\bar{x}), \quad \bar{x}(t = 0) = \bar{x}_o \tag{1}$$

and the complete evolution of the trajectory of the implement, and, therefore, the range, are uniquely specified once the initial condition $\bar{x}_o$ is chosen. (In general, the state vector $\bar{x}$ consists of the positions, orientations, velocities, and angular velocities of the thrown object.)

This characterization is useful since it relates the range to a set of conditions at a time when they are able to be influenced by the thrower, and also because it is possible to calculate either analytically or numerically the optimal set of initial conditions $\bar{x}_o$ which will maximize

Table 1
SOME PHYSICAL CHARACTERISTICS OF THE SHOT, HAMMER, DISCUS, AND JAVELIN

Properties	Shot	Hammer	Discus	Javelin
Mass (Kg)	7.260	7.260	2.0	0.80
Vol (ℓ)	0.70	0.70	0.90	1.25
Density (kg/ℓ)	10.37	10.37	2.22	0.64
Typical velocity (m/sec)	15	30	25	30
Max vacuum distance (m)	22	94	66	94
Projected area (m^2)	0.0095	0.0138	0.039	0.063
Inverse mass (kg^{-1})	0.143	0.143	0.50	1.25
Drag coefficient	0.47	0.7	1.0	1.2
"Aerodynamicity" (F_{aero}/F_{grav})	0.0086	0.075	0.764	5.33

the range. The problem for the thrower, then, is to produce this set of optimal conditions. We will discuss separately the launch and flight phases for each of the four throws. In all of the throws, because of the relative simplicity of the flight phase, much more is known about it than about the launch phase.

III. COMPARISON OF THE AERODYNAMICS OF THE JAVELIN, DISCUS, HAMMER, AND SHOT

Although the four throwing implements are affected equally by gravity, the javelin is by far the most aerodynamic. Our intuition that this might be the case is borne out by examining Table 1 in which they are compared. The first and third rows show that there are large variations in mass and density among the objects. The large variations in mass and in the rules governing the events result in sizable variations in achievable initial velocities when thrown by humans (row 4). A measure of the "aerodynamicity" is the ratio of the maximum possible aerodynamic forces which might act during flight to the constant gravity forces:[23]

$$\beta_{max} = \left(\frac{F_{aero}}{F_{grav}}\right)_{max} = \frac{\frac{\rho v^2}{2} AC}{mg} \tag{2}$$

where ρ = air density (1.23 kg/m^3), v = velocity, A = maximum projected area, C = aerodynamic coefficient, m = object mass, and g = acceleration due to gravity. The "aerodynamicity" can also be interpreted as the maximum acceleration in g's possible from aerodynamic forces during flight.

Equation 2 can be decomposed in a different way as a product of five factors:

$$\beta_{max} = \left(\frac{\rho}{2}\right)\left(\frac{v^2}{g}\right) A \left(\frac{1}{m}\right) C \tag{3}$$

atmospheric constant   throw distance in a vacuum   maximum projected area   inverse mass   shape

which measure, respectively, the contributions of air density, mass specific initial kinetic energy, size, inverse mass, and shape. The last four of these are shown in rows 5 to 8 of Table 1. In each of these last four factors, the javelin is greater than the discus and the discus is greater than the shot. The final row of Table 1 shows that the javelin, according to the measure of Equation 2, is roughly seven times as aerodynamic as the discus, the discus is more than ten times as aerodynamic as the hammer, and the hammer is approximately ten times as aerodynamic as the shot.

A clearer understanding of the effect of the "aerodynamicity" on trajectories may be obtained by examining the equation of motion for the flight of an implement thrown under windless conditions:

$$m \frac{d\bar{v}}{dt} = -m\bar{g} + F_a \bar{I}_a \qquad (4)$$

where F_a is the aerodynamic force magnitude, $\bar{v}$ is the velocity of the object, m is the object mass, $\bar{g}$ is the gravity vector, and $\bar{I}_a$ is a unit vector in the direction of the aerodynamic force (which, in general, varies during flight). Equation 4 can be written in perhaps its simplest form as

$$\frac{d\bar{v}}{dt} = -g(\bar{I}_g - \beta \bar{I}_a) \qquad (5)$$

When the aerodynamicity β is zero, the trajectory is parabolic. Thus, β_{max} is a measure of how much the trajectory departs from a purely gravitational one. When the body is spherical (shot), the aerodynamic force direction $\bar{I}_a$ is opposite to the velocity vector $\bar{v}$ and the drag force always decreases the range. In the cases of the nonspherical discus and javelin, however, the aerodynamic force can have a component (lift) perpendicular to the velocity vector, which may be used advantageously to overcome the effects of drag and extend the range beyond that achievable *in vacuo*. Thus, as the aerodynamicity varies by nearly three orders of magnitude from 0.0086 to 5.33 in Table 1, aerodynamic forces evolve from a small perturbation to a major determinant of the motion.

The general implications of Table 1 are the following. Range of the shot is not appreciably limited by drag and, thus, the trajectory of the shot may be modeled relatively accurately by neglecting drag. The zero drag assumption is less accurate for the flight of the hammer, however, and aerodynamic forces *must* be included in any model for the trajectories of the javelin and discus.

Further, for asymmetric shapes like the javelin and discus, aerodynamic forces are a function of not only the magnitude of the relative wind speed, but also the attitude of the body relative to the relative wind direction. Thus, initial attitudes and rotations of the body during flight must also be considered. In the case of the discus, its asymmetric shape makes it possible to compensate for the decreases in range due to drag, by analogous increases in range due to lift generated by appropriate discus attitudes during flight. Indeed, it has been shown by Soong[41] and also by Frolich[9] that these two factors may nearly cancel, resulting in a range in air nearly equal to that in a vacuum. The even more aerodynamic characteristics of the javelin make it possible for lift to outweigh drag substantially and for the (old) javelin to be thrown roughly 18% further in air than in a vacuum.[22] Having made these general comparisons between the flight phases of the four throws we now turn to specific events.

IV. SHOT PUT

A. Flight phase

Lichtenberg and Wills[29] have made the most comprehensive and detailed analysis of the flight of the shot put. In the first part of a two-part paper they treat the problem neglecting air resistance and derive an expression for the range R in terms of the release angle θ, release height h, and initial velocity v.

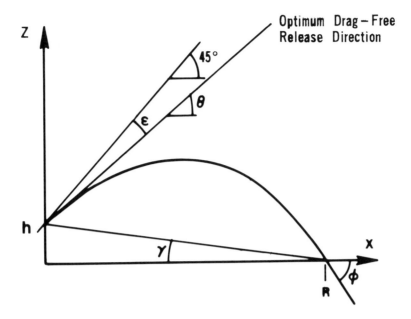

FIGURE 1. Drag-free trajectory of the shot. The optimal drag-free release angle is smaller than 45° due to non-zero release height, h. The deviation ϵ from 45° is exactly half the angle γ.

$$R = v^2 \cos \theta [\sin \theta + (\sin^2 \theta + 2gh/v^2)^{1/2}]/g \tag{6}$$

They then show that the optimal drag-free release angle θ_m which maximizes Equation 6 can be computed from

$$\sin^2 \theta_m = (2 + 2gh/v^2)^{-1} \tag{7}$$

By eliminating variables they also show that the maximum range R_m can be expressed as a function of only two variables as either

$$R_m = h \tan 2\theta_m \tag{8a}$$

or

$$R_m = (V^2/g) \cot \theta_m \tag{8b}$$

where R_m is the range attained with the optimum release angle θ_m and the given release height h and velocity v. The terminology is also shown in Figure 1.

Although it should not be necessary to point out something this fundamental, the reader should note the *quadratic dependence of the range on release velocity* in Equation 6. This functional form can be derived from purely dimensional considerations and must be considered to be the single most basic fact about throwing. Even in the events where aerodynamic forces play a larger role, throwing is essentially a struggle against gravity and the dependence of range in all throwing is roughly quadratic in velocity. We shall return to this point several times in the sequel.

In two subsequent articles in the same journal with the same title, Palffy-Muhoray and Balzarini[36] and Bose[2] show that the drag-free optimum release angle results of Lichtenberg

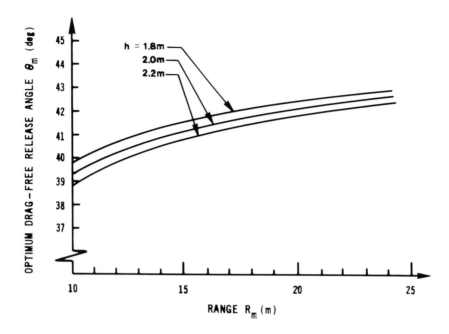

FIGURE 2.   Optimal shot drag-free release angle from Equation 9 vs. range for three values of release height. When drag is included the optimal release angle is smaller still, but only by approximately 0.1°.

and Wills[29] may be obtained without resort to calculus, using vector analysis and only high school algebra, respectively. Young[54] later used only geometry to produce the same results. Palffy-Muhoray and Balzarini[36] also note the interesting fact that when the shot travels along the "path of maximum range, the initial and final velocities are perpendicular," i.e., $\phi = 90° - \theta$ in Figure 1.

Figure 2 plots the optimum release angle θ_m given by Equation 8a vs. range R_m for three release heights, h = 1.8, 2.0, and 2.2 m, which likely bound actual release heights for most shot putters today. The main point here is that the deviation (by more than 5° for short ranges and tall putters) of the optimum release angle from 45° (the optimum in a vacuum) is due to the geometric fact that the shot is released from a non-zero height h. Notice that when h = 0, Equation 8 predicts $\theta_m = 45°$.

In an earlier purely descriptive paper devoid of mathematics, Ecker[8] described the implications of optimum release angle and noted that "the optimum angle can be (obtained) by bisecting the angle formed by a line drawn from the shot at release to the eventual landing point and a vertical line drawn through the shot." Although Ecker[8] did not offer any proof, this rule of thumb can be shown to be exactly true. Equation 8a can be rewritten as

$$\tan 2\theta_m = \frac{R_m}{h} = \cot \gamma \tag{9}$$

which implies that

$$2\theta_m = 90° - \gamma$$

or

$$\theta_m = 45° - \frac{\gamma}{2} \tag{10}$$

Thus, the deviation of the optimum release from 45° as a result of the non-zero release height h (see Figure 1) is given by

$$\epsilon = 45° - \theta_m = \frac{\gamma}{2} \qquad (11)$$

This fact was apparently first noted by Garfoot,[10] who perhaps was the source for Ecker.[8]

Equation 8 has appeared often in the shot-putting literature, apparently earliest in Garfoot[10] and later in Hay[18] and Zatsiorsky et al.,[55] and even incorrectly in Soong,[42] and clearly enjoys fairly widespread appreciation. The optimal release angle in Equation 7 has also appeared previously.[10,42]

What is less widely appreciated, however, is an assumption made in the derivation of Equation 7 and its implications. Equation 7 holds only when the velocity v is assumed to be an independent variable and *not a function of θ,* i.e., when the thrower can achieve the same release velocity independent of the release angle. If, on the other hand, the thrower can throw faster at lower angles, (which is probably the case when $\theta \simeq 40$ to 45°), then the optimum release angle must be found using constrained optimization techniques. In this case θ_m will turn out to be somewhat smaller than that predicted by Equation 7. Indeed, the measurements of mean release angles by Dessureault,[7] Groh et al.,[17] and McCoy et al.[31] lie roughly in the range of 36 to 37° and may be due to this dependence of release velocity on release angle. Apparently, no studies have ever been done to investigate this effect which is certain, in any case, to be thrower specific.

Equation 7 is the most accurate (and indeed the only exact) analytical result available for range in any of the throws. In this case, it is particularly easy to appreciate the commonly made assumption discussed above that the release velocity is independent of θ and the implications of this assumption on the calculation of the optimum release angle θ_m. However, even though the remaining three throws (hammer, discus, and javelin) are affected enough by aerodynamics to prevent a closed-form expression for the range in terms of the release conditions (the range must then be calculated by numerical integration of the equations of motion) and its subsequent functional optimization, the concept is still true:

> The optimal release conditions other than velocity depend crucially on how the maximum achievable release velocity is functionally related to the other release conditions.

Parenthetically, the series of shot put papers cited thus far illustrate some of the difficulties which are more generally found throughout the field of sport biomechanics today. Precise quantitative results, when they are available at all, tend to be generated by physicists or engineers and published in physics or engineering journals, and usually in a style more intelligible to physicists and engineers than athletes and coaches. Thus, they are not very accessible to the practitioners. Furthermore, the material which can be found in the coaching and athletic journals is a very mixed bag, is seldom stated quantitatively, and thus is usually not quantitatively verifiable. The bisection rule of thumb of Ecker[8] discussed above is the exception rather than the rule. It is thus very difficult, in the coaching literature, to separate what to believe from what to take with a grain of salt, sometimes even within the same paper.

In the second part of their paper, Lichtenberg and Wills[29] deal with the effects of air resistance. They derive an expression for the decrease in range dR_m due to drag. When there is no wind this expression reduces to

$$dR_m = -av^3/3g^2 \sin^2 \theta_m \cos \theta_m \qquad (12)$$

where a, a small parameter, is given by

$$a = CA\rho\nu/2m \tag{13}$$

and ν is a constant, approximate or "effective" velocity over the whole flight. Notice that their parameter a is approximately related to the aerodynamicity β by

$$a \approx g\beta/\nu \tag{14}$$

Dividing Equation 12 by Equation 8b we can express the percent reduction in range due to air drag as

$$\frac{dR_m}{R_m} = -\frac{a\nu}{3g \sin \theta_m \cos^2 \theta_m}$$

and using the definition of a in Equation 13 we deduce that

$$\frac{dR_m}{R_m} \approx -\frac{CA\rho\nu^2}{2mg} \frac{1}{3 \sin \theta_m \cos^2 \theta_m}$$

$$\approx \beta \frac{1}{3 \sin \theta_m \cos^2 \theta_m}$$

$$\approx \beta \quad \text{when} \quad \theta_m \approx 42° \tag{15}$$

Thus, the aerodynamicity, when it is small, is a good approximation to the percent reduction in range due to drag, regardless of the initial velocity.

Using this rule of thumb, from inspection of Table 1 we expect a reduction in range of the shot of approximately 0.8% due to drag. Lichtenberg and Wills[29] calculate that air drag decreases the range of a 21 m put only by 15 cm, agreeing very closely with the estimate from Table 1. This result has been also independently verified at different velocities by Garfoot[10] and Soong.[42]

Finally, Lichtenberg and Wills[29] derived an expression for the deviation μ of the optimum release angle from the optimum drag-free value θ_m which satisfies Equation 8a.

$$\mu = a\nu(\cos \theta_m - [\sec \theta_m]/3)/g$$

$$\approx \beta(\cos \theta_m - [\sec \theta_m]/3) \tag{16}$$

Their conclusion was that drag has a negligible effect on the optimal release angle, decreasing it by less than 0.1°, thus justifying the results obtained from the original drag-free analysis.

In summary, if we assume constant release velocity, the optimum release angle for a thrown object acted on only by drag (i.e., the shot and hammer) deviates from 45° for two reasons: (1) release occurs at non-zero height h (this deviation is given by Equation 11) and (2) drag acts on the body (this deviation is given by Equation 16). Both of these terms *decrease* the angle from 45° so that it can *never* be optimal to throw the shot or hammer at an angle exceeding 45°. In the shot put, the first effect ϵ is considerably larger than the second μ (by a factor of 20 or 40). They are more nearly equal in the hammer throw to be discussed below, because ϵ decreases with increasing range R_m while increased hammer aerodynamicity increases the second, μ. Summarizing, the optimum release angle is given by

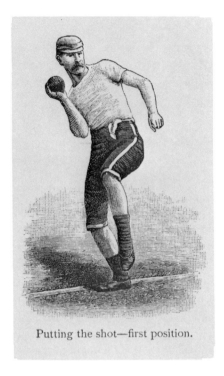

Putting the shot—first position.

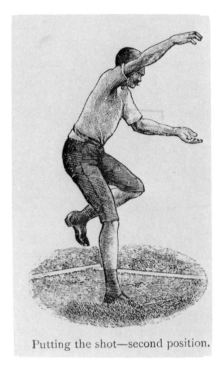

Putting the shot—second position.

FIGURE 3.   Putting the shot; the first and second positions (From Shearman, M., *Athletics and Football,* Longmans, Green, London, 1887. With permission.)

$$\theta^* = 45° - \epsilon - \mu \tag{17}$$

B. Launch Phase

The question of what the optimum technique should be during the launch phase to attain the optimum release conditions has existed for at least 100 years and probably since the event began to be standardized in the middle of the 19th century. Figure 3 portrays the beginning and ending positions of the technique recommended by Shearman[39] who wrote that "the main point to learn in weight-putting is to 'get one's weight on' . . . that is . . . to employ mere arm-work as little as possible, and to get the impetus for propulsion from a rapid spring and turn of the body.[77] Although the details of the launch have unquestionably undergone rather dramatic evolution in the last century, Shearman's synopsis is still reasonably valid.

A very complete review of the biomechanics of the shot put has been written by Zatsiorsky et al.[55] Although Equation 8 appears in their paper, it is used mostly to motivate a consideration of actions during the launch phase rather than to study the flight or to refer to optimum release conditions. We shall not attempt to improve on or repeat the review of Zatsiorsky et al.,[55] which contains a discussion of movements of body segments, lower extremities, and arms, as well as analyses of ground-reaction forces and the forces applied to the shot deduced from the inverse dynamics method.

V. HAMMER THROW

A. Flight Phase

Drag is considerably more significant in the flight of the hammer than in that of the shot. This is true mainly because the velocities are roughly twice as great. Two other factors,

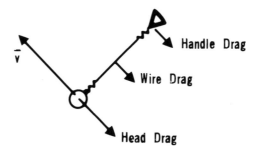

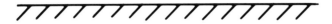

FIGURE 4.   Schematic diagram of the hammer in flight. The drag due to the wire hand handle, when it is perpendicular to the relative wind, can equal that of the head.

however, are that the projected area can be approximately 50% larger, and that the effective drag coefficient is also roughly 50% larger, because most of the handle and the cable (see Figure 4) are cylindrically ($C = 1.2$) rather than spherically ($C = 0.47$) shaped. Calculations show that the "effective" drag coefficient is roughly $C = 0.70$ in the flight position shown in Figure 4. Using this value, Equation 2 predicts that the aerodynamicity in the hammer throw can be approximately 8.7 times that of the shot.

Of course, the exact effects of drag are time-varying along the trajectory and depend on the attitude of the wire and handle relative to the flight path. When the wire and handle are oriented perpendicular to the relative wind (the worst case as shown in Figure 4), my calculations show that the drag due to the wire and handle is slightly greater than that of the head. When the handle trails the head in its wake, however, it is likely that the handle contributes very little to the total drag. Thus, as the handle moves erratically around the head during flight, the drag varies by approximately a factor of two.

Even accounting for the fact that the handle doubles the drag perhaps only approximately $7/10$ of the time, the effective aerodynamicity of the hammer is probably approximately ($1.7 \times 8.7)/2 = 7.4$ times that of the shot. Thus, $\beta_h \approx 0.064$, and from Equation 15 we would expect approximately a 6.4% reduction in range due to drag, a decrease of approximately 5.7 m in a 90-m throw.

Because the vacuum range of the hammer is roughly 90 m, and assuming (Dapena[5]) a shoulder level release height of 1.6 m, we might expect the optimum release angle to be much nearer 45° than it is in the shot put. The optimum release angle can be calculated (again assuming a constant release velocity which is independent of the release angle) by using Equation 17. The first geometric effect ϵ is basically inversely proportional to range and for a 90-m throw and a release height of 1.6 m is approximately (Equation 11).

$$\epsilon \cong \frac{1}{2}\frac{1.6}{90} \text{ rad} = 0.51°$$

The second small perturbation, μ, due to drag, is more than nine times larger than the corresponding term in the shot and is now larger than the geometric factor ϵ. Assuming $\beta_h = 0.064$ and $\theta_m = 44.49°$, we calculate using Equation 16 that $\mu = 0.90°$ and the optimum release angle for the hammer including both geometric and drag reductions is, in this example, $\theta^* = 45 - 0.51 - 0.90 = 43.59°$.

Dapena and Teves[4] studied and estimated the effects of drag on the hammer during flight. They found that air drag causes increasing effects on the length of the throw at an increasing rate with the length of the throw, a conclusion which is in agreement with the analysis presented above, that β is quadratic in velocity and thus roughly proportional to the range.

The major conclusion for the hammer, then, is that speed of release is the single most important release variable. A second conclusion is that insofar as is possible, the hammer should be released so that the handle trails the head, since the drag penalties from the wire and grip are potentially so large.

B. Launch Phase

Although there is relatively little literature dealing with the hammer throw, several studies have investigated the production of release velocity during the launch phase. Hammer speed increases gradually from roughly 10 to approximately 25 m/sec during the course of the throw, but exhibits oscillations of gradually increasing amplitude (approximately 2 m/sec at release) about the trend at the also gradually increasing turning frequency of the thrower (Dapena[5]). Two factors apparently account for most of the fluctuations in speed: gravity[5] and motion of the thrower-hammer center of mass across the circle.[6]   As yet there have been no experimental studies of the hammer throw incorporating force plates to better understand and measure the contribution of the role of the feet-ground forces on the attainment of release velocity. This appears to be a productive area for future research.

VI. DISCUS THROW

A. Flight Phase

As the aerodynamicity of the thrown object increases, the flight phase becomes more interesting and complex. The dearth of published papers regarding the hammer is in sharp contrast to a plethora of papers on the discus.

The first published scientific study of the discus was made by Taylor[44] in 1932 and was motivated by a desire to take into account the effect of wind on record throws. Wind-tunnel tests were performed to measure the lift and drag characteristics, but these results were not included in the paper. The study also used these experimental data to compute several flight trajectories, including assumed headwinds, and concluded that "the wind under certain conditions can help a throw to such an extent that it is unfair to allow it as a record."

Nearly 50 years later, similar, but more complete experimental studies were done by Cooper et al.,[3] and Ganslen.[12] Both of these studies contain published lift and drag coefficients as well as some conclusions regarding their effects on flight trajectories. Aerodynamic characteristics have also been measured by Kentzer and Hromas[27] and Tutevich.[53] Drag and lift coefficients as a function of angle of attack (the angle between the discus plane of symmetry and the relative wind vector) from all four of these authors are compared in a single figure (Figure 2) by Frolich,[9] and appear to be reasonably consistent.

Perhaps the most complete and rigorous studies of the discus are those of Soong[41] and Frolich.[9] Soong[41] draws on the scientific and engineering fluid mechanics literature (e.g., Atsumi[1] and Stilley[43]) for the aerodynamic data which form the basis of his computer simulations.

A major contribution of Soong[41] was the realization that sizable aerodynamic *torques* (as well as forces) act. These torques cause major attitude changes of the discus during flight and the inclusion of these torques in the model affects the results significantly. Specifically, the pitch attitude of the discus (together with the direction of the velocity vector) is the single most important determinant of the lift force. A rolling moment can precess the spin angular momentum, changing the pitch attitude of the discus to a possibly more advantageous position near the end of the flight when the benefits of large amounts of lift substantially

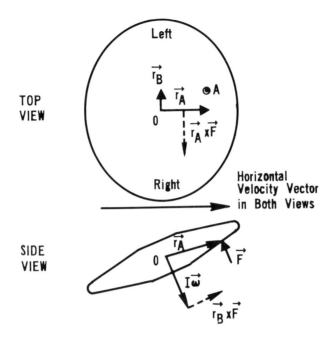

FIGURE 5. Aerodynamic torques can change the orientation of the axis of rotation of the discus during flight. The lift force, F, acts at the center of pressure, A, which is not necessarily at the center of the discus. For a discus with a positive angle of attack as shown here, the largest torques are due to the fact that the c.p. lies somewhat in front of (by distance r_A) the geometric center 0. Thus, the lift exerts a torque about the c.m. of magnitude r_AxF which causes the angular momentum vector H = Iω to precess in space and results in the right edge of the discus (as seen from the rear) to tilt slowly upwards in flight. A smaller effect is due to the relative wind speed being greater on the left side than the right because of the spin of the discus. This causes a lateral displacement of the c.p. to the left (by distance r_B). Thus, the lift also exerts a moment r_BxF which causes the front edge of the discus to tilt slowly upward during flight. This tilt can change the angle of attack and thus the magnitude of the lift later in the flight. This figure is adapted from Figure 3 in Frolich.[9]

outweigh the drawbacks due to the correspondingly large drag (see Figure 5). Unfortunately, Soong's otherwise very precise analysis falls short in certain practical areas. For example, he assumes a spin of the discus of 36.9 rev/sec, roughly five times the value of spin experimentally observed by Taylor.[44] This excessively large spin correspondingly underestimates, by a factor of five, the effect of the rolling moment in causing changes in pitch attitude.

In his paper, Frolich[9] first discusses qualitatively the effects of the three aerodynamic torques in yaw, pitch, and roll. They act to slow the spin, rotate the discus counterclockwise (the left edge moves down) as viewed from the thrower's perspective, and rotate the front edge upward, respectively. These torques are illustrated in Figure 5, which is adapted from Figure 3 of Frolich.[9] Although it is acknowledged by Frolich that the torques "are not negligible", they are nonetheless assumed to be zero in the numerical calculations and the discus attitude remains constant throughout the flight. Thus, even though Frolich[9] calculates "optimal" release conditions, it is very probable that a greater range can be obtained by somewhat different release conditions, if the gradual pitch-up caused by the rolling aerodynamic moment is accounted for in the equations of motion.

As the cost of computation has declined so dramatically during the last three decades, investigators have been willing to use more and more complex mathematical models of the dynamics of flight behavior and to draw more and more complicated conclusions. Yet the major failing of the study of Soong[41] was that too few conditions were investigated and no systematic optimization was included, although this certainly might have been done. It would seem that investigators are still too reluctant to use computational resources on a scale comparable to the human resources invested.

Indeed, this indictment can be made of all discus studies so far. They uniformly fall short in the systematic search for the optimum set of release conditions, being generally distracted by the wind, density, gravity, and other relatively peripheral effects over which the thrower has no control. While it is true that the wind can exert a major effect on the range, it makes little sense to search for optimal wind conditions, or to treat the wind in the same spirit as release conditions which *can* be determined by the thrower.

For example, Frolich[9] motivates the constant-discus-attitude (zero aerodynamic torque) simplifying the assumption discussed above, at least partly because "it is not practical to search for optimum combinations of eight variables." Yet when the list of eight variables

1. Initial rotation speed
2. Initial pitch orientation
3. Initial roll orientation
4. Initial release angle
5. Initial speed
6. Release height
7. Down-range wind magnitude
8. Cross-range wind magnitude

is examined carefully, only the first four are optimizable in any case. Numbers 5 and 6 are not optimizable because larger is always better and 7 and 8 are under noone's control, not even the weatherman! A four-dimensional optimization is not that impractical and should be the next major advance in the theory of discus flight.

Finally, it is necessary to point out once again that, as in the studies of the shot put, all the discus investigations above, including the optimization studies of Frolich,[9] assume that the release velocity is independent of the other release conditions.

In spite of the fact that much space has been devoted to a somewhat critical discussion of the papers of Soong[41] and Frolich,[9] these are unquestionably the best discus studies in the literature and contain together more insight and information than all others combined. They are strongly recommended for the reader who wishes to gain a high degree of understanding of the dynamics of discus flight.

At this point we make a brief digression. Several of the discus references and a review by Hay[18] contain considerable discussion of the significance of the angle of attack at which the maximum lift-to-drag ratio occurs. This is a concept which is used in aircraft design for problems like maximizing the steady cruising range of an aircraft, but it is absolutely irrelevant in a discussion of the (very) transient behavior of a discus (or for that matter the javelin, where similar comparisons have been made). Indeed, the concept has generated a great deal of confusion in spite of the fact that it has never explained any aspect of the discus or the javelin throws. Instead, much effort has been expended to resolve the "apparent conflicts" (Hay [18]) which arise in the confusion. It would be a welcome relief for the term, which was apparently first introduced to the discus community by Ganslen[12] and to the javelin literature in Ganslen[13] and which has enjoyed remarkable staying power in spite of its lack of relevance, to disappear quietly but entirely from the discus and javelin literature.

Several papers discuss the measurement of various release parameters in the discus throw. The most comprehensive of these, by McCoy et al.,[31] examined a total of 67 throws for four male (46 throws) and three female (21 throws) throwers, more trials than in any other such experimental study. Indeed, data were presented on at least 12 trials for five of the seven subjects and included throw distance, release angle, release height, release velocity, and trunk angle at release. Unfortunately, although the authors realized the necessity to

Table 2
RELEASE PARAMETERS IN THE DISCUS[31]

No. of throws	Female athlete	Release height (m)	Release angle (°)	Release velocity (m/sec)	Distance (m)
13	LG	1.49	32.1	24.7	55.34
		(0.12)	(2.0)	(0.5)	(1.92)
5	LD	1.61	36.7	24.9	60.82
		(0.03)	(1.4)	(0.7)	(1.74)
3	KP	1.43	35.7	22.8	55.32
		(0.05)	(1.1)	(0.7)	(1.88)

Note: Values in parentheses are standard deviations.

measure the attitude "angle of the discus . . . at release as well as throughout the flight," no information was presented on discus attitude.

One interesting result of the study of McCoy et al.[31] was precise estimates, for the first time, of how accurately and repeatedly elite discus throwers can control release parameters. For example, for the five throwers with more than 12 trials, the average release angle standard deviation was 1.94°. Furthermore, apparently, throwers also perform fairly consistently near their upper velocity limit. The average release velocity standard deviation for the same set of five throwers was 0.76 m/sec, less than 3% of the mean release velocity of 25.5 m/sec.

According to the interpretation of Figure 7 in Frolich,[9] *if the means of release angle and attitude are at optimal values,* a 2° standard deviation in both release angle and discus attitude will maintain more than 68% (±1 standard deviation) of the throws within 1 m of the optimum distance. On the other hand, if the mean values of release angle and attitude are significantly different from the optimum values, such repeatability merely guarantees that the performance will be repeatedly substandard. It thus becomes immediately clear how beneficial it might be for throwers to have such information about release conditions, not published in a journal 1 or 2 years hence, but made available to them rapidly enough to use this information in a feedback scheme to modify their mean values toward the optimum. Such a feedback scheme has been developed for the javelin throw (Hubbard and Alaways[24]) and is presently being tested.

A case in point occurs in the female throwers in Table 2 from the paper of McCoy et al.,[31] a portion of which is abstracted here in Table 2.

Subject LD attains a mean distance of 60.82 m, more than 5 m farther than LG and KP even though her mean release velocity is only 0.2 m/sec (probably much less than the measurement error) higher than LG. The reason for KP's poor performance evidently lies in her substantially lower release velocity of 22.8 m/sec. It is nearly equally evident that LG's poor performance results from the fact that her mean release conditions are not optimal for her (relatively high) release velocity. In the absence of any information about discus attitude, it is impossible to say which release conditions are the culprits, but it is clear that LG might benefit dramatically from immediate, precise, quantitative information about all her release conditions.

In a later study by some of the same authors, Gregor et al.[16] recorded the performance of all discus medalists at the 1984 Olympics. Again, however, discus attitude information is absent. Discus angles of attack have been reported by Lockwood[30] and Terauds,[48] but in each case only one throw by each thrower was analyzed, so it is impossible to gain any statistical confidence in the results. More studies are needed which are comprehensive in the sense that they focus on a relatively large number of throws by a selected group of elite

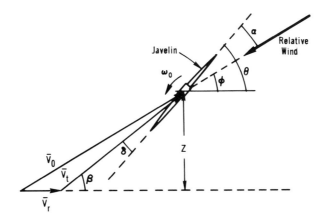

FIGURE 6. Javelin release geometry. Note a difference in terminology from Figure 1. The release angle, ϕ, between the velocity vector and the horizontal does not necessarily equal the javelin attitude angle, θ. When there is no wind, the difference, α, is the angle of attack, the most important variable on which the aerodynamic forces and moments depend. All angles change substantially and continuously during flight. Total javelin velocity is the sum of run-up velocity, v_r and throw velocity, v_t. Thus, a javelin thrown through the point can still have an initial angle of attack even when no transverse vibrations are induced and $\delta = 0$.

athletes, as in McCoy et al.,[31] and which are more complete in that they measure all relevant variables, including discus roll and pitch, release attitude, as well as velocity and release angle, and perhaps even spin rate.

B. Launch Phase

A good summary of the techniques generally thought to result in good throws is contained in Hay,[18] which discusses initial body positioning, preliminary swings, transition to the turn, the turn, and delivery.

VII. JAVELIN THROW

A. Flight Phase

The development of our understanding of the flight of the javelin has followed a course similar to that of the discus, but delayed somewhat in time. Ganslen and Hall[11] were the first to study experimentally the aerodynamic characteristics of the javelin, which had evolved rapidly and dramatically in the late 1950s to a design which then remained nearly constant until 1985.

Ganslen and Hall[11] first measured the lift and drag forces which act on the javelin as a function of angle of attack, α, defined as the angle between the javelin long axis and the relative wind vector as shown in Figure 6. Note that the terminology used in Figure 6 is different from that used in Figure 1. In work truly advanced and unusual for its time, Ganslen[13] later attempted unsuccessfully to use the theory of cross-flow aerodynamics to predict the aerodynamic characteristics (lift, drag, and pitching moment) of the javelin, given its shape. Lift and drag forces are not too sensitve to shape and thus are relatively easy to predict. They are a fairly direct function of platform area, dynamic pressure, and a cross-flow drag coefficient which is reasonably straightforward to estimate, since the javelin cross section is so nearly cylindrical. The pitching moment, however, is a different matter. I have made similar, equally unsuccessful attempts at predicting pitching moments using the cross-flow theory and known javelin shape, and now believe that a full three-dimensional solution of the inviscid Navier-Stokes equations will be required.

The payoffs for the successful solution of this problem are obvious, since such predictive capability would allow one to design an optimal javelin. A fascinating series of correspondence (Millikan[34] and Royce[38]) with aeronautical researchers at Cal Tech documents Ganslen's attempts to make the shape-aerodynamics connection. Meanwhile, back in the real world, javelin design was proceeding by trial and error with the resultant refinement of the so-called 'aerodynamic' javelin, whose characteristics are described more completely below.

Somewhat later, Terauds[45] did an experimental study of 14 different javelin models, which included measuring their aerodynamic characteristics in constant - velocity wind - tunnel tests as well as experimentally launching javelins under controlled conditions to study their flight characteristics. Data from this study were also later published separately in Terauds.[46] This work is very important since it is the last published experimental data on which theoretical predictions of javelin flight behavior and optimization of release conditions can be based. A little known aspect of Terauds'[45] work is the fact that, apparently due to the limitations of the wind tunnel and force balance equipment used, all the data were gathered at free stream velocities (89.4 m/sec) and Reynolds numbers roughly a factor of three larger than those corresponding to typical world-class release velocities. Although this was not felt to be a problem by Terauds, it still has not been verified experimentally that the Reynolds number dependence of the shape of the lift, drag, and (especially) pitching moment curves is negligible. This must be regarded as an extremely important item for resolution in the next series of javelin wind-tunnel experiments, whenever they may occur.

Terauds'[46] experimental data for three aerodynamic javelins are shown in Figure 7. Analogous to the sensitivity and difficulty which were found in the attempts at theoretical prediction of lift, drag, and pitching moments, the experimental lift and drag curves in Figure 7A are quite repeatable, but the pitching moments shown in Figure 7B vary considerably more from javelin to javelin. It is presumably the small variations in the shapes of the three javelins which cause the quite different pitching-moment profiles, while at the same time perturbing the lift and drag curves nearly imperceptibly. Each pitching-moment curve of an old "aerodynamic" javelin has three equilibrium points (two stable and one unstable), which is evidence that the center of pressure (CP) moves back and forth, first behind, then in front of, and then again behind the center of mass (CM) as the angle of attack is increased. Three of these, (H-70, H-90, and SSE) are shown in Figure 7B.

The practical implication of the largest equilibrium angle of attack (which is also stable) is that the javelin is capable of generating sustained large amounts of lift at angles of attack near 30°, since there is a restoring action of the pitching moment to that angle of attack in flight. A concomitant implication is that the javelin attitude dynamics are unstable in the neighborhood of the second equilibrium (near 10°) and that positive pitching moments are produced for angles of attack between 10 and 30°. This pitching-moment shape was a feature of virtually all javelin designs, until the javelin construction rules were changed by the IAAF in 1984 as discussed further below.

Athough both Ganslen[13] and Terauds[45] had all the information required (aerodynamic forces and moments) for the prediction of flight trajectories and in-depth computer studies, apparently neither of them took this next logical step. In the first theoretical and numerical study of the flight of the javelin, Soong[40] derived equations of motion and investigated the effects of various throw parameters including initial javelin attitude angle, flight-path angle, position of the center of pressure, d, and wind speed. The results showed how range, time of flight, and entry angle changed as a function of these parameters.

While it is true that in any mathematical model of this sort many assumptions and approximations must be made, two of Soong's assumptions were somewhat unrealistic and had the largest effect on his results. These assumptions were that:

1.   The initial velocity attainable by the thrower is independent of throwing angle (the initial javelin velocity was held constant at 30.45 m/sec in all calculations)

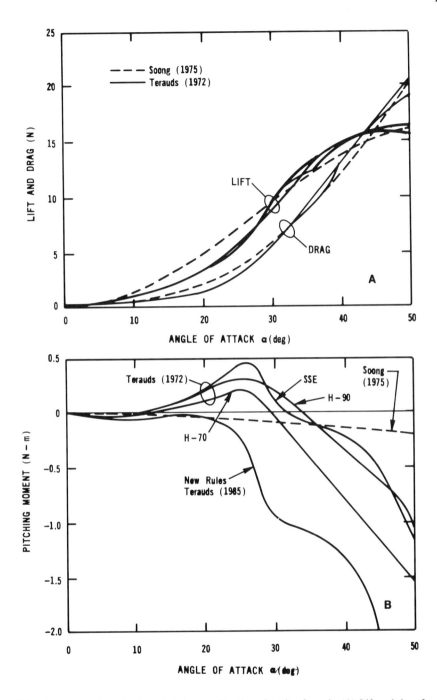

FIGURE 7. Javelin aerodynamic characteristics as a function of angle of attack. (A) Lift and drag forces are nearly the same from javelin to javelin, depending mostly on planform area. (B) Pitching moments, on the other hand are a strong function of javelin shape and vary markedly from javelin to javelin. Old "aerodynamic" javelins are characterized by three equilibrium angles of attack, but the New Rules javelin has a monotonic decreasing profile.

2. The pitching moment is the moment of the lift and drag acting at the center of pressure *which remains at a fixed distance, d from the CM even as the angle of attack changes*

Given the preceding assumptions, among Soong's conclusions were that (1) the initial release angle (ϕ in Figure 6) is more influential on distance than is initial javelin attitude, θ; (2) the optimum throw angle for the NCAA official javelin (which was calculated by Soong[40] to have d = 25.7 cm) was approximately 43° and would decrease to near 35° when d = 0.8 cm; and (3) shifting the center of pressure to d = 0.8 cm could result in a dramatic increase in range of approximately 16 m to 106 m.

Red and Zogaib[37] questioned the validity of the first assumption above. They presented experimental results from three throwers which showed that the attainable initial velocity decreases markedly with throwing angle. They then incorporated this dependence into a numerical solution of the equations of motion similar to that in Soong.[40] Their results showed that the throwers' inability to throw as fast at larger throw angles implied that the optimum throw angle remains aproximately 37°, independent of d.

To the author's knowledge, the work of Red and Zogaib[37] is the first and only study ever done for any throwing event in which the dependence of release velocity on release angle was measured. As such, it is a very important paper, one which should serve as an impetus for similar such studies for the other throwing events, although the experimental techniques might be improved somewhat. As pointed out in the discussions of the shot, hammer, and discus above, this sort of information is essential before meaningful optimization studies can be done.

The remaining limitations common to the models of Soong[40] and Red and Zogaib,[37] namely,

1. The unrealistic assumption of a *constant* center of pressure location
2. The assumption of zero pitching-angular velocity (rotation about the javelin short axis)

were removed by Hubbard and Rust.[20,21] In Hubbard and Rust,[20] the lift, drag, and pitching moments measured by Terauds[45,46] were included in a computer-simulation model. It was shown that most javelin pitching-moment profiles are not adequately approximated by a fixed center of pressure, and that the optimal release conditions for a given javelin depend on its particular aerodynamic characteristics.

Hubbard and Rust[21] presented a model which included non-zero initial pitching-angular velocity (ω_o in Figure 6). They gave a complete description of the evolution of the javelin orientation and other states during a typical good throw. They concluded that a good throw with the old aerodynamic javelin consists of two parts (see Figure 8B). The first portion has small angles of attack, lift, and drag, and flows continuously into a second part during which angle of attack, lift, and drag all increase to relatively large peaks before becoming smaller again. In this way, early drag is minimized while the substantial lift which can prolong ground contact is programmed correctly for the end of the flight. The correct magnitude for the pitching-angular velocity plays a very important role in allowing this trade-off to occur and, indeed, correctly chosen, can result in an increase in range of 4 m (roughly 4% at world-class distances).

The final drawback of the work of Soong,[40] and Red and Zogaib[37] was that their conclusions about optimal release conditions were drawn based on far too few simulations. They did not investigate thoroughly the complete initial condition space, neglecting entirely the pitch-ing-angular velocity (which was assumed to be zero) and relying instead on a somewhat sketchy sampling of the release angle-angle of attack space. Hubbard[22] for the first time, removed all restrictions and allowed all three optimizable initial conditions (release angle, angle of attack, and pitching-angular velocity) to assume arbitrary values. Nonlinear optim-

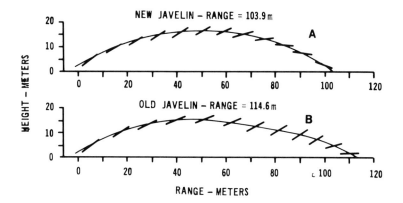

FIGURE 8. Comparison of flight of (A) new rules and (B) old javelins when thrown with the same release velocity, v = 31.1 m/sec. The optimal trajectory of the old javelin included large angles of attack (and thus, large lift) near the end of the flight. The changed pitching-moment profile of the New Rules javelin now makes such late lift impossible, and thus, the optimal range of the new javelin has been decreased by more than 10%.

ization techniques were then used to calculate the optimal set of release conditions (ϕ_o, θ_o, ω_o), given a release velocity and release height.

Included in the optimization calculations of Hubbard[22] was the additional realistic assumption, first verified by Red and Zogaib[37] and discussed extensively previously, that maximal achievable release velocity varies inversely with release angle. The best fit of Red and Zogaib[37] to their experimental data predicts that, in the neighborhood of a release angle of 35°, a decrease in release angle of 10° results in an increase in release velocity of approximately 1.27 m/sec. Expressed quantitatively this becomes

$$v = v_{nom} + 0.127* (\phi - 35°) \tag{18}$$

On first glance, 0.127 m/sec/° seems to be a very small sensitivity indeed, being a change of only 4 or 5% in velocity for a 30% change in angle. It cannot be overemphasized, however, how important a role this apparently small sensitivity plays in the ultimate optimization calculations. Figure 9, adapted from Hubbard,[22] shows contours of constant range as a function of angle of attack and release angle, assuming zero pitching-angular velocity. Shown in Figures 9A and 9B are the two cases where the velocity-release-angle sensitivity is assumed to be 0 and 0.127, respectively, all other variables being held constant. As is clear from the figure, *the difference in only this one assumption changes the optimal release angle from 42 to 30 °!* This example shows how important the release-velocity characteristics of the thrower are and how important it will be in the future to investigate this phenomenon more carefully, in all the throwing events.

When the javelin is released with other than a fork grip, the major component of the angular velocity is its spin about the long axis of symmetry. This spin has been measured to be as large as 22 rev/sec by Terauds.[49] Because the mass moment of inertia is so small about this axis (less than 1/1000 that about its short axis), however, there is very little associated angular momentum in this direction and, thus, it is believed by this author that the spin has very little, if any effect on the flight, even though Hay[18] states that spin "is generally considered to have a beneficial stabilizing effect."

B. New Rules Javelin

Javelin experts debated for nearly a decade (for example, see Held[19] and Ganslen[14]) before the IAAF finally voted in 1984 to change the rules for construction of the javelin. Several factors motivated this change:

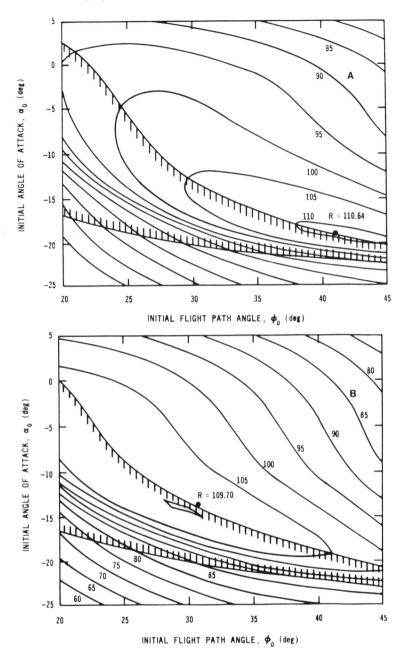

FIGURE 9.   Contours of constant range vs. angle of attack and release angle (A) Release velocity independent of release angle. (B) Release velocity decreases with release angle according to Equation 18. Both (A) and (B) assume *zero* initial angular-pitching velocity, ω_0. Flat throws occur for initial conditions between the hachured lines. The inclusion of the relatively small dependence of release velocity on release angle given by Equation 18, causes a large change in the optimal release conditions.

1.   The world record had increased to nearly 105 m, making it increasingly difficult to hold the event inside the typically 100-m-long stadia throughout the world
2.   The pitching-moment characteristics of the old aerodynamic javelin described above, implied that the old javelin was unstable in yaw as well as pitch, frequently causing erratic and dangerous throws which endangered spectators and officials
3.   The optimal release characteristics for the old javelin resulted in many nearly flat throws, placing large pressure on officials to determine whether a throw was fair or not

The rule change, which took effect in April 1986, essentially moved the CM forward while restricting the shape, thus effectively prohibiting the center of pressure from being moved forward as well. Thus, it is now practically impossible (although the manufacturers continue to try) to obtain a pitching-moment-angle of attack profile with a positive section between 10 and 30° as shown in Figure 7. Instead, the pitching-moment profile is guaranteed to be monotonic decreasing.

Also shown in Figure 7B (and labeled New Rules) is an estimate, from Appendix C of a recent book by Terauds,[51] of the pitching-moment profile for a javelin which conforms to the new rules. Although the data in this Appendix are presented to three significant decimals in the same format as the wind-tunnel experimental measurements in Terauds[45] and are entitled "Javelin Aerodynamic Test", the data were in fact, not measured in wind-tunnel tests at all (Terauds[52]). Instead they are merely three significant digit "estimates" of what the actual lift, drag, and pitching-moment curves of the new rules javelin might be. Although this is misleading, to say the least, these estimates are probably not too inaccurate and have been used for the lack of any actual experimental data in computer simulations of the flight of the new rules javelins (Hubbard and Alaways[25]). Indeed, except for an unpublished study made by a University of Washington undergraduate student, P. Bogataj, in 1984, there have been no actual wind-tunnel tests of any javelins whatsoever since those reported in Terauds[45] in 1972. In order for continued optimization studies such as those in Hubbard[22] to be possible for new versions of the new rules javelin, it is essential that actual wind-tunnel tests be conducted on the new javelin designs.

C. Launch Phase
Good discussions of throwing techniques prior to and during the launch phase may be found in Hay[18] and in Terauds.[51] The latter book has entire chapters devoted to the grip, carry, run and transition, and the throw, respectively.

Investigators have often measured various javelin-release conditions. Many of these studies have dealt, in some form or another, with the launch phase. Ikegami et al.[26] and Miller and Munro[33] both focused on the acceleration phase of the throw, which lasts only 150 msec. Ikegami et al.[26] give data from throwers of three experience levels. The information about the acceleration phase in Miller and Munro[33] is considerably more accurate and detailed, however, because a 200-Hz (rather than a 60-Hz) camera was used. Indeed, although not explicitly stated in the paper, the accelerations presented appear to include effects from the vibrations of the javelin induced by the pulldown during the throw, perhaps the first time this has been observed. Miller and Munro[33] also computed release angle, release velocity, and angle of attack for 27 throws of 8 male throwers, including as many as 6 throws for one thrower. This paper contains the most comprehensive data in the experimental-javelin literature.

Two papers by Terauds[47,49] both focused on throwers in international or Olympic competition so that the skill of the throwers was very high, but relatively fewer throwers were analyzed. Of all the above experimental-javelin papers, however, that of Miller and Munro[33] contains the best discussion of the accuracy (or lack thereof) with which the various mea-

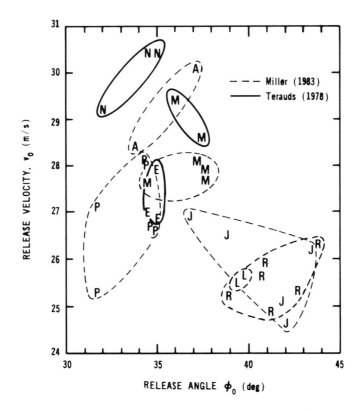

FIGURE 10.   Measured javelin release velocity vs. release angle for nine throwers from two sources. Individual throwers' data are encircled. Thrower repeatability varies. Too little data for each thrower over too small a range of release angles exists here to measure the important, thrower-specific sensitivity of release velocity to release angle referred to in the text.

surements can be made; a necessary part of any presentation of experimental data. For example, they estimated that the javelin-release velocity magnitude and direction were accurate to only 1 m/sec and 1° (4 and 3%), respectively.

Figure 10 shows release velocity plotted against release angle using experimental data of Miller and Munro[33] and Terauds.[49] The data-points are identified by letters corresponding to each thrower. From the figure it is possible to estimate the consistency with which a given thrower is able to control these two release conditions. Apparently, it is possible to control release angle within a degree or two, but it is hard to believe that all the throwers portrayed are throwing with optimal release conditions for their achievable velocities, even if they are reasonably repeatable.

Gregor and Pink[15] have reported the release conditions for the world-record throw by Petranoff which occurred in May 1983. Another paper (Terauds[50]) which discusses this same throw, among others, was the first paper ever to report measurements of javelin initial pitching-angular velocity at release. Apparently, this is because the importance of this variable to the flight was only recently discovered (Hubbard[22]) and also because it is extremely difficult to measure this quantity accurately. In Terauds[50] and also in Terauds[51] are presented the results of a throw with the following release conditions:

Release velocity	30.17 m/sec
Release angle	31°
Angle of attack	7.5°
Pitching-angular velocity	−53°/sec
Range	88.48 m

The difficulty of accurately determining the pitching-angular velocity is underscored by these data. The value of $-53°$/sec above seems highly unlikely, since computer simulations show that a javelin released with these conditions can only travel approximately 54 m. The trajectory is extremely pathological, exhibiting a negative angle of attack during the last half of the trajectory. The javelin noses down so much that it goes end-over-end and has an entry angle of approximately 100°, striking the ground with the tail further from the thrower than the tip!

The main problem in the calculations is that the determination of (linear and angular) velocities from camera or video position data involves differentiation or differencing. The sizable vibrations present in the javelin at release can cause correspondingly sizable motions of the points on the javelin whose positions are being differenced to compute the velocities. Thus, the vibratory motions act as noise and, unless they are either filtered or accounted for explicitly in the calculations, can result in unrealistic numbers such as the one above. Even when care is taken to minimize the adverse effects of the vibrations, typical measurement inaccuracies can result in uncertainties for the pitching-angular velocity as large as 6°/sec (Hubbard and Alaways[24]).

Most recently, a study of selected throwers at the 1984 Olympics has appeared (Komi and Mero[28]). This paper has data for 11 men and women throwers, but for only one throw each. Again, the standard data (release angle, velocity, and angle of attack) are presented, but most of the paper is devoted to a discussion of measurements of other biomechanical parameters during the launch phase such as positions and velocities of the elbow angle, knee joint, and whole body CG (center of gravity).

The paper of Komi and Mero[28] is somewhat disappointing in its demonstration of a lack of understanding of fundamentals. For example, a major conclusion in the abstract is that "despite great variation in throwing distance in women (55.88 m to 69.56 m) the release velocities were in **the** relatively small range (20.73 m/sec to 23.62 m/sec)." This statement entirely misses the absolutely basic point discussed earlier that *the dependence of range in all throwing is roughly quadratic in velocity*. The range of velocities observed (23.62/20.73 = 1.139) should be expected to lead to a *larger* range of distances (1.139*1.139 = 1.298) than that observed (69.56/55.88 = 1.245), not smaller. An additional disappointment is that so little data are presented for each thrower.

A single major criticism can be leveled at almost all experimental studies of the javelin thus far (and, indeed, at the experimental studies of the other throws). This is that there have been almost no carefully designed, exhaustive experiments with the variables which are hypothesized to have an influence, carefully and precisely controlled and containing many throws from a single thrower.

Rather, the investigators have chosen major international competitions (e.g., the Olympics) where the circumstances are almost certain to preclude careful experimental technique and certainly preclude thoughtful experimental design. In addition, in most cases not enough throws have been analyzed to gain the statistical confidence necessary to make regression studies valid and meaningful. Nevertheless, regressions have often been done, sometimes with a clear paucity of data. *Linear* regression coefficients have generally been reported between velocity and range in spite of the fact that *range is quadratic in velocity*. A much more logical procedure would be a linear regression between the square of release velocity and the range.

As an illustration of this point, Figure 11 shows the results of optimization studies which have been done for the new rules javelin (Hubbard and Alaways[25]). Optimal release conditions were calculated using the techniques described in Hubbard and Rust[21] and Hubbard.[22] Shown in Figure 11 is the resulting optimal range vs. release velocity which was calculated for velocities in the range $20 < v_o < 35$ m/sec together with a second-order polynomial regression fitted to the data.

R = 1.248 + 0.0397v + 0.1088v^2   r= 1.00

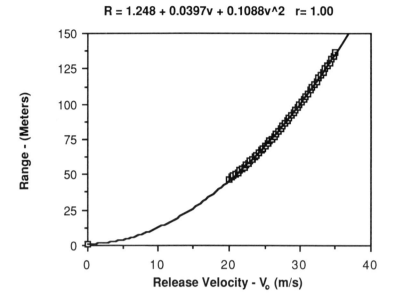

FIGURE 11.   Optimal range vs. release velocity for the New Rules javelin. A polynomial regression shows that the main dependence of range on velocity is quadratic with a coefficient, 0.1088, nearly exactly that which would be predicted (1/g) from a drag-free analysis.

$$R = 1.248 + 0.0397\, v_o + 0.1088\, v_o^2 \tag{19}$$

For an initial velocity near 30 m/sec, the optimum release angle from Equation 7 is 44.4°, and if there were no aerodynamic forces whatsoever, the vacuum range would be given nearly exactly by Equation 8b.

$$R = v_o^2/g = 0.1041\, v_o^2$$

Thus, the appearance of a linear coefficient in Equation 19 and the departure of the quadratic coefficient in Equation 19 from 0.1041 are measures of the contribution of aerodynamics to the range. In this case, the quadratic coefficient is clearly very close to that expected from gravity alone. For $v_o = 30$ m/sec the linear and quadratic terms add 1.19 and 4.23 m, respectively, to the range achievable in a vacuum.

Although optimizations over a similar wide range of velocities have not been done for the old javelin, we can state with reasonable certainty that even larger quadratic and linear coefficients would have resulted than those in Equation 19. Thus, the main effect of the rule change has been to severely limit the effects of the javelin's potentially very large aerodynamic contribution to range. Notice, however, that when $v_o = 30$ m/sec even the new rules javelin can be thrown approximately 5% further in air than in a vacuum.

ACKNOWLEDGMENT

This work was partially supported by a grant from the U.S. Olympic Committee.

REFERENCES

1. **Atsumi, S.,** Pressure distribution on a wing with circular plan form, *J. Aeronautical Sci.,* p. 499, October 1973.
2. **Bose, S. K.,** Maximizing the range of the shot put without calculus, *Am. J. Phys.,* 51, 458, 1983.
3. **Cooper, I., Dalzell, D., and Silverman, E.,** *Flight of the Discus,* Division of Engineering Science, Purdue University, Lafayette, 1959.
4. **Dapena, J. and Teves, M. A.,** Influence of the diameter of the hammer head on the distance of a hammer throw, *Res. Q.,* 53, 78, 1982.
5. **Dapena, J.,** Pattern of hammer speed during a hammer throw and influence of gravity on its fluctuations, *J. Biomech.,* 17, 553, 1984.
6. **Dapena, J.,** Factors affecting the fluctuations of hammer speed in a throw, in *Biomechanics IX-B,* Winter, D. A. et al., Eds., Human Kinetics Publishers, Champaign, Ill., 1985, 499.
7. **Dessureault, J.,** Selected kinetic and kinematic factors involved in shot putting, in *Biomechanics VI-B,* Assmussen, E. and Jorgensen, J., Eds., Human Kinetics Publishers, Champaign, Ill., 1978, 51.
8. **Ecker, T.,** Angle of release in shot putting, *Athletic J.,* 50, 52, 1970.
9. **Frolich, C.,** Aerodynamic effects on discus flight, *Am. J. Phys.,* 49, 1125, 1981.
10. **Garfoot, B. P.,** Analysis of the trajectory of the shot, *Track Tech.,* 32, 1003, 1968.
11. **Ganslen, R. V. and Hall, K. G.,** *Aerodynamics of Javelin Flight,* University of Arkansas, Fayetteville, 1960.
12. **Ganslen, R. V.,** Aerodynamic and mechanical forces in discus flight, *Athletic J.,* 44, 68, 1964.
13. **Ganslen, R. V.,** Javelin aerodynamics, *Track Tech.,* 30, 940, 1967.
14. **Ganslen, R. V.,** A critique of javelin behavior and design influencing international design specifications, *Track and Field J.,* 14, 13, 1982.
15. **Gregor, R. J. and Pink, M.,** Biomechanical analysis of a world record javelin throw: a case study, *Intl. J. Sport Biomech.,* 1, 73, 1985.
16. **Gregor, R. J., Whiting, W. C., and McCoy, R. W.,** Kinematic analysis of Olympic discus throwers, *Intl. J. Sport Biomech.,* 1, 131, 1985.
17. **Groh, H., Kuboth, A., and Baumann, W.,** De la cinétique et de la dynamique des movements corporels rapides, étude concernant les phases finales du lance du poids et du javelot, *Sportarzt,* 10, 1966.
18. **Hay, J. G.,** *Biomechanics of Sports Techniques,* 3rd ed., Prentice-Hall, Englewood Cliffs, N.J., 1985.
19. **Held, D.,** Proposed rule change on flat javelin landings, *Track Tech.,* 78, 2478, 1980.
20. **Hubbard, M. and Rust, H. J.,** Javelin dynamics with measured lift drag and pitching moment, *J. Appl. Mech.,* 51, 406, 1984.
21. **Hubbard, M. and Rust, H. J.,** Simulation of javelin flight using experimental aerodynamic data, *J. Biomech.,* 17, 769, 1984.
22. **Hubbard, M.,** Optimal javelin trajectories, *J. Biomech.,* 17, 777, 1984.
23. **Hubbard, M.,** Javelin trajectory simulation and its use in coaching, in *Proc. Intl. Symp. Biomech. Sports,* Academic Publishers, Del Mar, Calif., 1984b.
24. **Hubbard, M. and Alaways, L.,** Rapid and accurate estimation of release conditions in the javelin throw, in press, 1988.
25. **Hubbard, M. and Alaways, L.,** Optimal release conditions for the New Rules javelin, *Intl. J. Sport Biomech.,* 3, 207, 1987.
26. **Ikegami, Y., Miura, M., Matsui, H., and Hashimoto, I.,** Biomechanical analysis of the javelin throw, in *Biomechanics VII-B,* Morecki, A. et al., Eds., University Park Press, Baltimore. Md. 1981, 271.
27. **Kentzer, C. P. and Hromas, L. A.,** *Discobulus,* 4, 1, 1958.
28. **Komi, P. V. and Mero, A.,** Biomechanical analysis of Olympic javelin throwers, *Intl. J. Sports Biomech.,* 1, 139, 1985.
29. **Lichtenberg, D. B. and Wills, J. G.,** Maximizing the range of the shot put, *Am. J. Phys.,* 46, 546, 1978.
30. **Lockwood, H. H.,** Throwing the discus, in *Athletics,* Pearson, G. F. D., Ed., Thomas Nelson and Sons, Edinburgh, 1963.
31. **McCoy, R. W., Gregor, R. J., Whiting, W. C., Rich, R. G., and Ward, P. E.,** Kinematic analysis of elite shotputters, *Track Tech.,* 90, 2868, 1984.
32. **McCoy, R. W., Whiting, W. C., Rich, R. G., and Gregor, R. J.,** Kinematic analysis of discus throwers, *Track Tech.,* 91, 2902, 1985.
33. **Miller, D. I. and Munro, C. F.,** Javelin position and velocity patterns during final foot plant preceding release, *J. Hum. Movement Stud.,* 9, 1, 1983.
34. **Millikan, C. B.,** Letter to R. V. Ganslen dated August 20, 1954.
35. **Moore, K.,** Talk about a change of pace, *Sports Illustrated.* 65, 52, 1986.
36. **Palffy-Muhoray, R. and Balzarini, D.,** Maximizing the range of the shot put without calculus, *Am. J. Phys.,* 50, 181, 1982.

37. **Red, W. E. and Zogaib, A. J.,** Javelin dynamics including body interaction, *J. Appl. Mech.,* 44, 496, 1977.
38. **Royce, W. W.,** Letters to R. V. Ganslen dated November 23, 1959 and January 13, 1960.
39. **Shearman, M.,** *Athletics and Football,* Longmans, Green, London, 1887.
40. **Soong, T. C.,** The dynamics of javelin throw, *J. Appl. Mech.,* 42, 257, 1975.
41. **Soong, T. C.,** The dynamics of discus throw, *J. Appl. Mech.,* 43, 531, 1976.
42. **Soong, T. C.,** Biomechanical (analyses and applications) of shot put and discus and javelin throws, in *Human Body Dynamics: Impact, Occupational and Athletic Aspects,* Ghista, D. N., Ed., Clarendon Press, Oxford, 1982, 462.
43. **Stilley, G. D.,** Aerodynamic analysis of the self sustained flare, AD-740117, Naval Ammunition Depot, Crane, Ind., October 1972.
44. **Taylor, J. A.,** Behavior of the discus in flight, *Athletic J.,* 12, 9, 1932.
45. **Terauds, J.,** A Comparative Analysis of the Aerodynamic and Ballistic Characteristics of Competition Javelins, Ph.D. thesis, University of Maryland, College Park, 1972.
46. **Terauds, J.,** Wind tunnel tests of competition javelins, *Track and Field Q. Rev.,* 74, 88, 1974.
47. **Terauds, J.,** Javelin release characteristics, *Track Tech.,* 61, p1945, 1975.
48. **Terauds, J.,** Technical analysis of the discus, *Scholastic Coach,* 47, 98, 1978.
49. **Terauds, J.,** Computerized biomechanical analysis of selected javelin throwers at the 1976 Montreal Olympiad, *Track and Field Q. Rev.,* 78(1), 29, 1978.
50. **Terauds, J.,** Biomechanics of Tom Petranoff's javelin throw, *Can. Track and Field J.,* as cited in Reference 51, 1983.
51. **Terauds, J.,** *Biomechanics of the Javelin Throw,* Academic Publishers, Del Mar, Calif., 1985, 121.
52. **Terauds, J.,** personal communication, December 14, 1985.
53. **Tutevich, V. N.,** *Teoria Sportivnykh Metanii,* Moscow, 1969.
54. **Young, W. M.,** Maximizing the range of the shot put using a simple geometrical approach, *Am. J. Phys.,* 53, 84, 1985.
55. **Zatsiorsky, V. M., Lanka, G. E., and Shalmanov, A. A.,** Biomechanical analysis of shot putting technique, *Exercise Sport Sci. Rev.,* 9, 353, 1981.

Chapter 7

SKI-JUMPING, ALPINE-, CROSS-COUNTRY-, AND NORDIC-COMBINATION SKIING

Kazuhiko Watanabe

TABLE OF CONTENTS

I. INTRODUCTION

Recent developments in sports biomechanics, which cover many sports including skiing, could have a strong impact on coaching and training methods. A knowledge of sports biomechanics has in the past been applied to ski coaching and to training, and in some cases this has led to an improvement in performance. In an actual ski competition, athletes can sometimes only win the event by adopting principles of skiing techniques which are based on biomechanical investigation. For example, in the history of ski jumping, there has been a big change in body motion during the air phase which was strongly influenced by the results of biomechanical investigation. It is not surprising, therefore, that in recent years biomechanical information has become more attractive for many coaches. These powerful developments in sports biomechanics will bring significant benefits to top athletes and also to beginners for their safety and recreational enjoyment.

In this chapter I shall introduce some articles which relate to coaching and training for top athletes and also for recreational skiers. One of the goals of biomechanical study in skiing should be to present an excellent coaching and training system for skiers.

The following items will be covered: ski jumping, alpine skiing, cross-country skiing, nordic combination, basic skiing movement, and safety. Lastly, the idea of integrating the diverse research concerning ski science into an effective coaching and training system will be presented.

II. SKI JUMPING

A. Approach Phase

Recently, top athletes have adopted an "arms in back" position during the approach phase. Traditionally, the "arms in front" position was a very popular one, but this changed just before the Lake Placid Winter Olympic Games in 1980. After the Games there were few athletes who produced the "arms in front" position.

One question which was asked by coaches and athletes was which is the better technique? However, there were quite a bit of data on this point. Among the top nine Japanese athletes, six preferred the "arms in back" position in generating the vertical component of the force during simulated jumping.[1] However, statistically there was no significant difference between them. It seems that the "arms in back" position has the merit of allowing the jumper to adapt more quickly to the next flight position in the air. At the takeoff point, the simulated jumping experiment showed that the EMG activity of the deltoid muscle was already finished in the "arms in back" position (which meant that the arms were adapting to the next phase in the air), but was still active in the "arms in front" position. It would seem that in the "arms in back" position, there is the possibility of adapting to the flight position more quickly as seen in Figure 1.

The effect of arm position on the line of gravity was almost the same, but with the "arms in back" position the EMG activity from the tibialis anterior was larger than in the "arms in front" position. These results suggested that the action of this muscle was necessary to move the jumper's center of gravity (CG) from a backward to a more natural position.

From a historical standpoint, the jumping form has been produced by shifting from a more natural behavior of the human body to a more unusual and difficult one. In young jumpers or in the training of beginners, there may be a possibility that the "classic" approach style of the "arms in front" position would have merit for those jumpers who need to develop a stable jump skill in basic training.

The hands position should also be mentioned when considering approach speed. It is recommended that the hands be kept tightly along the trunk, thereby reducing air resistance.

With regard to foot spacing, the vertical jump test and simulated jumping were performed

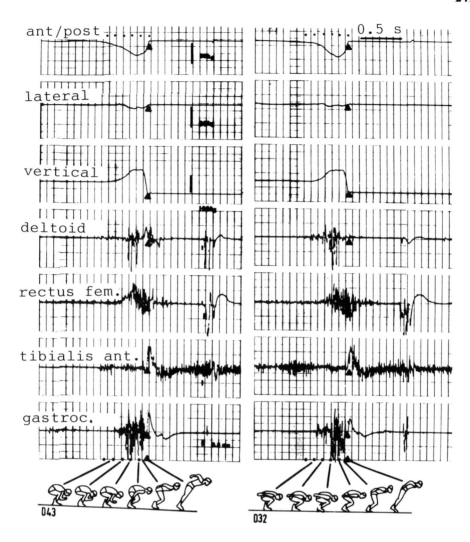

FIGURE 1. Comparison of different arm actions for the approach motion of simulated jumping. On the right side, jumping with the arms in the backward position allowed easier adaptation to flight phase because the EMG activity of the deltoid finished well before take-off.

by using a Kistler force plate and a 16-mm high-speed movie camera.[2] The foot spacing was set at five conditions: 0, 10, 20, and 40 cm, and free. The free foot space was between 10 and 20 cm (14.3 cm on average) for all athletes. There were no statistically significant differences in simulated jumping, either in production or in the initial vertical-jumping velocity, except for the 40-cm spacing. In the case of 40-cm foot spacing, the vertical jumping performance was clearly decreased, but the 20-cm foot spacing also showed a slight tendency towards decreased vertical jumping performance on average. In an actual condition at Lake Placid just prior to the Olympic Games, we measured foot spacing of 14.0 cm in the 70-m class and 17.8 cm in the 90-m class. From observations of jumping tests in the laboratory, we have shown that some athletes produce large differences in jump performance for different foot spacing, while highly skilled jumpers are relatively constant.

B. Take-Off Phase

In the take-off phase, there is a key strategy for successful jump performance. The actual jumping action should be produced at the moment of highest speed. Some studies have reported the motion analysis of take-off during an actual competition. Most of these were accomplished by using a 16-mm high-speed camera.[3,4] The analysis of take-off motion will be divided into the following categories: timing, spacing, and grading. These factors relate to each other for producing a skilled take-off motion.

1. Timing

Komi et al.[4] pointed out that the better jumpers initiate the movement closer to the edge of the ramp, while completing the take-off in less time. Watanabe[5] reported on a laboratory experiment. A small steel ball was dropped from a height of 2 m and 2 m in front of the jumpers. The ski jumpers (24 top Japanese athletes) were requested to initiate their take-off motion just at the moment the ball touched the ground, and the peak value of the jump power production and timing error were measured. When subjects jumped and concentrated mainly on timing, the jump power decreased by 59% and the jump height also decreased to 40% compared with their maximum free-jumping height. When the subjects jumped with timing and also aimed for maximum power production, the values decreased much less, to 96% in jump power and 82% in height, whereas timing errors increased by nearly 30%.

These results suggest that when a jumper produces his maximum strength or maximum power, the timing skill will be decreased and vice versa. One useful suggestion for a jumper's training is that he should aim to utilize the maximum jumping power, because a large part of this power could be easily canceled if he concentrated too hard on timing.

One question arising from a film analysis of take-off motion concerns the motion of the knee joint. Which is better, the knee joint extended fully at the edge of the jump apron or not? There are few clear experimental data for answering this point. However, it should be mentioned that based on the best jumper's motion analysis, the knee was sometimes slightly short of full extension at the edge of the apron. When a jumper has fully extended his knee joint, his vertical acceleration will have reached a peak and his ability to modify his posture for the next flight phase will be limited. In coaching jumpers, especially young jumpers, it might be better to regard the edge not as a "line", but as an "area" of jumping to facilitate good concentration and thus produce nearly maximum jump power and a better position in the air.[5]

2. Spacing

Many jumpers and coaches want to know the best take-off angle for the best performance. However, little research has been done on this point. Some coaches believe the best take-off angle to be 45° and a little smaller. Top athletes produced a take-off angle of almost 45° in simulated jumping on the ground with an "eye closed" condition, simulating a 90-m jump (Figure 2).[5]

In expanding on this point, Watanabe[6] experimented with a simulated jump from different surface conditions (frictional coefficients in the range of 1.0 to 0.03) and compared the jump performance (distance) and power production on a Kistler force plate. The nearest frictional condition to snow was $\mu = 0.03$ in the case of the subject on roller skates. The subjects produced their maximum jump power at an angle of 85° and the values ranged from 80° to vertical jumping because of the slippery conditions. Thus, there exists a very large gap between the take-off angle in actual conditions and simulated take-off. It might be important to pay more attention to the mental image of athletes for training even if there is a large gap between this image and scientific observation.

Watanabe[7] compared the take-off motion for seven top Japanese athletes and eight from other countries during the 90-m World Cup competition in Sapporo in 1980 (Figure 3). The trajectories of their centers of gravity were compared to each other. The Japanese team produced angles of 6.2 ± 0.9°, whereas the others produced values of 4.6 ± 0.9° against the ground when they were 1 m in front of the edge of the apron. These values were

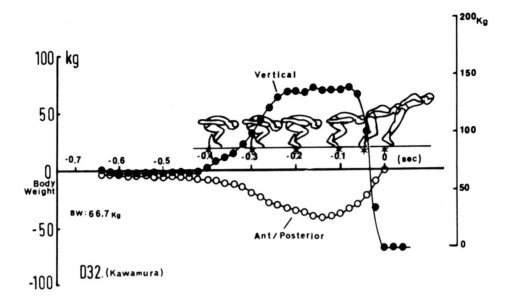

FIGURE 2. Simulated jump on a force plate. The force production in the antero-posterior- and vertical directions was measured from one of the top Japanese jumpers with his arms in the backward position.

(A) H. YAGI

(B) A.KOGLER

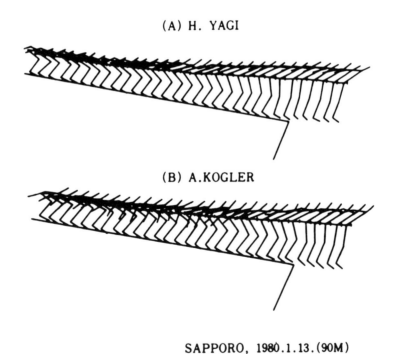

SAPPORO, 1980.1.13.(90M)

FIGURE 3. The trace of the center of gravity is compared for two top jumpers by the use of a high-speed camera in an actual competition.

statistically different at the 0.01 level. The average velocity was 25.5 ± 0.2 m/sec for the Japanese team and 25.4 ± 0.2 m/sec for the others. These results suggest that the Japanese jumpers produced a slightly higher CG position at take-off. More attention should be paid to the difference of the image of jumpers between the actual (dynamic) condition and the simulated (static) condition.

3. Grading

Grading means the regulation of jumping power during take-off. An important objective is to generate vertical velocity of the body during take-off, thus facilitating flight arch in the next phase. For most coaches and jumpers, the main interest is in training the leg muscles to increase the vertical component of jump power and continuing jump power with skill. For increasing jump power, the use of elastic energy of the muscle has been proposed. Recent ideas and experimental data have suggested the usefulness of producing more energy,[8-10] but more investigation will be required to apply this basic physiological theory to an actual training system of jumping. The force production in simulated jumping has been measured in the laboratory.[14,15] In an actual condition, Tveit et al.[16] demonstrated the force measurement at the heel and toe in a 70-m jump hill using a telemetry system. They pointed out that during a force production pattern of take-off there is a shift of force from the heel to the toe in the take-off itself, both in a simulated jump and in an actual condition. The more clear-cut results were obtained in simulated jumping. When comparing the force production in the simulated jump, almost 100 kp was produced, but in an actual condition the figure was only 25 kp. They concluded that the coaching and training target should be focused on a reasonable aerodynamic position before take-off, rather than paying too much attention to vertical acceleration. Sagesser et al.[17] devised a force-measuring system for ski jumping using strain gauge force plates. A total of six force plates were mounted on the apron covering a distance of 6 m. By using this system, the time interval between the maximum force and the last moment of contact was measured and compared. A correlation between the jumping time and jump performance (distance) was produced and the best jump of each subject had a take-off time between 40 and 43 msec. As pointed out by Baumann,[18] less than 20% of the variance of the jumping length can be explained by the variance in the take-off parameters. Many reports have stressed the importance of the take-off phase, namely, the vertical component of acceleration which promises a big arch in the next phase. Hochmuth,[19-24] in his series of reports on ski jumping, and Komi et al.[4] also favor this viewpoint.

Recently, the relative contribution of jump power to the jump distance seems to have decreased. The reason for this may be related to changes of the jump style in the air phase, and also to the increase in importance of this phase to the jump performance. Nevertheless, the take-off phase is still a factor in jump performance, and jump power itself plays an important role in jump performance. The important point for jump power would be how to regulate the power production, that is, "grading".

Recently, the jump power meter or force plate has become popular in the laboratory, and in the future these systems will be used effectively for training and coaching by monitoring the power produced by jumpers.

C. Flight Phase

1. Best In-Flight Position

Which position is best in the flight phase? In attempting to answer this vital question, as far back as 1926, Straumann started his scientific investigations which have led us to the challenging area of sports biomechanics in ski jumping.[25-29] In 1927, Straumann presented his findings on optimum posture during the in-flight phase using a model of a jumper in the wind tunnel. He pointed out that the trunk should be bent forward for getting a larger lift component and minimizing the drag component. Comparison of the posture in an actual competition among the top jumpers was performed by a traditional research technique.[30] However, it was some time before the more basic scientific information, which required more advanced scientific methods, was available for the development of the optimum posture. This investigation was performed by Tani et al.[31-34] They recognized the significance of Straumann's theory that during the in-flight phase the body should be kept bent forward, and they also stressed that the arms should be kept extended backwards to achieve a better

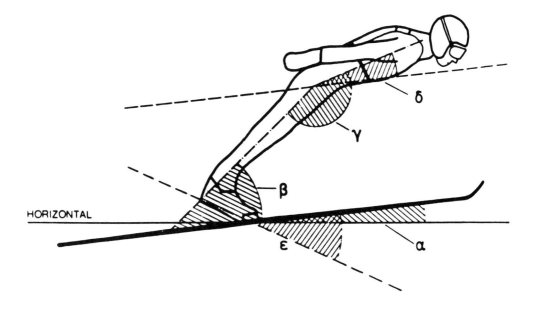

A

Author	ε	β	γ	δ
NAGORNYJ (1955)	10°-30°	50°	150°	-20°
HOCHMUTH (1958)	30°-40°	70°	130°	-20°
TANI/IUCHI (1971)	20°-30°	20°	158°	2°
BAUMANN (1978)				
all trials	35°-50°	25°-40°	130°-150°	+10°-20°
best 10 trials	30°	22°	150°	8°

B

FIGURE 4. (A) Body angles during the flight phase (Adapted from Baumann[3]). Table (B) indicates body angles for the "Optimum" flight position, which have been reported by different investigators.

performance. This evolutional theory was adopted first by the European teams and has spread throughout the world. Recently, the question concerning the arm position during the flight phase has been presented by coaches. The reason for this is that the suggested optimum arm position is sometimes difficult to keep in the air even for the top athletes. Watanabe[35] performed a wind-tunnel experiment which focused on arm position, using a life-sized model wearing actual ski equipment. The arms of this model were positioned against the body from 0° (touching the body) and extended to 90°. In this flight phase of ski jumping, the lift-to-drag ratio (SL/SD) is a useful indicator, since an increment in this value produces an improvement in the jump performance. He concluded that the recommended position of the arms was close to the body for providing the optimum lift-to-drag ratio. The training target for coaches and athletes was presented as quite a severe condition from these experiments. The optimum flight position has been summarized in Table 1 and Figure 4 which was originally presented by Baumann.[3]

In Figure 5, two jumpers are compared just after takeoff. The shadowed jumper has a lower arch 0.45 sec after take-off. The main difference between the two athletes is that the

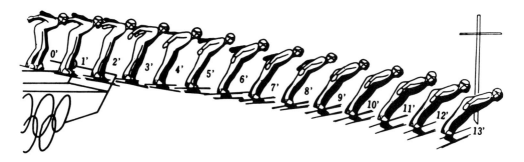

FIGURE 5.   A comparison of the motion for two jumpers in the 90 m event. The shaded jumper adapted his arm position relatively later in the flight phase.

elite jumper finishes his take-off phase much quicker than the other[36] (take-off speed: 91.7 and 91.7 km/hr, respectively).

Baumann[3] pointed out that in the approach, an "egg-shaped" position produces 50% less air resistance than the "half-standing" position. Assuming a tangential velocity of 26 m/sec and an inclination in the apron of 10°, the tangential velocity could be decreased by 0.3 m/sec during the last 5 m. This negative effect can be exacerbated if the arms are not close to the body. How quickly the jumper adapts to the optimum flight position would be an important factor for getting the best jump performance in the flight phase.

2. Jump Skill in the Air

It has sometimes been pointed out that there exists little relationship between take-off velocity and jump distance.[37] This statement stresses the importance of jump skill in the air. From an EMG analysis during flight in the air and to landing, in the case of the excellent jumper, the activity of rectus femoris and tibialis anterior increased gradually until he reached the take-off line. On the other hand, in the case of the less-skilled jumper, the EMG pattern indicated that he found it hard to keep his movements under voluntary control.

In the air to landing, the excellent jumper kept his skis still just before landing by maintaining the activity from tibialis anterior right up to the moment of landing. On the other hand, the less-skilled jumper was not able to maintain his EMG activity until the landing.

The more physiological information such as EMG, should give us some useful information for coaching. In order for the jumper to maintain a stable posture, the pitching moment is quite important aerodynamically. The whole system, including the jumper's body and his ski equipment, can sometimes be disturbed in the air by many factors. One dominant factor was investigated by Ward-Smith and Clements[38] who used a wind-tunnel experiment, and suggested that if it were possible to avoid tumbling at low incidence angles, maximum jump length would be achieved at an angle of 8°. They studied the aerodynamic effects on the ski jumper by using a treadmill, suggesting that these effects might be closely related to the jumping skill just before landing. They also postulated that the jumper can accommodate an out-of-balance pitching moment of 5 N·m given a safe region of incidence angles between 35 and 55°.

III. ALPINE SKIING

A. Ground-Reaction Force Measurement During the Turn

The measurement of force production during a ski turn was originally performed by Nishiwaki et al.[39] in 1956. An ordinary binding was fixed to a metal plate that was supported by four strip springs. The plate was 25 mm above the ski surface. The bending of the four springs (toe and heel in both sides of each ski) was recorded on a tape of stylus paper that was driven by a rotating drum coupled with a miniature electric motor. The time marks were also recorded. Seven expert skiers practiced a number of turns using ski equipment fitted with the apparatus (total mass was 5.5 kg including batteries). Continuous recording during a double turn was performed with the subjects. This apparatus opened the way for analyzing ski turns mechanics, and the group performed the following applications of ski research.[40] By analyzing the parallel turn continuously, they showed that the delay in switching the edge of the inside ski behind the outside one is usually less than 0.1 sec, while in a stem turn it is longer, sometimes as long as 0.5 sec. The device has been further developed by Ohnishi and Sakata[41] and applied to measure more clearly an exerted force during the turn.

A more refined method was demonstrated by Fukuoka[42,43] who measured the force production during a turn and knee joint movement, simultaneously, by telemetry and 16-mm high-speed cinematography. This experiment demonstrated that we are standing on the threshold of an electronics era in sports science. In this report, the timing of motion and the force production were analyzed precisely.

The electronic measurement of force production in skiing using strain gauges was also applied to other conditions. Iizuka and Miyashita[44] applied this technology to analyze skilled and unskilled skiers running over a bump. Miura et al.[45] also demonstrated the difference between skilled and unskilled skiers by studying the distribution of force at the boots. Hull and Mote [46] demonstrated the complete excitation between the boots and ski which was measured during skiing. The signal was transmitted by FM radio waves to a receiving station approximately 3 km away. Three skiing maneuvers (snowplow, stem turn, and parallel turn) were tested. Torsion and bending component amplitudes, measured at the boot sole, are approximately equal to the static ultimate strength of the tibia during both elementary skiing maneuvers and falls. These studies, which aim to improve skiing safety, are supported by a strong experimental facility and are still going on. Since the area of skiing safety is beyond the original aim of this review chapter, I would like to highlight just a few relevant papers.[47-50]

In order to analyze the actual conditions during turns, a more simple method of collecting data for coaching and training was developed. Ikai[51] measured the ground-reaction force during a turn by using a high-speed camera. A special course was constructed with a radius of 14.2 m and the camera was set at the center of the circle. The subjects were top Japanese alpine skiers. One athlete recorded 1150 N of maximum force during a turn from the ground at a speed of 12.8 m/sec: this value was 81% of his maximum leg strength. Theoretical calculations have also been performed for the Swedish team.[52] The same idea and method was applied to an actual course at the Sapporo Pre-Olympic Games. The turn course was selected at Gate No. 4, in a downhill course, where the radius was 19.0 m. The ground-reaction forces were measured at 2070 N on average for the ten top skiers. The turn speed was measured at 22.4 m/sec on average. Recently, a high-speed video system (200 frames per sec) has been devised and applied to motion analysis of some sports including skiing. In the future, faster feedback of data to coaches and athletes will be possible, including both the motion analysis and the ground-reaction forces. The measurement of ground-reaction forces during turns in an actual condition should be performed more often, since a reasonable training system would include both weight training and the training of skiing skill.

B. Running Speed and Posture

In alpine skiing, skiing speed is obviously a very important factor. The jump motion during skiing is of interest to researchers and coaches, because it easily generates significant air resistance and postural disturbances when passing over a bump. The skiing speed was compared by a method of high-speed cinematography (64 frames per sec) as demonstrated by three top Japanese alpine skiers.[53] The three skiers went down a straight course of 29°

Subj. H.C.

Subj. Y.M.

Subj. E.O.

Sapporo

1970. 3.26

Distance 130m

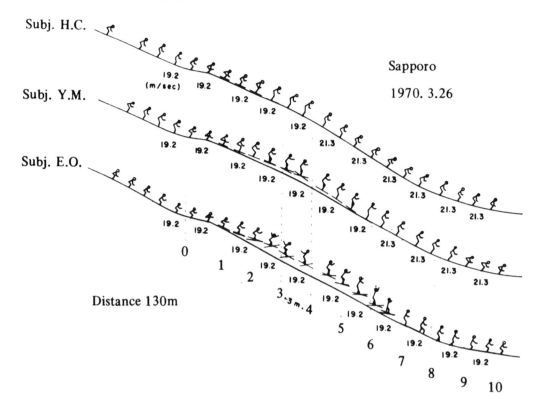

FIGURE 6.   Comparison of postural disturbance and running speed in alpine skiing for three top Japanese athletes.

average gradient and the length of the course was 130 m. The bump was set up 100 m from the starting point. Vertical poles with marked numbers were set along the course every 3 m to analyze the speed of the skier, and two cameras were set at a distance of 110 m apart along the course. The same speed of 19.2 m/sec was recorded for all skiers before the jump. The most stable skier, when passing over the bump, increased his speed to 21.3 m/sec at the 12-m mark from the bump. The skier whose posture was not severely disturbed by the bump obtained a speed of 21.3 m/sec when he was 18 m from the bump. In contrast, the skier whose posture was severely disturbed (the arms were outstretched and the trunk was extended in the air) did not obtain a speed of 21.3 m/sec even 30 m after the bump. These results remind us that there exists a close relationship between postural changes and the running speed of skiing (Figure 6).

We have also performed experiments for evaluating the aerodynamic effect on an alpine skier by using a wind tunnel, as the air resistance obviously acts as a speed-reducing factor.[54] Three wind velocities were chosen for the experiment (10, 20, and 30 m/ sec), and two top athletes served as subjects. Among the various kinds of postures, our results showed that at a wind speed of 30 m/sec, air resistance was 116 N in the "egg-shaped" posture, and 194 N in the "half-standing" posture. The effect of posture on running speed was clearly demonstrated by these results. Further attention was given to the effect of the arms. The contribution of the arms was calculated to be more than 50 N at 30 m/ sec. The arms are sometimes easily extended reflexively when the skier passes over a rough part of the course in an actual race, so these values will not be negligible.

We have also demonstrated the effect of postural changes on the running speed directly by using a coil-magnet system at Syowa Station in Antarctica.[55,56] A straight ski course of 100 m, with an average gradient of 12°, was constructed. The subjects, with a small magnet fixed on one leg, ran closely down past the coils placed every 5 m along the course. The electric signal, which was induced from the coil-magnet system when the skier (magnet) passed the coil, was used to measure the speed of the skier. Two members of the Japanese Antarctic Research Expedition who were well-trained skiers, acted as subjects. Running speed was measured in three different postural conditions: (1) standing, (2) egg-shaped, and (3) starting in the egg-shaped posture and then standing erect in the latter half of the course. Velocities were measured 65 m from the starting point for each postural condition: subject A, (1) standing 7.6 m/sec, (2) egg-shaped 8.6 m/sec, (3) egg-shaped, followed by standing erect 8.2 m/sec; subject B, (1) 7.8 m/sec, (2) 8.9 m/sec, (3) 8.4 m/sec, respectively. These results demonstrate the dramatic effect that posture can have on running speed.

How to keep a reasonable posture even on a rough course is another important matter which relates biomechanical and physiological factors. These points will be discussed later on in the section on basic movement.

IV. CROSS-COUNTRY SKIING

In cross-country skiing, two types of scientific approach have been followed: a physiological approach emphasizing the cardiovascular system, and biomechanical studies in which the main emphasis has been running skill.

Research on cross-country skiing has traditionally been performed in Scandinavian countries. As early as 1945 Pallin[57] used film analysis and calculated the variation in loading on the ski during the diagonal stride sequence. Other biomechanical approaches to cross-country skiing have also been tried.[58-67]

Prior to the Sapporo Olympic Games a research project on cross-country skiing was performed.[60] In that experiment by Kuroda et al., the main emphasis was to compare the running techniques of the Japanese skiers and the best skiers from other countries. In this report, the results of physical fitness tests including body size and motor performance were also presented for the Japanese athletes. In addition, $\dot{V}O_2$ maximum was measured as 4.76ℓ/min (74 mℓ/kg· min) in males on average; the largest value was 5.33 ℓ/min (78 mℓ/kg· min). In females, the corresponding value was 3.38 ℓ/min (60 mℓ/kg· min) on average. The $\dot{V}O_2$ of the male Swedish national team, for example, was 84 mℓ/kg·min on average, a difference of 10 mℓ/kg·min. A training program was initiated to minimize the gap between the Japanese and foreign teams with particular reference to the cardiovascular component. Most of the attention was placed on developing the $\dot{V}O_2$ maximum and the cardiovascular system for skiing performance, and the measurements were taken during an actual competition, or for artificial conditions, in the summer season. The heart rate and respiratory rate were recorded by a telemetry system, and $\dot{V}O_2$ maximum was also measured.

Besides these experiments, the running technique for the ''diagonal'' method was analyzed by film in an actual race using a 35-mm cine camera at 24 frames per sec. A total of 15 athletes were filmed during the flat part of the course of 15-, 30-, and 50-km races, and comparisons were made of the Japanese and the top foreign athletes. Primary measurements were the angle of the trunk bending forward against a vertical line and hip, knee, ankle joint angles, and the pole angle against the horizontal line. These measurements were compared for one cycle of running, and the data were fed back to coaches for training purposes . In 1978, Nigg and Waser[61] reported a more precise film analysis of cross-country skiing during an actual competition in Lahti (Finland) for 15-, 30-, and 50-km races. They divided the skiing cycle into five phases; last use of the stick, last push-off of the leg, first use of the stick, stop on the front foot, and initial position as adopted by Soliman.[62] This precise analysis was filmed on a 16-mm high-speed camera and analyzed by a computer system. Most of the analysis described the changes of the body angle or joint angles at the described running phases. This work provided us with a useful comparison of the differences in skiing

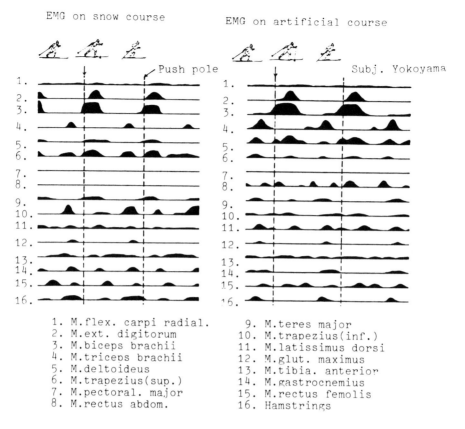

FIGURE 7.   Comparison of EMG activity during cross-country skiing on snow and on an artificial course. Further details are contained in the text.

skill, but for coaching, more appropriate information, especially on the production of propelling power, will be required. Kuroda[60] reported an EMG analysis using Japanese athletes three males, three females) in which the EMG was recorded by an on-line system from 16 parts of the body and simultaneously filmed on a 35-mm cine camera for motion analysis. One example of the recording is shown in Figure 7. The left side shows the EMG recording on snow and the right side is on a plastic artificial course. The data for the biceps brachii suggest that skiing on the artificial course is not the same condition as the snow. Therefore, skiing skill on an artificial course will have to be carefully controlled for training purposes, because athletes will sometimes run the risk of learning unusual techniques. It is possible that the merit in training on an artificial course is to recruit many of the muscles for propelling the body forward, and thus increasing muscle strength.

Ekström[63] reported on a biomechanical application for analyzing running techniques. He measured continuously the force distribution in the horizontal and vertical directions and the pressure of poles simultaneously by a telemetry system, comparing the diagonal stride and double-poling. He stressed that in diagonal skiing on a flat surface, the ski is stationary for 20 to 40 msec during each stride, which has also been shown previously by other authors,[64,65] The relative speed in a diagonal skiing stride (Figure 8) was compared and the same values as Komi et al[66] were obtained. He showed that when one ski has zero speed, the other has maximum speed in the stride. The force-interplay between the ski and the ground begins when the back leg is swung forward and thereby moves the ski to the ski track. At this point, a maximum forward propulsive force of 50 N was measured. In double poling, the skier pushes himself forward only with the force built up in the ski poles. Immediately after

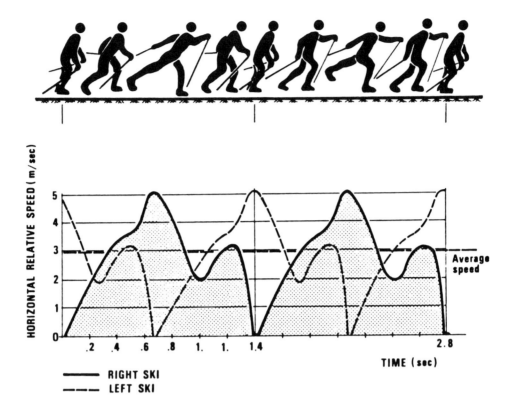

FIGURE 8. Relative speed in the diagonal skiing stride. When one ski has zero speed, the other has maximum speed in the stride. In the diagonal skiing stride, there is a momentary phase when the continuous forward movement comes to a halt. This is one of the major differences when compared to the new skating technique.

the vertical force is reduced the horizontal push-off force is built up to provide propulsion in the track. The maximum force in each pole measured at 210 N in this experiment. These results could be very useful for devising a training program for improving muscle strength and skiing skill. Dal Monte et al.[67] performed an analysis of the diagonal stride technique in cross-country skiing and measured the acceleration of the skis and of the athlete's body, and the forces applied by the arms to the ski poles. These research techniques should also provide useful information for coaches. Recently, another useful running technique has been developed in competition and is called the "skating" technique. Very little research, from a scientific standpoint, has been done on the skating technique in cross-country skiing. It has been reported that the American, Bill Koch, copied this new running technique from the Europeans. He trained in this technique himself, refined it, and in 1981, finished a flat 50-km race in 2 hr. He skated the whole way with one ski in the track, pushed backward with poles, and pushed out sideways with the other ski. It would appear that the main advantage of this technique is that the ski never stops, whereas this happens momentarily during the kick phase of the diagonal stride. Skating skill in uphill, downhill, and on a flat course, should be studied separately. An interesting point to study might be how to use the elastic component of muscle during the skating technique. This new running technique should be an encouragement for researchers in cross-country skiing, aside from the traditional emphasis on energy dependent training and coaching.

V. NORDIC COMBINATION

There are quite a few scientific studies on Nordic combination skiing. Usually, combination skiing is understood by many to be a "mixed" item, a combination between jumping and cross-country skiing. However, there is still some debate whether the best training should also be mixed. One question is sometimes raised by coaches. Which part should be trained first, or, in other words, which part should be dominant for getting the best performance? There is probably nobody who has the data to answer this question at the moment. There are even no clear data whether the ski jumper's muscular training should emphasize the fast-twitch or slow-twitch fibers, from a histochemical standpoint. It is probably reasonable to recommend to athletes and coaches that the combined skier should be trained in distance skiing first, from the physical fitness standpoint. A lack of physical resources is a fatal weak-point for performing in this sport, which could, indeed, have a negative effect on the jumping performance. Naraoka[68] performed an experiment for training the Nordic combination ski team in Japan in which the main thrust was to increase the running performance. A general physical fitness test was performed, and energy consumption during running on an artificial course was measured. The heart rate was monitored continuously in different running conditions and finally the training regime was presented. Watanabe[14] compared physical fitness values of Nordic combination skiers with those of the jumpers and found no significant differences between them. In the future, it is suggested that more research should be directed towards this interesting sports item both from a biomechanical and physiological point of view.

VI. BASIC MOVEMENTS

A. Field Studies

Concerning research on basic movements in skiing, some reports which emphasize biomechanics, have been performed. Changes were demonstrated in the knee angle and the weight on the ski during swinging motion by a telemetry method.[43] The force distribution of the boot was studied for various postures during normal and snowplow skiing, by using a force transducer on the ski.[45] For the extremes of the forward and backward leaning postures, the angle of the CG from the ankle joint ranged between 25 and 30° from the vertical line. It was assumed that a skier could maintain stability within this range. The range of stability, the range of the point of application of the force, and the magnitude of torque during forward and backward postures, tended to be greater for the highly skilled skier than for the intermediate skier.

In another study, the body position during the turn was analyzed, and the CG was estimated for the skier at specific points during turns, for comparison of long skis and short skis.[69] Furthermore, Sodeyama et al.[69] demonstrated that for the skilled skier, by maintaining the CG further forward during a turn, the path became narrower and the speed increased. In the less-skilled skier, the path was wider and the speed decreased.

Iizuka et al.[44] compared skilled and unskilled skiers when passing over a bump by analyzing their postural behavior by using a 16-mm high-speed camera and a specially designed transducer on the ski, which was previously described in this chapter. They pointed out that the most significant difference in the "over-bump" motion between the skilled and unskilled skier was observed in their body rotation before the summit. Their results showed that when the skilled skier ascended the bump, the ski/body angle gradually decreased and his body was rotated forward. However, the unskilled skier first increased the ski/body angle, and his body was rotated backward when he hit the bump. Miyashita et al.[70] did further experimentation on this point by using EMG, and pointed out that the highly trained skier takes up a "ready" posture toward the bump as compared with the beginner.

Watanabe et al.[71] performed a motion analysis experiment using children during the running over a bump. A straight course with a bump (18 cm high) was constructed. Coils were buried in the snow for analyzing the speed of the skier, since signals were emitted when the skis passed over the coils. EMG activity was detected from seven muscles by telemetry and a high-speed camera was also used. Each child attempted ten trials on the same experimental course. These children showed an adaptation process, since the integrated EMG patterns became smaller with successive trials. This tendency was most clearly shown for the upper arm position. It was speculated that the skier would be able to inhibit the involuntary postural distribution after the trials. The postural distribution was understood to be the postural reflex action which was produced when passing over the bump. This postural disturbance might have originated from the labyrinthine organ, a reflex which was induced when passing over the bump.

How do we understand the term "skilled movement" in skiing? In various sports, there are many cases of athletes who have to control their posture by maintaining an optimum position while adapting to a given situation. In attempting to understand the postural control skill, it has been speculated that the "skilled" performer sometimes produces a fundamental reflex pattern even in his voluntary action.

Fukuda[72] described the tonic neck reflex which appears by rotation of the head and consists of extension of the jaw and flexion of the contralateral extremities, thus forming a basic pattern of human movement. By using this reflex, the postures assumed in various sports such as archery, shot-put, and high jump, are timed to coincide with the application of maximum muscular strength.

The tonic neck reflex was investigated by Ikai[73] and Tokizane et al.,[74] and it was established that this reflex has the possibility of producing increased power even in a normal healthy person. Fukuda[72] also extended this idea and applied it to the dynamic posture of skiing. When the skier produced the turning motion, the motion resembled the lumbar reflex in healthy subjects which had been detected by the EMG method of Tokizane et al.[74] These ideas were originally investigated using laboratory animals.[75-77]

From these basic investigations and the careful observation of sports movements, it might easily be argued that the postural reflex is a fundamental motor pattern which undoubtedly plays an important role in sports motions. However, in sports movements, the rules sometimes extend beyond the biological limits of human beings. It may thus be possible to find some negative postural reflex pattern used in a sports situation. Watanabe[78] pointed out that the term "postural change" or "postural compensation" is often used in biology, but in sports it sometimes means a "disturbed" posture. This is because the change in posture sometimes has a negative effect on the sports performance. One example of this negative effect of the "postural change" is an increase in air resistance in alpine skiing (also in ski jumping) when passing over a bump or through a gap. Hence, one of the important targets for improving skiing performance has been to concentrate on the postural reflex control system, and it has also been important for arranging the training program.

How does one control posture to improve performance? The answer will probably come from concentrating on two research areas. The first is an investigation of the nature of the "disturbance" itself, while the second is from an investigation of a method to inhibit or control the "disturbance" in a voluntary manner. For these reasons, it is suggested that some of the following investigations should be carried out:

B. Laboratory Studies

There are many research fields which do not necessarily relate biomechanics and skiing performance. Nevertheless, there are so many important articles concentrating on the basic movements of skiing. This information will play an important role in giving basic scientific guidance to coaches, trainers, and athletes for finding a reasonable way to construct their training program.

1. Adaptation to Horizontal Acceleration

One of the main thrusts of this point is to find out the postural control mechanism in a disturbed or perturbated condition. Nashner[79] using a healthy person, disturbed the standing posture with three different conditions: (1) antero-posterior sway; (2) rotation of the base, thus rotating the ankles directly at 6°/sec; and (3) by ankle rotation produced in equal proportion to the sway rotation stabilizing the ankles during the induced antero-posterior sway. By using EMG methods, he ruled out the possibility that the fixed pattern of postural stability of agonist and antagonist activity in the lower legs caused the mechanical coupling of rotatory movements among the joints of the body.

Nashner et al.[80] presented a model of rapid postural adjustments of standing humans, a method which seems to have some merit in trying to understand the role of leg and trunk muscles for controlling standing posture.

Watanabe[81] used a shift-board apparatus to move the subjects suddenly forwards or backwards. This apparatus was aimed at simulating the horizontal acceleration of skiing. The experiments were designed to give an unexpected shifting disturbance to the subject who was standing still on the platform (shift board). The platform was moved backward and forward at a given speed (36 cm/sec) and through a distance of 10 cm. In this experiment, EMG activities were detected from the following muscles: tibialis anterior, gastrocnemius, rectus femoris, biceps femoris, rectus abdominus, erector spinae, sternocleidomastoid, and biceps brachii. The time-latency of each muscle activity was recorded at 50 msec or less from stimulus, but most of them were 70 to 90 msec. These latencies were understood to be the involuntary reflex action after their time-latency. This reflex was originally induced from the rotation of the ankle joint when the board was shifted forwards or backwards. When the shift-board stimulus given to the subject was, for example, forward, the ankle was rotated in such a way that the tibialis anterior was stretched. Thus, the action was interpreted as the stretch reflex, which gave an original impulse (input) to the other muscles via the central nervous system. An interesting observation was that the activated muscle activity decreased with successive stimuli of the shift board.[82,83]

These results suggest to us one possibility for controlling the disturbed posture. Fujiwara and Ikegami[84] demonstrated postural response in an upright stance to floor vibration. A vibration table with a force plate, on which the subjects stood with eyes open or closed, was vibrated sinusoidally in an antero-posterior or right-to-left direction with 2.5-cm amplitude and various frequencies (0.1, 0.5, and 1.5 Hz). In the future, it is possible that simulated training may include a disturbed course, controlled by computer and modeled from an actual course. Another experiment using the same shift-board method showed that the integrated EMG activity was successively decreased following a number of trials. The intertrial interval was set randomly, approximately 1 min apart. With regard to the time-latency of the EMG responses, these can be considered as a reflex action, and can be attributed to the stretch reflex, which originates from the extension of the ankle joint when shifting the board.[82] In the vibration mode of 0.5 and 1.0 Hz, the stability of standing posture was much higher in the trained than in the untrained subjects, and also when comparing eyes open with eyes closed.

The development of stability of posture is another important point for coaching, especially when applied to children. Concerning this point, Watanabe[85,86] demonstrated the development of postural control by using a shift-board apparatus. Children of 12 years of age produced almost the same values of adaptability against the sudden shifting disturbance as adults. Shumway-Cook and Woollacott[87] also presented the development of postural control in children between 15 and 31 months, and a group between 7 and 10 years, using an antero-posterior shifting apparatus with rotational disturbance of the ankle. They showed that postural synergies underlying stance balance, appeared to be present in very young children (15 months), though not in adult-like form. The children between 15 and 31 months exhibited fairly consistent large amplitude postural responses which were also of longer duration. Rotational trials showed that appropriate adaptation of postural synergies to altered environments, was found in some 4 to 6 year olds, though the adaptational process required longer exposure to altered input than was seen in the 7 to 10 year olds or adults.

2. Adaptation to Vertical Acceleration

Besides being subjected to horizontal disturbances, perturbations in the vertical direction are sometimes experienced in ski jumping and in alpine skiing as well. In this situation, the labyrinthine organ plays an important role in controlling the posture by integrating the information from the other sensory organs, including visual, auditory, and cutaneous.

Vidal et al.[88] used a monkey which experienced a sudden fall (90 cm) while sitting on a chair, and they investigated the muscle response from the lower limbs. Melville Jones and Watt[89] used healthy human beings and subjected them to unexpected falls onto a force plate from a bar which they gripped. The disturbance from platform to toe, varied from 2.5 to 20.3 cm. The EMG response commenced 74 msec after starting the fall, independent of height differences. It was suggested that this response in the leg muscles should be interpreted as a reflex originating in the otolith organ. In addition, a possible mechanism for the control of repetitive hopping and, perhaps, running movements, and involving this reflex, was postulated.

Greenwood et al.[90] also studied unexpected falls, using healthy subjects. The subject was suspended in a parachute harness by a rope passing through freely running pulleys to a metal plate held by an electromagnet. The distance of the subject's toes above the landing platform could be varied by an electric winch. The EMG activity in the soleus during unexpected falls was found to be more complex than that described by Melville Jones and Watt.[89] After a silent period of approximately 80 msec an initial peak of activity lasts until approximately 200 msec after release. In falls from a sufficient height, a second peak of activity occurs before landing. The initial peak of activity is found in muscles throughout the body and is absent during falls in which the subject releases himself. This initial peak of activity was understood to be a startle response to the release. The second peak of activity was found in muscles of the lower limbs. This activity was understood as relating to the timing of landing and concerned with the voluntary control of landing.

Another experiment, performed by Watanabe[91] in a laboratory setting, was more similar to the actual condition of skiing over a bump. The subject stood still on a plate and was given a free-falling stimulus, the falling distance being 12.5 cm. The behavior of the subject was recorded by EMG methods. In the case of the free-falling condition, the subject produced an EMG pattern of an arm extension motion. The EMGs were recorded from deltoid, biceps brachii, triceps brachii, and tibialis anterior muscles. The latency times of selective muscle actions from a falling stimulus, were measured. Most of them were approximately 60 to 65 msec. It might be that the extension of the arms was originated mainly from the labyrinthine organ when the body fell.[91] A similar result for the time-latency of the muscle activities from the stimulus, was observed when compared to the shift-board experimental condition.

One of the main purposes of research in motor learning is to find a way to answer the question of how to become skilled in motion, in this case, how to become skilled in skiing. These results from some experiments which suggested that inhibiting the postural reflex motion to get a more skilled or stable posture, could help us understand skilled motions in skiing and other sports.

3. Control of Posture in Disturbed Conditions

In summary, to answer the question of how to control the reflex action which has a negative effect on performance, the following process will now be recommended. One method is to adapt to the condition by considerable practice or experience. This training method would concentrate on practice in different conditions to expand the subject's experience level. In such a process, training to control the postural disturbance mainly involves the feedback control system including a memory of the specific condition.

The other method is an "anticipatory" postural control against the disturbed situation. This control system relates to a so-called "feedforward" system. The importance of this system for sports skill acquisition cannot be overemphasized. With regard to this point, some initial work has been done, but more research should be performed to produce a training program which stresses the "quality" of the memory.

VII. CONCLUSIONS

I have briefly presented my idea of a basic movement study in skiing, but we should realize that the science of skiing is not only supported by biomechanics. There is a considerable volume of research which relates to skiing and belongs to different research fields. I would like to present a schema of skiing research as an integrated science which was originally presented as the introduction of the Japanese scientific approach to skiing research. In this chapter, I have presented some articles which hopefully will lead to a better understanding of skiing. At present skiing research is mainly supported by biomechanists and physiologists. However, the basic sciences of physics and engineering have also performed an important role; for example, the mechanics of the ski itself[93-95] and the mechanics of ski boots.[96,97] The study of ski bindings[98,99] has recently been extended to research on designing an electronic safety-binding system.[100,101] In addition, a unique idea has been presented for skiing safety.[102]

The study of snow conditions has also contributed to our knowledge in this field,[103] while studies in the medical field which concern skiing safety are also very important and useful. In this area, an international symposium has been convened since 1974, and their activity was summarized in the conference proceedings: *Skiing Safety II*[104] *and Skiing Trauma and Safety*.[105] The study of skiing turns by using a skirobot, could also give us considerable insight into understanding this mechanism.[106,107]

Biomechanical and histochemical research has also contributed to the design of training and coaching programs.[109-112] These research data will require further rearrangement and integration before they can be directly applied by coaches.

Fundamental research from divergent fields has the possibility of providing support for each field and being integrated into a goal of ski-research activity (Figure 9). The results are not only of value to the champion skier, but also to the recreational skier and to the student of skiing in physical education. In the future, a more developed and organized research system should be constructed internationally to develop winter sports science, including ski science, for the benefit of people who live in a cold environment.

257

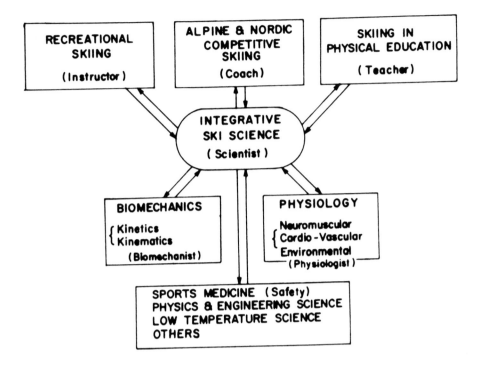

FIGURE 9. A proposed schema of skiing research as an integrated science.

REFERENCES

1. **Watanabe, K.,** Ski jump, "Taikyo Jiho", *J. Jpn. Amateur Athletic Assoc. (in Japanese),* 4, 18, 1980.
2. **Watanabe, K.,** Skiing research in Japan, *Med. Sci. Sport Exercise,* 13, 205, 1981.
3. **Baumann, W.,** The biomechanics of ski-jumping, *Proc. Int. Symp. Sci. Skiiing (Zao, Japan),* 1979, 70.
4. **Komi, P. V., Nelson, R. C., and Pulli, M.,** Biomechanics of ski-jumping, *Stud. Sport Phys. Educ. Health (Univ. Jyväskylä),* Finland, 1974, 5.
5. **Watanabe, K.,** Motion analysis of take-off, Taiiku no Kagaku, *J. Health Phys. Educ. Recreation,* 33, 884, 1983.
6. **Watanabe, K.,** Maximal jump power production in different frictional conditions (in Japanese), *Annu. Rep. Sports Med. Sci. Jpn. Amateur Athletic Assoc.,* 8, 279, 1985.
7. **Watanabe, K.,** Comparison of center of gravity tracing during take-off between the national and foreign jumper (in Japanese), *Annu. Rep. Sports Med. Sci. Jpn. Amateur Athletic Assoc.,* 7, 349, 1984.
8. **Asmussen, E. and Bonde-Petersen, F.,** Apparent efficiency and storage of elastic energy in human muscles during exercise, *Acta Physiol. Scand.,* 92, 537, 1974.
9. **Cavagna, G. A., Komarek, L., Citterio, G., and Margaria, R.,** Power output of the previously stretched muscle, in *Biomechanics II,* S. Karger, Basel, 1971, 159.
10. **Cavagna G. A. and Kaneko, M.,** Work and efficiency in human locomotion, *J. Physiol.,* 268, 467, 1977.
11. **Komi, P. V. and Bosco, C.,** Utilization of stored elastic energy in leg extensor muscles by men and women, *Med. Sci. Sports,* 10, 261, 1978.
12. **Komi, P. V.,** Elastic potentiation of muscle and its influence on sports performance, in *Biomechanics and Performance in Sports,* Baumann, W., Ed., Verlag Karl Hofmann, Schorndort, W. Germany, 1983.
13. **Gollnick, P. O., Armstrong, B., Saubert, C. W., Piehl, K., and Saltin, B.,** Enzyme activity and fiber composition in skeletal muscle of untrained and trained men, *J. Appl. Physiol.,* 33, 312, 1972.
14. **Watanabe, K.,** Data report of physical fitness test (1981 — 1984), in *SAJ Data Reports,* Vol. 3(1:B), Ski Association of Japan, Tokyo, 1985.
15. **Dillman, C. J., Campbell, D. R., and Gormley, J. T.,** Force platform testing of ski jumpers, *J. U.S. Ski Coaches Assoc.,* 3, 35, 1980.

16. **Tveit, P. and Pedersen, P. O.,** Forces in the take-off in ski jumping, in *Biomechanics VII-B,* 1981, 472.
17. **Sagesser A., Neukomm, P. A., Nigg, B. M., Ruegg, P., and Tvoxler, G.,** Force measuring system for the take-off in ski jumping, in *Biomechanics VII-B,* 1981, 478.
18. **Baumann, W.,** The take-off in ski-jumping and its influence on the jumping length, in *Biomechanics VI-B,* Asmussen, E. and Jørgensen, K., Eds., University Park Press, Baltimore, 1978, 85.
19. **Hochmuth, G. and Stark, J.,** Aerodynamische Berechnungen von Skiflugkurven, ihre Anwendung auf den Schanzenbau und das wissenschaftliche Springertraining, *Theor. Prax. Körperkultur,* 2, 1953.
20. **Hochmuth, G.,** Über die Absprungmechanik beim Skispringen, *Theor. Prax. Körperkultur,* 1956.
21. **Hochmuth, G.,** Untersuchungen über den Einfluss der Absprungbewegung auf die Sprungweite beim Skispringen. Ein Beitrag zur Sporttechnik des Skisprunges, Ph. D. thesis, Dresden, University of E. Germany, 1958.
22. **Hochmuth, G.,** Untersuchungen über den Einfluss der Absprungbewegung auf die Sprungsweite beim Skispringen, *Wiss. Z. DHfk (Leipzig),* 1, 1958/59.
23. **Hochmuth, G.,** Die zweckmassigste Absprungtechnik beim Skispringen, *Theor. Prax. Körperkultur,* 8, 505, 1959.
24. **Hochmuth, G.,** Biomchanischer Skisprungtest, *Wiss. Z. DHfk (Leipzig),* 2, 233, 1959/60.
25. **Straumann, R.,** Vom Gletisprung und seinem Einfluss auf den Schanzenbau, *Der Winter,* Heft 20, 1926/27.
26. **Straumann, R.,** Vom Skiweitsprung und seiner Mechanik, *Ski Schweizer Jahrbuch,* 1927.
27. **Straumann, R.,** Vom Skisprung zum Skiflug, *Sport,* 63, 7, 1955.
28. **Straumann, R.,** Der moderne Skisprung, *Sport,* 63, 7, 1955.
29. **Straumann, R.,** Ski jumping style, flight paths and their evaluation, *Sport,* 9, 1964.
30. **Nashimovich, V. K.,** The technique of flight and landing, *Theor. Pract. Phys. Cult.,* 1,67, 1973.
31. **Tani, I. and Mitsuishi, S.,** Aerodynamics of ski-jumping science (in Japanese), 21, 117, 1951.
32. **Tani, I. and Mitsuishi, S.,** Aerodynamics of ski-jumping. I. in *Scientific Study of Skiing in Japan (in Japanese),* Hitachi Co., Tokyo, 1971, 57.
33. **Tani, I., Iuchi, M., and Watanabe, I.,** Aerodynamics of ski-jumping, II, in *Scientific Study of Skiing in Japan (in Japanese),* Hitachi Co., Tokyo, 1971, 64.
34. **Tani, I, and Iuchi, M.,** Flight-mechanical investigation of ski jumping, in *Scientific Study of Skiing in Japan (in Japanese,),* Hitachi Co., Tokyo, 1971, 33.
35. **Watanabe, K.,** Aerodynamic investigation of arm position during the flight phase in ski jumping, in *Biomechanics VIII-B,* Matsui, H. and Kobayashi, K., Eds., Human Kinetics Publishers, Champaign, Ill, 1983, 856.
36. **Watanabe, K.,** Measurement of air resistance by using wind tunnel experiment, *Jpn. J. Sport Sci.,* 1, 413, 1982.
37. **Watanabe, T., Kasaya, A., and Kawahara, Y.,** Kinematic studies on ski-jump, in Proc. Int. Congr. Winter Sports Med., Sapporo, 1972, 98.
38. **Ward-Smith, A. J., and Clements, D.,** Experimental determination of the aerodynamic characteristics of ski-jumpers, *Aeronaut. J.* December, 384, 1982.
39. **Nishiwaki, N., Hagi, S., and Hirata, M.,** Continuous measurement of live load on each ski during skiing turns. I. Method of experiment, in *Scientific Study of Skiing in Japan,* Hitachi Co., Tokyo, 1971, 8.
40. **Hosaka, N., Nishiwaki, N., and Hagi, S.,** Continuous measurement of live load on each ski during skiing. II. Analysis of results, in *Scientific Study of Skiing in Japan,* Hitachi Co., Tokyo, 1971, 17.
41. **Ohnishi, T. and Sakata, I.,** Recording live load on each ski during a turn, in *Scientific Study of Skiing in Japan* , Hitachi Co., Tokyo, 1971, 25.
42. **Fukuoka, T.,** *Zur Biomechanik und Kybernetik des alpinen Schilaufs,* Limpert, Frankfurt, W. Germany 1971.
43. **Fukuoka, T.,** Changes in the knee angle and in the load of the ski during swing motions in alpine skiing, *Biomechanics II,* 1971, 246.
44. **Iizuka, K. and Miyashita, M.,** Biomechanical analysis of skiing over a hump: comparison of the skilled and unskilled skier, in *Science in Skiing, Skating, and Hockey,* Terauds, J. and Gros, H. J., Eds, Academic Publishers, Del Mar, Calif., 1979, 49.
45. **Miura, M., Ikegami, Y., Kitamura, K., Matsui, H., and Sodeyama, H.,** Force distribution at the boot for various postures during normal and snowplow skiing in *Science in Skiing, Skating, and Hockey,* Terauds, J. and Gros, H. J., Eds., Academic Publishers, Del Mar, Calif., 1979, 23.
46. **Hull, M. L., and Mote, C. D.,** Analysis of leg loading in snow skiing, *J. Dyn. Syst. Meas. Control,* 100, 177, 1978.
47. **Kuo, C. Y,. Louie, J. K., and Mote, C. D.,** Field measurements in snow skiing injury research, *J. Biomech.,* 16, 609, 1978.
48. **Mote, C. D., and Louie, J. K.,** Accelerations induced by body motions during snow skiing, *J. Sound Vib.,* 88, l07, 1983.

49. **Louie, J. K., Kuo, C. Y., Gutierrez, M.D., and Mote, C. D.,** Surface EMG and torsion measurements during snow skiing: laboratory and field tests, *J. Biomech.,* 17, 713, 1984.

50. **Lieu, D. K., and Mote, C. D.,** Mechanics of the turning snow ski, in *Skiing Trauma and Safety: 5th Intl. Symp.,* ASTM STP 860, Johnson, R. J., and Mote, C. D., Eds, 1985, 117.

51. **Ikai, M.,** Alpine skiing, in *Scientific Report of Sapporo Olympic Games,* Japan Amateur Athletic Association, 1972, 157.

52. **ALPRINT,** Rep, No. 17, Series of Idrottsfysioligi, Trygg, Hansa, Stockholm, 1977.

53. **Ikai M., Watanabe, K., and Fukunga, T.,** Motion analysis and telemetering electromography of alpine skiing, Intl. Congr. of Winter Sports Medicine, Sapporo, 1972, 106.

54. **Watanabe, K. and Ohtsuki T.,** Postural changes and aerodynamic forces in alpine skiig, *Ergonomics,* 20, 121, 1977.

55. **Watanabe, K. and Ohtsuki, T.,** The effect of posture on the running speed of skiing, *Ergonomics,* 21, 987, 1978.

56. **Watanabe, K.,** Measurement of the speed of skiing throughout the turn by the "coilmagnet system", in *Science in Skiing, Skating and Hockey,* Terauds, J. and Gros, H. J., Eds., Academic Publishers Del Mar, Calif., 1979, 41.

57. **Pallin H.,** Löpmotsåndet vid skidåkning, in *Raben and Sjogren,* på skidor, Stockholm, 1945, 16.

58. **Beresin, G. W.,** Der Bewegungsrhythmus des Diagonalschrittes bei unterschiedlichen Gleitbedingungen, *Theor. Prax. Körperkultur (Leipzig),* 18, 975, 1959.

59. **Moeser, G. and Tschirnich, B.,** Vergleichende Untersuchung über den Bewegungsablauf des Diagonalschrittes im Skilanglauf auf Schnee und auf künstlichen Laufbahnen, *Theor. Prax. Köperkultur (Leipzig),* 11, 977, 1962.

60. **Kuroda, Y.,** Ski distance, in *Scientific Report of Sapporo Olympic Games,* Japan Amateur Athletic Association, 1972, 103.

61. **Nigg B. M. and Waser, J.,** *Skilanglauf,* Juris Druck und Verlag, Zurich, 1978.

62. **Soliman, A. T.,** Filmanalyse des Diagonalschrittes in der Ebene, Laboratorium für Biomechanik, ETH Zurich, 1977.

63. **Ekström, H.,** Biomechanical research applied to skiing, Linkoping Studies in Science and Technology, Dissertation No. 53, 1980.

64. **Waser, J.,** Filmanalyse bimechanischer Parameter beim Skilanglauf, *Leistungssport* 6, 476, 1976.

65. **Hixson, E.,** *The Physician and Sport Medicine Guide to Cross Country Skiing,* McGraw-Hill New York, 1980.

66. **Komi, P. V., Normal, R., and Caldwell G.,** Horizontal Velocity Changes of World Class Skiers Using the Diagonal Technique, working paper of Department of Biology and Physical Activity, University of Jyväskylä, Finland, 1980.

67. **Dal Monte, A., Fucci, S., Leonardi, L. M., and Trozzi, V.,** An evaluation of the diagonal stride technique in cross-country skiing, *Biomechanics VIII-B,* Matsui, H. and Kobayashi, K., Eds., Human Kinetics Publishers, Champaign, Ill., 1983, 851.

68. **Naraoka, K.,** Nordic combination, in *Scientific Report of Sapporo Olympic Games,* Japan Amateur Athletic Association, 1972, 57.

69. **Sodeyama, H., Miura, M., Ikegami, Y., Kitamura, K., and Matsui, H.,** Analysis of the body position of skiers during turns, in *Science in Skiing, Skating and Hockey,* Terauds, J. and Gross, H. J., Eds., Academic Publishers, Del Mar, Calif., 1979, 33.

70. **Miyashita, M. and Sakurai, S.,** Biomechanical analysis of skiing over a hump, in Proc. Intl. Symp. Sci. Ski. Zao, Japan, 1979, 96.

71. **Watanabe, K., Ohtsuki, T., Akashi, M, Hirai, T., Matsuo, A., Tamukae, M., Yamaguchi, T., Seki, T., and Yada, H.,** Analysis of disturbed posture in skiing, in *Science of Human Motion,* Kyorin Shoin, Publishers, Tokyo, 1983, 248.

72. **Fukuda, T.** *Statokinetic Reflexes in Equilibrium and Movement,* University of Tokyo Press Tokyo, 1984, 72.

73. **Ikai, M.,** Effect of alcohol on the postural reflex in normal persons, *Nat. Sci. Rep. Ochanomizu University,* Japan, 1, 118, 1951.

74. **Tokizane, T, Murao, M., Ogata, T., and Kondo, T.,** Electromyographic studies on tonic neck, lumber and labyrinthine reflexes in normal persons, *Jpn. J. Physiol.,* 2, 1951.

75. **Magnus, R.,** *Körperstellung,* Julious Springer Verlag, Berlin, 1924.

76. **Magnsu R.,** Croonian lecture: animal posture, *Proc. R. Soc. London Ser. B,* 98, 339, 1925.

77. **Sherrington, C.,** *The Integrat Action of the Nervous System,* Yale University Press, New Haven, 1961.

78. **Watanabe, K.,** Postural disturbance and its control: the meaning of posture in the "situation" of sports (in Japanese), *Proc. Biomechan.,* 6, 15 1982.

79. **Nashner, L. M.,** Fixed pattern of rapid postural responses among leg muscles during stance, *Exp. Brain Res.,* 30, 13, 1977.

80. **Nashner, L. M. and Woollacott, M.,** The organization of rapid postural adjustment of standing humans: an experimental conceptual model, in *Posture and Movements,* Talbott, R. E. and Humphrey D. R., Eds., Raven Press, New York, 1979, 243.

81. **Watanabe, K.,** The study on the standing posture: the latent time of postural control, *Jpn. J. Phys. Fitness Sports Med.* 24, 118, 1975.

82. **Watanabe, K. and Asahina, K.,** Studies on postural controllability. I. Methodology, *Rep. Res. Cent. Phys. Educ.,* 2, 273, 1974.

83. **Nashner, L. M.,** Adapting reflexes controlling the human posture, *Exp. Brain Res.,* 26, 59, 1976.

84. **Fujiwara, K. and Ikegami, H.,** The characteristics of postural response in upright stance to the floor vibration, *Jpn. J. Phys. Educ.,* 29, 251, 1984.

85. **Watanabe K.,** Development of postural control from 4 to 12 years of age and its characteristics, in *Biomechanics VI-A,* Asmussen, E. and Jorgensen, K., Eds., 1978, 176.

86. **Asahina, K. and Watanabe, K.,** Studies on postural controllability. II. Changes in postural controllability with age from 4 to 12 years, *Rep. Res. Cent. Phys. Educ.,* 3, 149, 1975.

87. **Shumway-Cook, A. and Woollacott, M. H.,** The growth of stability: postural control from a developmental perspective, *J. Motor Behav.,* 17, 131, 1985.

88. **Vidal, P. P., Lacour, M., and Berthoz, A.,** Contribution of vision to muscle responses in monkey during freefall: visual stabilization decreases vestibular dependent reponses, *Exp. Brain Res.,* 37, 241, 1979.

89. **Melville-Jones, G. and Watt, D. G. D.,** Muscular control of landing from unexpected falls in man, *J. Physiol.,* 219, 729, 1971.

90. **Greenwood, R. and Hopkins, A.,** Muscle responses during sudden falls in man, J. Physiol., 254, 507, 1976.

91. **Watanabe, K.,** Control of standing posture under a disturbance of horizontal acceleration by shift board in adults, in 6th Int. Symp. on Ski Trauma and Skiing Safety (Naeba, Japan), Abstract, 43, 1985.

92. **Dufosse, M., Macpherson, J., and Massion, J.,** Reorganization of posture before movement, in *Preparatory States and Processes,* Kornblum, S. and Requin, J., Eds., Lawrence Erlbaum Associates, Hillsdale, N. J., 1984, 339.

93. **Ohnishi, T.,** Die physikalischen Eigenschaften des Schibretts, in *Scientific Study of Skiing in Japan,* Hitachi Co., Tokyo, 1972, 68.

94. **Lieu, D. K. and Mote, C. D.** Mechanics of the turning snow ski, in *Skiing Trauma and Safety,* Johnson R. J. and Mote, C. D., Eds., ASTM, Philadelphia, 1985, 117.

95. **ASTM Committee F27 on Snow Skiing,** ASTM Standards on Snow Ski, 1st ed., 1985.

96. **Schattner, R., Hauser, W., and Asang, E.,** Basic mechanics of boot/skier interaction, in *Skiing Trauma and Safety,* Johnson, R. J. and Mote, C. D., Eds., ASTM, Philadelphia, 1985, 151.

97. **Hauser, W., Asang, E., and Schaff, P.,** Influence of ski boot design on skiing safety and skiing performance in *Skiing Trauma and Safety,* Johnson, R. J. and Mote, C. D., Eds., ASTM, Philadelphia, 1985, 159.

98. **Ekland, A. and Lund, Ø.,** Comparison of the BfU and IAS binding adjustment systems for recreational skiers, in *Skiing Trauma and Safety,* Johnson, R. J. and Mote, C. D., Eds., ASTM, Philadelphia, 1985, 203.

99. **Brown, C. A. and Ettlinger, C. F.,** A method for improvement of retention characteristics in alpine ski bindings, in *Skiing Trauma and Safety,* Johnson, R. J. and Mote, C. D., Eds., ASTM, Philadelphia, 1985, 224.

100. **Hull, M. L.,** A survey of actively controlled (electronic) snow ski bindings, in *Skiing Trauma and Safety,* Johnson, R. J. and Mote, C. D., Eds., ASTM, Philadelphia, 1985, 138.

101. **Hull, M. L.,** A second generation microcomputer controlled snow ski binding system, in 6th Intl. Symp. on Ski Trauma and Skiing Safety, Naeba, Japan, Abstract, 39, 1985.

102. **Zucco, P.,** Evaluation and characteristics about a new soft skiing shoe, in 6th Intl. Symp. on Ski Trauma and Skiing Safety, Naeba, Japan, Abstract, 38, 1985.

103. **Nakaya, U., Tada, M., Sekido, Y., and Takano, T.,** The physics of Skiing: preliminary and general survey, in *Scientific Study of Skiing in Japan,* Hitachi Co., Tokyo, 1972.

104. **Figueras, J. M., Eds.,** Skiing Safety II, University Park Press, Baltimore, 1978.

105. **Johnson, R. J. and Mote, C. D., Eds.,** Skiing Trauma and Safety, ASTM Special Technical Publication, Philadelphia, 1985.

106. **Iizuka K., Kobayashi, T., and Miyashita, M.,** Skirobot for parallel turning, in 9th Intl. Congr. of Biomechanics Scientific Program, 1983, 109.

107. **Iizuka, K.,** Parallel turning by skirobot, *J. Sci. Phys. Educ.,* 33, 900, 1983.

108. **Hasegawa K. and Shimizu, S.,** Dynamics of turning performed by an alpine skiing robot, *Jpn. J. Sport Sci.,* 4, 971, 1985.

109. **Nygaard, E., Andersen, P., Nilsson, P., Erikson, E., Kjessel, T., and Saltin, B.,** Glycogen depletion pattern and lactate accumulation in leg muscles during recreational downhill skiing, *Eur. J. Appl. Physiol.,* 38, 261, 1978.

110. **Tesch, P., Larsson, L., Eriksson, A., and Karlsson, J.,** Muscle glycogen depletion and lactate concentration during downhill skiing, *Med. Sci. Sports,* 10, 85, 1978.
111. **Droghetti, P., Borsetto, C., Casoni, I., Cellini, M., Ferrari, M., Paolini, A. R., Ziglio, P. G., and Conconi, F.,** Noninvasive determination of the anaerobic threshold in canoeing, cross country skiing, cycling, roller- and ice skating, rowing and walking, *Eur. J. Appl. Physiol.,* 53, 299, 1985.
112. **Saibene, F., Cortili, G., Gavazzi, P., and Magistri, P.,** Energy sources in alpine skiing (giant slalom) *Eur. J. Appl. Physiol.,* 53, 312, 1985.

Chapter 8

TENNIS STROKES AND EQUIPMENT

Bruce C. Elliott

TABLE OF CONTENTS

I. INTRODUCTION

This chapter reviews the biomechanics literature published on tennis. A small number of papers, at present awaiting publication, have been reviewed in an attempt to ensure the current status of this chapter. Section II. reviews the literature on stroke production, Section III. looks at research on the equipment needed to play the game, while Section IV. reviews the literature on general mechanical principles related to tennis. Specific conclusions will be drawn from the literature where this is possible. Coaching theory based on subjective opinion will not be used to support a given line of thinking where the literature is either inconclusive or at variance. Books by Braden and Bruns,[1] Elliott and Kilderry,[2] and Groppel,[3] just to name a few, link science and subjective opinion in deciding teaching techniques that can be used by coaches. The applications from an instructor's manual by Brody[92] that relates science and tennis coaching, has not been able to be integrated into this chapter because of publication deadlines.

II. THE TENNIS STROKES

A. The Serve

The service is probably the most important stroke in tennis. As it is a closed skill, it is logical to assume that service technique can be improved through an understanding and then practice of the important components of the action.

1. Muscle Activity and Movement Patterns for Selected Overhead Sport Skills and the Tennis Serve

Many coaches and teachers believe that the similarity in joint and segment movements between selected overhand sport skills, particularly the overhand throw, and the tennis serve, enables a transfer of learning effect from the overhand skill to the serve. Gresner[4] stated that "serving is throwing, and to serve well one must be able to throw well."

Broer and Houtz,[5] in an electromyographic (EMG) study on one skilled performer, reported that the timing of the activity for a given muscle was relatively constant for the tennis serve, badminton clear, and overhand throw. Adrian and Enberg,[6] in a cinematographic study, however, reported intraindividual and interindividual differences for three college-age women in the movement pattern of the tennis serve, volleyball serve, and badminton smash. Their intercollegiate performer in all three sports showed greater intraindividual differences in the contact position than did the other two subjects. The movement patterns of the wrist and radio-ulnar joints of the striking arm of the overarm strokes in tennis, badminton, racquetball, and squash for college subjects, proficient in at least one of these sports, tended to replicate the pattern for the preferred skill. The amplitude of movement and angular velocity of the wrist were not similar for the seven subjects, particularly in the period just prior to impact. On the basis of the data presented by Adrian and Enberg[6] and Jack et al.,[7] it is probable that the differences in performing the overhand patterns studied may be as important as the similarities, especially at the highly skilled level.

A further EMG and cinematographic study by Anderson[8] of three skilled female throwers, three skilled tennis players, and three females skilled in both activities, supported the findings of Adrian and Enberg.[6]

Ten muscles (right upper, middle, and lower trapezius, pectoralis major, right anterior and posterior deltoid, right infraspinatus, right serratus anterior, and right and left external obliques), were tested in an attempt to verify the findings of Broer and Houtz[5] who tested all but the infraspinatus muscle in their study. The subjects used similar joint actions and, with some exceptions, activated the same number of muscles during the later stages of the preparation phase and during the force-production phase of throwing and serving. The posterior deltoid, infraspinatus, and the three parts of the trapezius muscle were active in eight of the nine subjects as the racket was raised during the preparation to throw or serve. Marked activity (greater than 50% of that muscle's peak level of activity) was evident in the pectoralis major, anterior deltoid, infraspinatus, right and left external obliques, serratus anterior, and lower trapezius in eight of the nine subjects during the force-production phase of both activities.

However, while all subjects, regardless of skill, tended to use the same muscles to execute the throw or serve, the range of segment movement together with the time and sequence of the muscle activity varied considerably. Rear and lateral films showed that all nine subjects had a greater degree of shoulder joint abduction, glenoid fossa upward rotation, and lateral trunk flexion away from the throwing limb during the force-production phase for the serve than in the throw, as they adjusted their upper-limb positions to make contact with the ball. No two subjects demonstrated the same sequential timing in the order in which muscles initiated activity during the preparatory phase in the two skills. In the force-production phase, subjects selected for their high skill levels in both throwing and serving showed greater variations in the order in which muscles either initiated or ceased activity than did subjects selected for their ability in just one of the two skills.

In EMG studies linked with cinematography, Miyashita et al.[9,10] studied three subjects (including a skilled male pitcher and skilled male tennis player) and investigated further the muscle activity patterns for the tennis serve and overhand throw. The results from the muscles tested (trapezius transversa, pectoralis major, sternocostalis, deltoid pars acromialis, infraspinatus, and long head of biceps brachii and triceps brachii) generally supported the data of Anderson.[8] The EMG patterns of the trapezius muscle, deltoid muscle, and biceps brachii muscle of the pitcher differed from those of the tennis player when serving, although the other muscle activity was similar. The trained pitcher exhibited similar EMGs to the tennis player during the overhand throw. There were clear differences in the EMG patterns of the tennis player and the untrained subject when serving and between the pitcher and the untrained subject when throwing. Miyashita et al.[10] also reported that EMGs from skilled performers were characterized by silent periods between the bursts of activity for selected muscles.

Research would thus tend to indicate that if performers can perceive these differences between the overarm throw and the serve, then the practice of throwing, or reference to the movements of the throw, may not be a good method to gain expertise in the tennis serve.[8] A pedagogical study with children as subjects, is now required to find if overhand throwing practice is of any assistance in the early stages of tennis serve development.

A comprehensive EMG study of the muscles of the trunk and limbs during tennis, is also needed. Such a study was completed by Van Gheluwe and Hebbelinck;[93] however, the results were not able to be integrated into this manuscript because of publication deadlines.

2. The Ball Toss

The height that the ball should be "pushed" in the toss has always proven a problem for beginners, as role models have used such a variety of heights. Plagenhoef[11] used high-speed photography to show that the great majority of highly competent servers strike the ball just after it has begun its drop (Newcombe and Talbert, 0- to 2.5-cm drop; Seixas, 2.5- to 7.5-cm drop; Ashe, 7.5- to 12.5-cm drop; Gonzales and Hoad, 15- to 22.5-cm drop). Beerman and Sher,[12] using Newtonian mechanics (ignoring the influence of air resistance), showed that a player has eightfold the time to contact the ball when it is thrown to the height of the "sweet spot" of the racket, than when the ball is thrown 1.2 m above this point. When the ball is tossed 1.2 m above the racket, the player has to make contact with a target moving at approximately 5 m/sec.[12]

3. Kinematics and Kinetics of the Serve

The primary consideration in any serve technique is rhythm. As the body provides the energy supply for the serve, it is important that the coordination of the body segments occurs in a sequence that produces an optimal racket position, trajectory, and velocity at impact. Better servers are those best able to coordinate the sequence of motion, often referred to as the "kinetic chain", which produces an ideal racket position at impact.[1,2,11]

Smith[13] reported that the weight distribution for five male varsity players in the starting position, was a very individual characteristic, with three subjects having their weight distributed in front of the rear foot, one was evenly balanced, and one had the weight predominantly placed on the front foot. Smith also found that this individual weight pattern was consistent for the flat and slice serves. During the backswing phase the center of gravity (CG) either moved back towards the rear foot or remained relatively constant for those who started with their weight near the back foot (75% of stance width from the front toe for flat serve). At contact, the line of the CG was 25 cm forward of the front toe in the flat serve and 41.5 cm forward of the front toe in the slice serve.

What body movements then drive the whole body CG forward and upward for impact? Elliott and Wood[14] used dynamometry and cinematography to evaluate foot-up (FU or platform thrust) and foot-back (FB) serve techniques. Six male and three female college-level tennis players were filmed both laterally and from above while serving from a Kistler force platform. While all subjects were competent in both techniques, four had a preference for the FU technique and five preferred the FB method. The impulse curves for the FU and FB service techniques, following the initial transference of weight, were different in pattern. Vertical ground-reaction forces were larger throughout the drive phase prior to impact for the FU group when compared to the FB group (Figure 1). The greater vertical impulse resulted in a significantly higher impact position and a better up-and-out racket trajectory for the FU technique when compared to the FB style. The FB technique produced larger horizontal reaction forces during the drive phase than the FU style and may, therefore, be more conducive to rapid movement to the net following the serve.

The sequence of upper-limb movements must be coordinated with the lower-limb drive if a successful serve is to result. Tennis texts[1,2,11] have advocated the flow of energy from the lower limbs to the trunk, and finally to the racket arm so as to produce an optimal velocity at impact. Van Gheluwe and Hebbelinck[15] and Elliott et al.[16] in three-dimensional cinematographic studies of skilled servers, reported that this summation of velocities did occur. The lower-limb drive not only began the summation process, but also assisted in increasing the range of racket movement during the loop of the racket down the player's back. At the time of maximum vertical velocity of the hip, the shoulder was accelerated upward and the racket and forearm recorded maximum negative velocities as the racket moved "down the back" of the server.[16]

The linear velocity of segment end-points (Table 1) shows how a gradual summation of velocity occurs. The times when the maximum end-point velocities were achieved were closer to the time of impact as the end-point velocity was closer to the racket.[15,16] The sagittal end-point velocities derived from three-dimensional coordinates for a female junior international graphed from near the completion of the lower-limb drive, are recorded in Figure 2. The end-point kinematics in this figure represent the magnitude of the resultant velocities and do not indicate the direction of the vertical and horizontal vectors. The summation process is evident in this figure as end-point velocity increases from the hip to the shoulder to the elbow to the wrist and finally to the racket. The timing of the forearm extension at the elbow (indicated by wrist end-point velocity) in the plane of the hit, may have been fractionally late with reference to upper-arm movement if an optimal result was to be attained. Impact, as with so many hitting activities, occurred after maximum racket velocity had been reached.

The role of forearm pronation in this summation process was identified by Jack et al.[7] An electrogoniometer recorded radioulnar rotation (pronation) of 900°/sec, 0.1 sec prior to

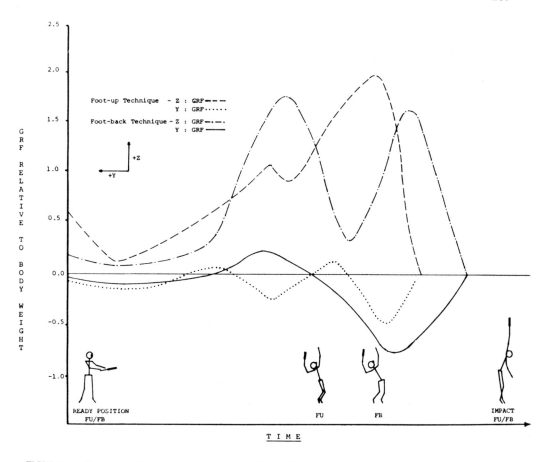

FIGURE 1. Vertical and horizontal ground-reaction forces (GRF) during the foot-up and foot-back service technique. (From the *Austral. J. Sports Sci.*, 3, 2, 1983. With permission).

Table 1
LINEAR VELOCITIES OF THE HITTING ARM IN
THE TENNIS SERVE (m/sec)

	Horizontal velocities[a] (n = 1, male international)		Resultant velocities[b] (n = 4; two college males [M], two college females [F])	
	Maximum	Impact	Maximum	Impact
Shoulder	3.3	2.6	2.7 (F) 3.3 (M)	0.7 (F) 0.8 (M)
Elbow	5.4	3.9	5.1 (F) 6.4 (M)	1.7 (F) 1.9 (M)
Wrist	8.1	6.1	6.3 (F) 7.8 (M)	2.1 (F) 2.3 (M)
Center of racket	Not reported	31.0	26.1 (F) 28.2 (M)	23.4 (F) 27.7 (M)

Note: Values shown are in m/sec.

[a] Modified from Van Gheluwe and Hebbelinck, 1983.
[b] Elliott et al., 1986.

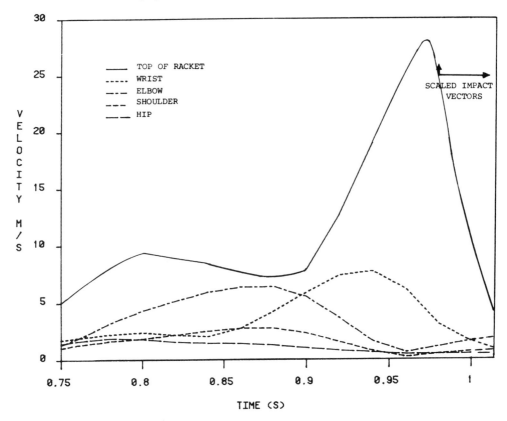

FIGURE 2.   Summation of resultant end-point velocities in the latter stages of the tennis serve.

impact for a skilled tennis player. Van Gheluwe and De Ruysscher[17] corroborated this result for three skilled tennis players filmed at 300 frames per sec. This study clearly demonstrated the marked pronation of the forearm during the follow-through phase of the stroke.

Jack et al.[7] further reported the angular velocity of the wrist as 1087°/sec just prior to impact for a skilled tennis player. This velocity had reduced to 600°/sec, 0.1 sec into the follow-through phase of the stroke. An optimal velocity for the racket is an end-result of the summation chain. Elliott and Wood[14] reported angular velocities of 1570°/sec, 0.02 sec prior to impact, in a cinematographic laboratory-based experiment on serving. These values were not as high as the on-court maximum racket - angular velocities of 1900°/sec for Connors and 2200°/sec for a fast serve action just prior to impact.[18] At impact, the body should be extended to produce an optimal hitting height. Elliott[19,20] reported that a more extended body position was attained as serve-maturity was achieved (Table 2).

Taylor,[21] in a combined EMG- and cinematography study, reported that the triceps muscle played a major role in positioning the racket for impact. Significant differences in the level of activity for the triceps muscle were recorded between the flat-and-twist serves and the slice-and-twist serves, but no difference in activity level was recorded between the flat and slice serves. No differences in activity levels were recorded for the anterior deltoid, middle deltoid, or posterior deltoid muscles for these three serve actions.

The path of the racket just prior to impact and its implications for rotation and trajectory of the ball, are very important and, therefore, will be discussed in a separate section.

4. Racket Trajectory Prior to and Following Impact

Research has shown that a serve is seldom hit flat at high speeds, because the height of the impact above the court for players of average stature is too low to allow the ball to clear

Table 2
BODY AND RACKET POSITION AT IMPACT

Body Segment/Joint/Racket	12 years				15 years				Adults			
	M	M	F	F	M	M	F	F	M	M	F	F
Racket[a]	96	91	94	100	92	91	94	92	90	90	94	90
Racket												
Wrist	186	183	221	222	197	199	216	210	202	180	213	180
Forearm												
Elbow	180	164	176	159	178	173	158	158	174	179	172	180
Arm												
Shoulder	178	186	184	151	200	188	174	170	177	197	164	195
Trunk												
Hip	166	149	129	151	153	169	151	139	155	158	157	161
Thigh												
Knee	173	169	165	156	180	175	175	167	178	173	174	172
Leg												
Ankle	126	150	156	160	143	145	138	141	140	140	142	145
Foot												

Note: Values shown are in degrees.

[a] Racket angle is given in degrees with respect to the right hand horizontal. All joint angles represent the angle between adjacent body segments reported in degrees.

the net and yet still land in the service court.[1,11,19] Braden and Bruns[1] stated that "to hit the ball hard, on a straight line, so that it clears the net by one to six inches and lands one inch inside your opponent's service line, the center of your racket must be ten feet in the air." A ball is therefore seldom hit flat at high speeds if a successful service is to result, but must be hit so that a degree of forward rotation can be imparted to the ball.[11]

Gravity, air resistance, and forward rotation of the ball all help to ensure that an appropriate trajectory occurs for a successful service. Gravity, to a greater or lesser extent depending on where the match is played, is always present. The influence of air resistance on forward velocity is demonstrated by the fact that a service velocity of 62 m/sec off the racket was reduced to 48 m/sec as the ball crossed the net,[22] or a velocity of 51 m/sec was reduced to 40 m/sec[23] just prior to impacting the court.

The influence of air resistance and the fact that tournament players hit even their flat serves with forward rotation, means that results from calculations ignoring these factors[24] must only be considered in very general terms. Golenko,[25] who considered air resistance in his calculations, produced nomograms relating height, velocity, and trajectory angle.

The need for such a large margin of error at the net is necessary, as Ariel and Braden[18] have shown that serving is a ballistic action where the racket follows an almost predetermined trajectory. Forward ball rotation will provide this extra margin for error at the net, and so coaches teaching the power serve have emphasized an up-and-out hitting action which produces this spin. Borg[26] categorized those actions where the racket moved squarely along the target line and hit the ball with no spin as "beginners' serves".

Elliott [19,20] investigated the service action of three groups of two males and two females using high-speed cinematography; one group was adult, one group was 15-year olds, and one group was 12-year olds. All subjects were tournament players deemed by professional coaches to have good service actions for their stage of development. All subjects were instructed to hit a fast serve from near the center mark on the baseline so that it would land in a 1.5-m² position in the left-hand corner of the deuce service court (only successful serves were analyzed).

The flat serve appears to be a misnomer for many highly skilled players. Table 3 shows that the four adults all served a fast power serve with an up-and-out action immediately preceding impact, which imparted forward rotation to the ball.

The highest forward rotation resulted from a 5° upward racket trajectory immediately prior to impact followed by a further 2° upward trajectory immediately following impact (Figure 3).

The group of 15-year olds lay between the other groups with regards to their service development, as the racket either moved straight through the ball or upward at 1° immediately prior to impact. No significant ball rotation resulted from an impact where the racket moved in a straight line both one frame prior to and following impact, a characteristic of the group of 12 year olds.

B. The Forehand and Backhand Drives

1. The Grip

The first problem all prospective tennis players must address is the manner in which the racket is held. The height that a tennis ball bounces is dictated by the coefficient of restitution between the ball and the court surface.[27] The grips taught for the forehand and backhand have therefore varied in accordance with the surface used for play. Western forehand and backhand grips are linked to the slower surfaces (such as clay), while eastern forehand and backhand grips are used on faster surfaces (such as cement).[2] Although the role of grip firmness in stroke production will be reviewed in a later section, it is appropiate at this stage to mention the work of Vogt,[28] who reported that tennis-playing ability did not increase following a wrist-strength training program of only 5 weeks.

2. Footwork

Integral to any discussion of footwork is the question of how a player can get to the ball as quickly as possible and then maintain balance in preparation for the subsequent stroke. Very little research has been directed at these questions, and so research findings from peripheral areas will be used to give some guidance in this area.

From a ready position the body must "unweight" itself by accelerating downwards towards the court. Deceleration of the body then applies stretch to the muscles which results in the subsequent storage of elastic energy in muscles and associated tissues.[29] This stored energy can then at least partially be used to assist the lower-limb drive in moving the player to the vicinity of the next stroke.

The timing of the split step in tennis is critical and must be coordinated with this concept of "unweighting".[30] Observation of experienced players shows their feet are off the ground at or just after the opponent's stroke. With proper timing, a player can visually determine the direction and depth of the opponent's shot when the feet touch the ground.[30] This is the time for the "unit turn". Papers by Abernathy and Russell[31] and Glencross and Cibich,[32] although not biomechanical, analyze the areas of reaction- and movement-times related to tennis, and cueing for different tennis strokes.

Table 3
RACKET AND BALL MOVEMENT PRE- AND POSTIMPACT IN THE TENNIS SERVE

	12 years				15 years				Adults			
	Males		Females		Males		Females		Males		Females	
Racket path												
1 Frame prior to impact (°)	Flat	1	Flat	Flat	1	Flat	Flat	1	3	5	2	4
Impact to 1 frame postimpact (°)	Flat	Flat	−4	−1	Flat	−5	−2	Flat	Flat	2	Flat	Flat
Ball movement												
Height of impact (m)	2.5	2.3	2.4	2.2	2.7	2.9	2.4	2.6	3.0	3.1	2.6	2.9
Velocity (m/sec)	32.0	30.3	33.6	31.4	43.3	44.0	37.0	38.1	48.6	50.0	43.3	47.0
Impact to 1 frame postimpact (°)	Flat	−1	−2	1	Flat	−1	−1	Flat	Flat	Flat	−1	Flat

Modified from Elliott.[19,20]

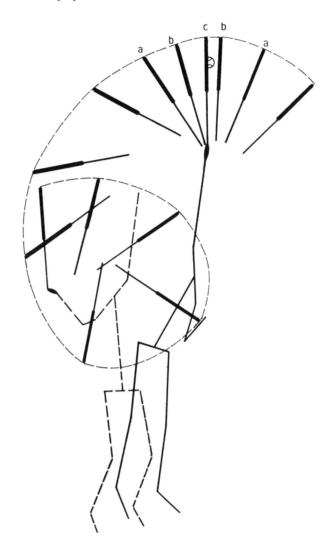

FIGURE 3. Path of the racket from the beginning of lower-limb extension to impact in a tennis serve. (A) 2 frames pre- and postimpact; (B) 1 frame pre- and postimpact; and (C) impact. (From *Sports Coach*, 6, 4, 1983. With permission).

If movement of any great distance is required to impact the ball the player must use the arms to run efficiently and to maintain balance. The racket is then taken back in preparation for ball impact.

Once the player is prepared to hit the ball, imaginary lines between the head and feet will ideally constitute a triangle with two equal sides and a base of varying length.[30] When further movement is required to reach the ball, the knee of the player's forward leg must be between the lead foot and a vertical line through the CG for a balanced hitting position.

3. The Kinematics and Kinetics of the Swing

Ariel and Braden,[18] in biomechanically analyzing the movement patterns of top-class tennis players, identified that a combination of ballistic and tracking modes existed in the groundstrokes of highly skilled tennis players, where high velocity with control was required. Ballistic movement characterized by preprogrammed neural control was therefore tempered with feedback from muscles, tendons, and skin receptors to modify movement patterns and cause a controlled impact situation (tracking mode).

Keating, in Braden and Bruns,[1] theoretically calculated that the racket head gains approximately 2.7 m/sec for every 30 cm it continuously moves during the backswing. The advantage of a circular backswing was corroborated by Pecore[33] in a cinematographic study of varsity women, where subjects using a circular backswing averaged higher racket head velocities at impact, when compared to players using a straight backswing. Plagenhoef[23] suggested that research had indicated that the length of the backswing should be altered so that the closing velocity of the racket and the ball did not exceed 44.7 m/sec.

The body must summate the velocities of different segments for a groundstroke in a similar fashion to the serve. This force-summation starts as the lower limbs generate a ground-reaction force by pushing against the court. Groppel[3] used high-speed cinematography to show that Connors did not leave the ground until the instant of impact, thus, the "jumping action" observed during his high-velocity groundstrokes does not contribute to the power of his strokes. The reaction from the ground does, however, initiate the gradual build-up of velocity for impact.

Van Gheluwe[34] and Ariel and Braden,[18] in three-dimensional cinematogaphic studies of skilled players, showed that this summation process does occur in the forehand drive. Table 4 shows how the linear velocities of different anatomical landmarks increased as the body segments approached the point of impact.[34] A peak angular velocity of 870°/sec for the elbow joint was reduced to 100°/sec at impact, while the wrist decreased from 350°/sec to approximately zero at impact. A wrist angle of 158° and minimal angular velocity at this joint, is supported in the coaching literature which advocates a laid-back and stabilized wrist at impact.[34] The velocity curves of various body segments (Figure 4) for Nastase hitting a forehand drive show that the summation effect is apparent.[18]

The need for both accuracy and power to be ingredients for a successful forehand, causes a reduction in racket velocity just prior to impact. Nastase slowed from a peak angular velocity of the racket of 1800°/sec to a velocity of 1450°/sec at impact, while Evert slowed from a peak value of 1660°/sec to 1075°/sec at impact.[18] The skilled performer in the study by Van Gheluwe,[34] also slowed from a peak linear velocity of approximately 36 m/sec at the end of the racket to 20 m/sec at impact.

The need for stability at impact was further reported by Van Gheluwe.[34] A stable head, a left shoulder that did not show appreciable movement away from the direction of the hit prior to impact (right-handed player), and a center of mass that rose gradually during the forward swing, were characteristics of the skilled subject.

The velocity curves of the various body segments were very similar for a forehand and backhand drive by Nastase[18] (Figure 4). In this stroke, Nastase again showed the need for control when his racket slowed from a peak angular velocity of 2250 to 1650°/sec at impact. Evert, with her two-handed backhand, slowed from 1800 to 1050°/sec at impact.

The trajectory of the racket during the forward swing is a major determinant of the type of spin imparted to the ball. Varying amounts of topspin or backspin are imparted to the ball in an endeavor to allow the ball to clear the net by a reasonable margin and yet land in the court (topspin); to upset an opponent's rhythm; and to control shot placement. The need for a margin of error at the net has been clearly established, since 66% of all points won in a study by Hensley[35] were a direct result of an opponent's mistake, while 75% of the errors made in a match were the result of the ball hitting the net.[36] Groppel et al.[37] used mathematical modeling and cinematography in an attempt to relate the factors of racket trajectory, racket and head orientation, and racket and ball velocities, to predict postimpact spin of the tennis ball. A graph was constructed through the use of analytical equations to provide coaches and teachers with a means for teaching spin production or the modification of spin production. A racket face "closed" by 10° produced a larger level of topspin for a given racket trajectory than did a vertical racket orientation.[37] This nomogram corroborated a trajectory angle for the racket of 45 to 55° if topspin was to be imparted to the ball.[23]

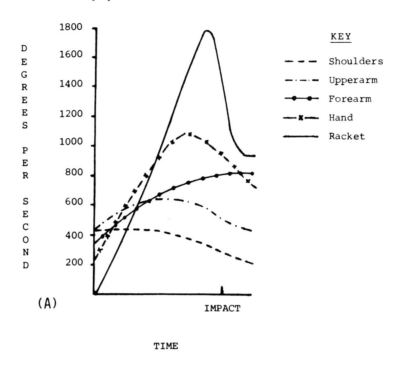

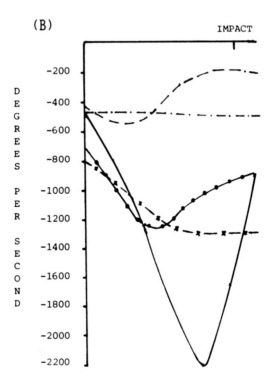

FIGURE 4. Overhead view of forehand (A) and backhand (B) drive. (Modified from Ariel and Braden[18]).

Table 4
LINEAR VELOCITY AT IMPACT IN THE DIRECTION OF THE HIT FOR THE FOREHAND DRIVE

Right hip	0.7
Right shoulder	1.2
Right elbow	4.0
Right wrist	8.5
Top of racket	20.0

Note: Velocity values are in m/sec and for a right-handed player.

Modified from Van Gheluwe.[34]

Blievernicht[38] showed that skilled players alter the impact position in an attempt to alter the direction of the hit. The ball was impacted in line with the front shoulder and 21 cm behind the front foot for a down-the-line return and in front of both the front shoulder and front foot (7.5 cm) for an cross-court return. The angle of the racket mirrored these positions with an angle range of 72 to 80° for down-the-line returns and 93 to 103° for across-court returns.

Hobart[39] and Holcomb[40] identified the joint action making the major contribution to the forward movement of the tennis racket in the forehand and backhand drives, as forward rotation of the pelvis at the hip joint of the forward leg. This result was partially corroborated by Young[41] who used cinematography to record the groundstrokes of advanced and novice players. Analysis of this film revealed that an increased ball velocity for the forehand was accompanied by an increase in the distance the racket moved on the forward swing of the advanced players, while the increased velocity on the backhand was accompanied by an increase in spinal rotation of both groups. Pecore,[33] in analyzing the backhand techniques of advanced and beginner varsity women, reported that advanced players were characterized by a firm wrist at impact, contact was made with the center of the strings, and they stepped into the ball and thus enlarged the base in the direction of the hit to allow a forward shift of the CG. Beginners were not able to position themselves at a comfortable distance from the ball and generally started the forward swing with the elbow leading the movement. An EMG and cinematographic study of the forehand drives of advanced and beginner players showed that the decrease in muscle activity in the advanced players was paralleled by an increase in racket velocity, which indicated an increase in the efficiency of the stroke.[42] Anderson[42] further reported that there was minimal variation in the EMGs recorded for each subject, but the variation between subjects hindered a rank-order of muscle involvement.

4. The One-Handed vs. the Two-Handed Backhand

A great deal of tennis literature has been devoted to this selection problem. This section will only report similarities and differences between these strokes that have been investigated in research studies. The efficient backhand requires the addition of forward body movement (linear motion), with the rotation of the trunk at the hip joints and the rotation of the racket limb about the glenohumeral articulation (angular motion). The linear velocity of the racket at impact is derived from the radius of rotation and the angular velocity of the hitting system plus any forward velocity of the body. For a high racket velocity, the radius of rotation must be kept as long as possible, and therefore the angular motion of the hitting limb should follow as large an arc as possible, a factor which would favor the one-handed technique.[43] The reduced moment of inertia of the two-handed technique may assist the player in attaining a higher angular velocity of the racket-limb system, thus counteracting the effect of a reduced hitting radius.[40]

The next obvious question then, is whether this reduction in lever length influences the reach of a player. Groppel[44] used high-speed cinematography to analyze the one-handed (18 subjects) and two-handed (18 subjects) backhands of skilled female tennis players. He showed that there was no difference in reach between the two strokes when the players were not forced to run or stretch for the ball. Theoretically, the one-handed backhand does have an advantage in reach if the player is required to stretch for a wide return.

One of the major reported benefits of the two-handed backhand is the fact that the coordination of body segments is made easier because of the reduced number of segments required to produce this stroke. Groppel[44] identified five distinct body segments that needed coordination for a one-handed backhand, while the two-handed counterpart only required two segments. The one-handed stroke needed the coordination of hip-turn, trunk-rotation, upper-arm rotation, slight forearm movement, and then hand and racket movement prior to impact. The two-handed backhand only required the coordination of the hips and the trunk-upper-limb-racket segment which acted as a single unit. He further reported that the two-handed backhand was characterized by greater trunk rotation, while hip rotation played a dominant role in the one-handed stroke. He concluded that the two-handed backhand should be the preferred stroke when hitting a tennis ball in such a position that the body is a comfortable distance from the ball.

A young beginner using a one-handed backhand will often have a problem holding the racket the required distance from the body and impacting the ball in front of the lead foot. Groppel[45] and Elliott[46] have both shown that wrist strength was needed to counteract the torque created about the long axis after off-center impacts. It is logical to assume that greater hitting-limb strength is required for the multilink model used in the one-handed backhand than in the two-link model of the two-handed backhand. No research study has specifically addressed this hypothesis, however.

Does the increased difficulty in a five-segment skill (one-handed backhand) compared to a two-segment skill (two-handed backhand) affect the ability to learn these skills and does the reduced strength requirement of the two-handed backhand complicate this effect? Schroeder et al.[47] taught college-age students a one-handed (56 subjects) or two-handed backhand (65 subjects) for two classes per week over an 8-week period. Teaching, although standarized, was not by the same instructors and a request that additional practice be limited could not be easily controlled. Significant improvements were recorded for both groups, although no significance was found between the modes of performance. Rhinehart[48] had earlier reported that there was no difference between the accuracy of the one-handed and two-handed strokes for beginners. These results would suggest that tennis students should be allowed their own preference in backhand development. A more rigidly controlled pedagogical study with young children is needed if advice to coaches is to be based on sound research evidence.

C. The Volley

The only biomechanical research done on the volley was a study of five professional players,[49] in which it was reported that the power in the stroke came from the legs thrusting the body forward, the turning of the shoulders and extension of the forearm at the elbow, or the movement of the upper limb as a unit from the shoulder.[49] No decision was possible to identify a single-volley technique based on the five professionals filmed.

III. EQUIPMENT DESIGN

A. Tennis Racket Selection: A Factor in Early Skill Development

It has been reported that a marked disparity often exists between the physical characteristics of young players and the rackets they use during class lessons or general play. Preliminary results suggested that an enhanced performance resulted when the physical characteristics of the player and the racket were optimized.[50-52]

Knuttgen,[50] who investigated the influence of varying racket lengths (64 to 74 cm) on the stroke performance of advanced and beginner college players, concluded that a shorter racket improved the accuracy of beginner players.

Ward and Groppel[51] investigated the influence of different length tennis rackets on the stroke mechanics of the forehand drive. Three 8-year-old children (one male, two female), who were unfamiliar with the game of tennis, were instructed in a clinic for 1 week with a long racket (standard size: 68.6 cm 370 g) and 1 week with a short racket (58.4 cm, 370 g). Filming of the forehand drive occurred at the end of each week of the coaching clinic. Identical procedures then followed with three further beginning children, who were taught using a short racket during week 1 and progressed to the long racket for week 2. The results of this study indicated that all the subjects swung more effectively with the smaller racket when compared to the larger implement. The children swung the shorter racket with a greater horizontal velocity (14.7 m/sec compared to 12.2 m/sec). They also swung the shorter racket with less vertical velocity (1.9 m/sec compared to 3.2 m/sec) and had a more vertical racket-face at impact than was produced when hitting with the longer racket. The path of the racket in the forward swing to the impact phase of the forehand stroke, for two subjects (one male, one female), clearly showed the inability of these subjects to control the moment of inertia of the longer racket during this phase of the stroke.

Elliott[52] investigated the influence of racket size on the learning of tennis skills in young children aged between 7 and 10 years, who had no previous tennis coaching or playing experience. Sixty children were matched for age, height, weight, and manual dexterity, and placed into groups for an 8-week, 16-session (50 min per session) coaching program. The first group was taught using junior rackets (66 cm, 310 g), the second with racquetball rackets for 4 weeks (44 cm, 247 g) and subjunior rackets for 4 weeks (61 cm, 265 g), and the third group used only subjunior rackets. The Hewitt revision of the Dyer backboard test[53] to assess general tennis ability, together with specific tests of stroke production, was administered at the end of the program. Group 1 was tested using junior rackets, while groups 2 and 3 used subjunior rackets. A two-way analysis of variance with post-hoc comparisons, was used to test for difference between groups.

It can be seen from Table 5, that tennis-playing ability, as measured by the Hewitt revision of the Dyer tennis test, was superior for the group taught using a subjunior racket. The superior performances of groups 2 and 3 over group 1 were recorded in tests of the service, forehand drive, and backhand drive. Only in the volley tests, where the swing moment of inertia (this concept will be fully discussed in Section III.B) of the racket was of minor concern to the stroke (minimal backswing), were the results not in favor of stroke production with the subjunior racket. It is evident that the higher swing moment of inertia of the junior racket, when compared to the subjunior racket, reduced the ability of the young children to master basic tennis skills.

Both studies[51,52] clearly demonstrated the need for racket size generally to be related to body size as indicated by age. Neither study, however, totally answers the problem of racket selection in relation to body size and strength. The position of these papers echoes sentiments expressed by Pruitt,[43] who concluded that designing rackets for the "average" individual is fundamentally unsound. Research data do, however, provide coaches and teachers with some information that can assist in the selection of a racket to suit an individual need.

B. The Racket

The tennis boom has been paralleled by an increase in the technology directed at equipment development, with the focal point being the ultimate "weapon" of the game, the racket. Early research into the flexibility of different rackets[54-57] reported that most aluminum rackets could be classified as very flexible, whereas wooden (or wooden composite) rackets varied from a very flexible to a very stiff classification. Brody[58] suggested, however, that much

Table 5
TENNIS PERFORMANCE TESTS

		Group 1 — junior rackets	Group 2 — racketball/subjunior rackets	Group 3 — subjunior rackets	*p*
Hewitt test	X̄	5.6[a]	6.5	7.2[b]	
	SD	1.8	3.4	4.2	<0.01
Forehand drive	X̄	8.9[a]	14.6	14.7	
	SD	5.8	6.9	7.6	<0.01
Backhand drive	X̄	2.3[a]	9.2	9.9	
	SD	1.8	5.6	6.7	<0.01
Forehand volley	X̄	7.4	6.0[b]	7.4	
	SD	2.1	2.8	2.3	<0.01
Backhand volley	X̄	5.2	4.8	6.3[b]	
	SD	2.6	2.7	2.6	<0.01
Serve	X̄	7.1[a]	13.3	13.8	
	SD	4.1	5.8	6.0	<0.01

[a]   A significant difference (0.01) between this and groups 2 and 3.
[b]   A significant difference (0.01) between this and the other two groups.

From Elliott, B., *Austral. J. Sports Sci.,* 1, 23, 1981. With permission.

more research was required in the area, as the half-period of oscillation of flexible rackets measured was approximately twice the contact-time of the ball on the strings. If this is the mode of oscillation that a racket undergoes when it strikes a ball, then all the energy that goes into deforming the racket is lost, as the ball has left the strings before the racket can begin to return to its pre-impact position. Brody[58] reported that if a hand-held racket oscillated with a node at the center of mass and not at the handle, then the oscillation period would be shorter and more easily related to the contact time of the ball. In a further study, Brody[59] concluded that an increase in the rebound coefficient would follow if more energy was absorbed by the strings (lower tension) and less energy was lost to the racket (stiffer frames).

Today, the use of materials such as graphite, Kevlar®, boron, and fiberglass has permitted the manufacture of a large number of different rackets. Laboratory testing of rackets has therefore been dominated by manufacturers and a laboratory supported by the *World Tennis magazine,* the *Journal of the United States Tennis Association.* A Racket Almanac of over 100 models tested for stiffness, stability, "power zone", and "playability" was presented in their 1984 December issue.[60]

Tennis players continually seek added power, control, and a reduction in the unpleasant vibrations produced by off-center impacts. Fisher,[61] in an interview with Howard Head, the inventor of the Prince® oversize rackets, reported him as saying that the development of this design was motivated by a desire to reduce the torque produced by off-center impacts. An increase in the polar or roll moment of inertia was achieved by increasing the distance of the mass from the central axis (perimeter-weighting) or by enlarging the rackethead. Blanksby et al.[62] reported that the oversize racket is "equal to, or superior than, conventional rackets where stroke accuracy of recreational players is concerned." This result was corroborated by Gruetter and Davis,[63] who investigated the differences between oversized and standard-sized rackets, using groundstroke, volley, service, and return of service tests of accuracy for college-age pupils. Both beginner- and intermediate-level performers scored higher when using the oversized racket.

The moment of inertia of a tennis racket about its principal axes influences how the racket plays and how it feels when it is swung.[64] The wider the head of the racket (the higher the polar moment of inertia about the Y axis, Figure 5), the less likely it is that the racket will twist in your hand for an off-axis impact.[64] This theoretical premise was supported experimentally by Elliott et al.[65]

Oversized rackets (higher polar moment of inertia) demonstrated lower vibration levels (measured using accelerometry) and higher rebound velocities (measured using stroboscope photography) than their conventional counterparts, when balls struck by the racket were compared along a line drawn perpendicular to the racket shaft and through the geometric center of the strings.[65] The Wilson® company has increased the polar moment of inertia by the addition of discrete masses to the frame in their Perimeter Weight System® rackets. Brody[64] showed how to calculate the moment of inertia using the torsional oscillator technique: $T = 2\pi\sqrt{I/K}$ where T = period of torsional oscillator, I = moment of inertia of racket about a specific axis, and K = torsional constant of the wire (determined using an object of Known I).

Brody[64] further reported how the torsional oscillation method was used to calculate the moment of inertia about the center of mass and then how the parellel-axis theorem (cf. Figure 5) enabled values to be calculated about an axis through the pivot-point on the handle. The moment of inertia about an axis in the horizontal direction of the hit is often referred to colloquially as the "swing weight", as it is a measure of how heavy a racket feels when it is swung (Figure 5, X axis). This measure, which greatly influences stroke production particularly of young children, was discussed in the previous section. The moment of inertia about the Z axis perpendicular to the plane of the racket, is of concern for players whose trajectory during the forward racket swing is very steep and who thus impart a great deal of either topspin or underspin to the ball. Measurements of the moments around the polar (Y) and swing (X) axes through the handle, but in the plane of the racket, show that the moment about the X axis is approximately 20 times the moment about the Y axis. Therefore, the moment about the axis through the handle, but perpendicular to the racket plane (Z), being the sum of the other two moments, will be only 5% greater than the "swing weight".[64]

If the ball hits the center of mass of a racket it will translate, but not rotate. If the ball hits the racket a distance from the center of mass, the racket will rotate and translate. The point where an impact produces the effect of the motion due to rotation exactly canceling the overall translation at the pivot point on the handle, is referred to as the center of percussion.[58,66] For a conventional racket held at the handle, the center of percussion is usually 5 to 6 cm closer to the throat of the racket from the geometric center of the strings.[58] This position was supported experimentally by Elliott et al.[65] where minimum vibrations and maximum rebound velocities were obtained for impacts 4 cm closer to the throat of the racket for a sample of two oversized, two conventional wooden, and two conventional aluminum rackets. Manufacturers have addressed this problem by varying the shapes of the racket head, in an attempt to create an "area of percussion" that is centrally positioned on the string surface.

Clarification is still required for the term "sweet spot" which is often used interchangeably with the center of percussion of a racket. If the "sweet spot" is the center of percussion, then it is a well-defined point (or pair of conjugate points) for a rigid body and the location of this point can be found by using the racket as a physical pendulum and measuring its period.[59]

$$S = \frac{Icm}{Md}$$

where S = distance from the center of percussion to the pivot point, I_{cm} = moment of

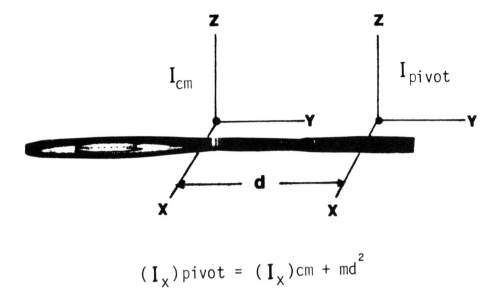

$$(I_x) \text{pivot} = (I_x) \text{cm} + md^2$$

FIGURE 5.   The axes of a tennis racket through the center of mass (cm) and the pivot point on the handle (pivot). (Modified from Brody[64]).

inertia about the cm, M = mass of the implement, and d = distance from the cm to the pivot point.[11,66]

If the "sweet spot" is the region on the racket face where the rebound coefficient (post impact ball velocity compared to preimpact velocity) is above some arbitrary value, then to reduce confusion, this area should be called the power zone and the point where the rebound coefficient is maximum, as the power point. Normally, stroboscope photography[65] or high-speed cinematography[67] has been used to identify the above locations. A further definition has the "sweet spot" as the point where racket vibrations or oscillations are a minimum. Sykes et al.[66] and Elliot et al.[65] used accelerometry to identify the point or area of minimal vibration, and Brody[59] used a "liquid potentiometer" and camera to observe modes of oscillation.

All three definitions of the "sweet spot" have merit and, in general terms, the points corresponding to them are located in slightly different places.[59] It is asumed that the ideal tennis racket would have all three of these points located in the center of the strung area.

C. String Type and Tension

String type, tension, and the interaction of tension and racket flexibility, have all been researched in an effort to provide greater insight into equipment characteristics. Gut strings have a slight advantage over synthetic strings in their ability to store energy from the incoming ball and then return this energy to the ball.[23,50,67-69] Pouzzner[70] concluded that 16-gauge gut strung at 222-, 258-, and 289-N tension was more resilient than nylon, and that both string types were more resilient as the tension was reduced. Nelson[71] referenced research findings of Kaminstein and reported that gut and nylon have almost identical coefficients of elasticity and elongation under strain. The small difference in the rebound coefficient is probably caused by the rougher texture of the gut which reduces string movement when compared with the synthetic material, and thus less energy is dissipated through friction.

The question that has often been posed relating string tension and rebound coefficients (velocity of the ball post-impact compared to pre-impact) is whether to string one's racket tighter for more control or for more power. Bosworth,[69] an acknowledged authority on the interaction of rebound coefficients and string tension, and racket flexibility and string tension, proposed the following guidelines for the selection of string tension.

1. String the racket at the upper end of the manufacturer's tension range for control and at or below the lower end of the range for power.
2. A stiff racket frame requires a higher tension than does a more flexible frame, if the tension is to complement the design characteristics of the frame.

These guidelines have, in fact, been substantiated by research findings. Ellis et al.[68] varied string tensions from 222 to 289 N for oversized and regular rackets of similar flexibility, while Groppel[67] varied tensions from 178 to 311 N in a single fixed racket. The higher rebound coefficients were obtained for the lower string tensions. The lower tensions allow the strings to deflect more during impact and therefore less energy will be lost from the ball, which will produce a higher rebound coefficient. Brody[58] further proposed that the greater the energy maintained in the strings, the greater would be the rebound coefficient, provided the time of ball-contact matched the half-period of oscillation of the strings. Groppel,[3] after filming impacts at 4500 frames per sec reported that an increase in string tension caused the ball to "flatten out", which in turn embedded the strings further into the nap of the ball, than would occur for lower tensions. This greater embedding led to greater ball control.

Baker and Wilson,[72] in a study where a clamped static racket was struck by balls with a preimpact velocity of 45 m/sec, reported that stiff rackets were not significantly influenced by differing string tensions (178 to 267 N). Medium and flexible rackets had the highest ball velocities after impact when strung at 222 N. Elliott[73] further investigated the interaction of string tension and racket stiffness using a pneumatically driven racket arm and a ball machine for center and off-center impacts. String tension had no significant influence on rebound velocity for a stiff racket with an inward ball velocity of 22.7 m/sec and a racket velocity of 6.8m/sec. Medium and flexible rackets produced the highest rebound coefficients for both center and off-center impacts when strung at 245 N when compared to 289 and 334 N. Flexible rackets should therefore be strung at lower tensions and stiff rackets should generally be strung at higher tensions.[2] However, if the player prefers a flexible racket and has problems with control, then a higher tension may be of assistance.

Putnam and Baker[74] compared the amount of spin imparted to a tennis ball during impact with conventionally and diagonally strung rackets. Multiple-image photography was used to record the impacts between a static racket, orientated vertically, and balls projected towards the racket at an angle of 45°. They showed that for similar pre-impact conditions, the angular impulse of the contact force applied to the ball (and hence the amount of spin) was not significantly different for the two string configurations.

D. The Tennis Ball

Rand et al.,[27] who recorded rebound height using stroboscopic photography, conducted an experiment designed to indicate which brand of tennis balls fatigued the quickest and what number of bounce impacts was required to cause fatigue. All brands tested rebounded higher after 800 impacts than when new, because the loss of nap increased the ball's coefficient of restitution and decreased its aerodynamic drag, and, in general, this superior performance was evident up to 3200 impacts. Rand et al.[27] reported that the major factor influencing rebound performance was the time out of pressurized conditions (i.e., the can). Five days out of a can produced deteriorations in rebound height for both the balls undergoing rebound testing and a control group that was not impacted.

Whereas a tennis court's dimensions are exactly stated, the composition of the surface material is not covered within the rules of tennis. This variety in surface types (clay, synthetic and rubber carpets, concrete, and grass, just to mention a few) is often classified as being "fast" or "slow". Brody[75] attempted to quantify the interaction of a tennis ball and a number of different court surfaces by investigating two physical characteristics, the coefficient of restitution and the coefficient of friction (sliding and rolling), during the impact between the ball and the surface. A court can be classified as "slow" when the ball changes from a sliding to a rolling mode during impact, such that the horizontal velocity after the bounce is reduced by 40%. This, however, does not happen for most tennis shots, with the possible exception of the lob. Since the majority of shots do not clear the net by more than 1 m, when the ball bounces it will remain in a sliding mode and the resulting loss of horizontal velocity will be proportional to the coefficient of sliding friction between the ball and the court surface. Brody[75] then calculated the coefficient of sliding friction for a number of surfaces to give some indication of court "speed" (wood, $\mu = 0.25$; Laykold,® $\mu = 0.49$; Supreme® court, $\mu = 0.61$).

E. The Tennis Shoe

Shoe manufacturers have invested huge sums of money and large amounts of time to produce shoes that are the state-of-the-art, whether used for hard or soft surfaces. Research, however, into the many aspects of tennis shoe design has paled into insignificance when compared to the research on their counterpart, the running or jogging shoe.

Tennis players, when walking, running, and jumping during practice or in a match, experience a shock on each contact with the court surface. The initial ground- (surface) reaction force (GRF) is transmitted by bones, cartilages, tendons, and muscles to the knee and hip joints.[76] The absorption of these forces signifies a load on the human body and it may be that excessive forces cause pain or even injuries.[77] The magnitude of this shock which can exceed three times body weight[76] depends on the technique used in the movement, the playing surface, and the structure and materials used in shoe design.

Movement technique that does not exacerbate the potential for injury, although essential to performance, will not be discussed in this chapter. Playing surface and the design characteristics of tennis shoes both play a major role in determining the amount of GRF experienced by the player.

The acceleration and GRF amplitudes for running and jumping were nearly twice the value on asphalt when compared to grass.[77] Nigg[76,77] recommended that synthetic surfaces should be developed with damping characteristics which decrease GRF and acceleration amplitudes.

Shoe designs that provide damping in the vertical direction, and yet permit translation and rotational movements in the horizontal plane, are essential if the body is to be protected from injury. The tennis shoe can dampen the GRFs if used on hard surfaces; however, if play is on a soft surface (grass) then the shoe will not further dampen the GRFs.[76,77] Nigg[76] reported that an adequate tennis shoe dampened the acceleration effect of running from 16 g (i.e., 16 times the acceleration due to gravity) to 10 g whereas a soft surface (grass) produced a reduction from 16 to 7 g (comparisons were made with a barefoot runner on an artificial and a grass surface).

Leuthi and Nigg[78] studied the influence of two different shoe designs on the occurrence of pain or discomfort over a 3-month period. Shoe design and individual movement patterns both influenced the occurrence of discomfort and pain. They concluded that lateral stability in shoe design must allow an optimal range of inversion of the foot to permit lateral movements in tennis.[78] The design characteristics which are essential for comfort, performance, and injury prevention are reported in Groppel[3] and Horan.[79]

IV. MECHANICAL CHARACTERISTICS RELATED TO TENNIS

A. Grip Tightness: Its Influence on Rebound Velocity and Reaction Impulse

Tennis coaches have believed that firmness of grip by the hand on the racket at impact was one of the most important factors in determining the effectiveness of a return.[1,36] The optimal effectiveness of a firm grip was supported by a theoretical review of the impact between a racket and a ball by Hatze,[80] who reported that a relationship existed between the tightness of the grip (indirectly represented by the torque applied at the handle to counteract impact) and the recoil impulse (impulse reaction to impact) occurring at the player's hand. He stated that the vibration level at the hand at impact can only be reduced by lowering grip tightness, which then would result in a 10 to 15% reduction in the impulse and, hence, in the power of the stroke.

Studies featuring central impacts on clamped or free-standing rackets by a ball fired from a ball machine, found that rebound coefficients (velocity of the ball post-impact compared to velocity pre-impact) were independent of the level of grip pressure.[28,81-83] A study by Missavage et al.[84] established the theoretical bases for the previous studies concerning grip firmness and its effect on the ratio of post- to pre-impact velocities. This model predicted that, for central impacts, there was no change in the ball: velocity ratio when a regular tennis racket was tightly clamped at the grip or a allowed to stand freely on its butt. They further reported that shortening the length and thus greatly increasing the stiffness of the racket, was required before the effect of grip firmness was noticeable. A paper by Liu,[85] using a mathematical model based on impact theory, provided further analytical support for the previous experimental findings. This model predicted that the rebound coefficient was principally a function of the coefficient of restitution which is practically independent of the condition of grip firmness. Elliott[46] also reported a nonsignificant difference in rebound coefficients for a change in grip pressures for central impacts with a pneumatically driven hitting-arm.

Baker and Putnam,[82] for a static impact, and Elliott,[46] for a moving racket at impact, both reported that there was no significant difference between the impulse applied by the racket to the ball under clamped or free-standing conditions.

An increase in reaction impulse and a decrease in rebound coefficient were generally reported for off-center impacts. Hatze[80] reported that theoretically, an off-center impact would be accompanied by an increase in recoil impulse, which need not be transmitted to the ball. Preliminary findings for off-center impacts (using photographic techniques) by Baker and Putnam[82] suggested that these impacts caused the frame to twist, and consequently reduced the impulse applied by the racket to the ball. This change in impulse was different for clamped and free-standing conditions.[82] These preliminary findings were supported by research into off-center impacts by Plagenhoef,[23] using photographic techniques and a racket instrumented with a pressure transducer, and Elliott,[46] using photographic techniques and a racket instrumented with tri-axial Kistler load cells. Plagenhoef[23] reported that the further away from the long axis an impact occurred, the lower was the rebound coefficient. An impact 2.5 cm above the center produced a 15% reduction in velocity compared to a central impact velocity, while an impact 5.0 cm above the center resulted in a 40% reduction in postimpact velocity.

Postimpact ball velocities were, however, less affected by off-center impacts along the long axis, where reductions of only 10% were reported for impacts near the end of the racket when compared to velocities from central impacts. These reductions in rebound coefficients for off-center impacts were accompanied by increases in the forces transmitted to the hand.[23] Elliott[46] also reported a reduction in rebound coefficient for off-center impacts. Significantly higher off-center coefficients were, however, associated with an increase in grip pressure as shown in Table 6. These higher rebound coefficients were the result of higher reaction impulses in the direction of the hit with an increase in grip pressure for impacts 5.0 cm above the center and 5.0 cm from the center to the distal end of the racket.[46]

Grabiner et al.[83] also investigated the relationship between resistance to rotation (about the longitudinal axis) and postimpact ball velocity following off-center impacts. They reported no significant differences between postimpact ball velocity for two extreme conditions of grip firmness (maximal pressure-clamped and free-standing). However, they suggested

Table 6
REBOUND COEFFICIENTS FOR
DIFFERENT IMPACT LOCATIONS WITH
DIFFERENT GRIP PRESSURES FOR
WOODEN RACKETS

Impact position[a]		Light	Medium	Tight	*p*
C	$\overline{X}$	0.64[b]	0.65	0.69	
(N = 6)	SD	0.08	0.07	0.06	NS
+5	$\overline{X}$	0.52	0.56	0.61[c]	
(N = 6)	SD	0.05	0.07	0.07	<0.01
A5	$\overline{X}$	0.41	0.48	0.52[c]	
(N = 6)	SD	0.04	0.04	0.05	<0.01

Note: Values are means ± S.D.

[a]   C, geometric center of the strings; +5, 5 cm from the center to the distal end; A5, 5 cm above the geometric center.
[b]   Rebound coefficients compare the postimpact velocity with the pre-impact velocity which was approximately 22.7 m/sec.
[c]   The posthoc comparison showed the significant difference to be between the light-grip and the tight-grip levels.

Modified from Elliott.[46]

that an interaction may be apparent between closing velocity of both ball and racket considered) and the influence of grip firmness. The closing velocity in this study was only 10.6 m/sec (well below what would be expected in a tennis match), but the increases in rebound coefficients for an increase in grip firmness for extreme off-center impacts, were reported for higher closing velocities (26.5,[82] 30,[46] and 38 m/sec[23]).

B. The Mechanical Characteristics of Impact

Gravity, the forces associated with the collision between the ball and the racket, and the forces exerted on the racket by the player's hand, all play a role in determining the trajectory of a racket during any stroke. The impulsive force at impact between the racket and ball, is conveyed from the point of impact to the racket rim, thence to the handle, and finally to the hitting limb of the player.[86] This section reviews research directed at racket vibrations and forces that occur during the tennis stroke, with specific emphasis on the impact between the racket and the ball.

Brannigan and Adali[86] used mathematical modeling to support the experimental results of Brody,[58] that the higher the string tension, the shorter the impact time (range 4 to 6 msec for a change of string tension from 150 to 350 N). This increase in string tension was accompanied by an increase in force on the frame.[86]

Ohmichi et al.[87] used two strain gauges attached to a wood and graphite racket to assess racket vibrations for different power strokes. Central impacts produced very low levels of vibration at impact; however, off-center impacts produced an increase, as did the difference between a softly hit shot and a powerful impact. All vibration levels were given in arbitrary units and, consequently, no values can be reported. Hatze[80] reported that an increase in grip pressure was accompanied by an increase in amplitude of the resulting vibrations at impact. While impact only lasts approximately 4 msec, the subsequent oscillation behaves as a sinusoidal function[86] and extends over a period of approximately 40 msec.[80]

The arm of the player experiences diminishing bilateral loadings with a frequency of approximately 330 Hz (caused by vibration of the string surface), followed by a vibration of approximately 83 Hz (caused by racket vibration).[88] These results supported the findings of Brannigan and Adali[86] who reported an initial racket frequency of 100 Hz, which was the second node of free vibration.

Rackets instrumented either with accelerometers or strain gauges, have been used to validate mathematical models of the forces associated with movement of a tennis racket and the racket/ball impact. Both the force and the moment of force behave like a sinusoidal function, the maximum amplitude of which, decreases almost exponentially. Reported forces for groundstrokes at impact for a free-swinging racket, have varied from 40 N (Brannigan and Adali,[86] using modeling), 68 N (Kacelson,[88] strain gauge instrumented racket), to 101 N (Kane et al.,[89] strain gauge instrumented racket). Fritz and Hartman[90] reported a peak force at impact of 166 N for a fixed racket instrumented with both accelerometers and strain gauges. Plagenhoef,[23] using an instrumented racket (strain gauges), reported a range of force levels from 124 to 248 N for center and off-center impacts.

Hatze[80] reported the magnitude of the maximum torque applied by the player during the swing phase of 13.2 and 9.4 N·m for the forehand and backhand strokes, respectively. This supported the work of Kane et al.,[89] who reported a torque of 10.8 N·m for the backhand stroke. Hatze[80] calculated a maximum torque level of 23 N·m for a forehand stroke at impact, which was later corroborated by Brannigan and Adali[86] who reported a maximum value of 20 N·m at impact.

The literature indicates that in analyzing the force-time characteristics of racket movement and impact, the curves corresponding to the same stroke performed by different players have the same general shape, but differ in detail.[87,89] McLaughlin and Miller[91] further warned that using a single-skilled subject to perform a skilled (conventional backhand) and unskilled movement (elbow-leading backhand) produced higher torque levels for the skilled performance than in the unskilled movement pattern, presumably because of the familiarity of the subject with the skilled performance.

ACKNOWLEDGMENT

I wish to acknowledge the assistance of Dr. Graeme Wood in the preparation of this chapter.

REFERENCES

1. **Braden, V. and Bruns, B.,** *Vic Braden's Tennis for the Future,* Little, Brown, Boston, 1977.
2. **Elliot, B. and Kilderry, R.,** *The Art and Science of Tennis,* Saunders College, New York, 1983.
3. **Groppel, J. L.,** *Tennis for Advanced Players and Those Who Would Like To Be,* Human Kinetics Publishers Champaign, Ill., 1984.
4. **Gresner, R.,** *Tennis,* W. B. Saunders, Philadelphia, 1975.
5. **Broer, M. R. and Houtz, S. J.,** *Patterns of Muscular Activity in Selected Sports Skills,* Charles C Thomas, Springfield, Ill., 1967
6. **Adrian, M. J. and Enberg, M. L.,** Sequential timing of three overhead patterns, in *Kinesiology Reviews,* Widule, C., Ed., AAHPER, Washington, D.C., 1971, 1.
7. **Jack, M., Adrian, M., and Yoneda, Y.,** Selected aspects of the overarm stroke in tennis, badminton, racquetball and squash, in *Science in Racquet Sports,* Terauds, J., Ed., Academic Publishers Del Mar, Calif., 1979, 69.
8. **Anderson, M. B.,** Comparison of muscle patterning in the overarm throw and tennis serve, *Res. Q.,* 50, 541, 1979.
9. **Miyashita, M., Tsunoda, T., Sakurai, S., Nishizono, H., and Mizuno, T.,** The tennis serve as compared

with overhand throwing in *Proc. Natl. Symp. Racquet Sports,* Groppel, J. L., Ed., University of Illinois, Champaign, 1979, 125.

10. **Miyashita, M., Tsunoda, T., Sakurai, S., Nishizono, H., and Mizuno, T.,** Muscular activities in the tennis serve and overhand throwing, *Scand. J. Sports Sci.,* 2, 52, 1980.

11. **Plagenhoef, S.,** *Fundamentals of Tennis,* Prentice-Hall, Englewood Cliffs, N.J., 1970.

12. **Beerman, J. and Sher, L.,** Improve tennis service through mathematics, *JOHPER,* September, 46, 1981.

13. **Smith, S. L.,** Comparison of selected factors associated with the flat and slice serves of male varsity tennis players, in *Proc. Natl. Symp. Racquet Sports,* Groppel, J. L., Ed., University of Illinois, Champaign, 1979, 17.

14. **Elliott, B. C. and Wood G. A.,** The biomechanics of the foot-up and foot-back tennis service techniques, *Aust. J. Sports Sci.,* 3, 3, 1983.

15. **Van Gheluwe, B. and Hebbelinck, M.,** The kinematics of the service movement in tennis: a three dimensional cinematographic approach, in *Biomechanics IX-B,* Winter D. A., Norman, R. W., Wells, R. P., Hayes, K. C., and Patla, A. E., Eds., Human Kinetics Publishers, Champaign, Ill., 1983, 521.

16. **Elliot, B. C. Marsh, T. and Blanksby, B.,** A three-dimensional cinematographic analysis of the tennis serve, *Intl. J. Sports Biomech.,* 2, 260, 1986.

17. **Van Gheluwe, B. and De Ruysscher, I.,** Pronation and endorotation of the racket arm in a tennis serve, presented at the *10th Intl. Congr. Biomechanics,* Umeå, Sweden, 1985, 277.

18. **Ariel, G. B. and Braden, V. K.,** Biomechanical analysis of ballistic vs. tracking movements in tennis skills, in *Proc. Natl. Symp. Racquet Sports,* Groppel, J. L., Ed., University of Illinois, Champaign, 1979, 105.

19. **Elliot, B. C.,** Spin and the power serve in tennis, *J. Hum. Movement Stud.,* 9, 97, 1983.

20. **Elliott, B. C.,** Spin and the power serve: a coach's perspective, *Sports Coach,* 6, 42, 1983.

21. **Taylor, C. D.,** An Electromyography and Cinematography Analysis of the Tennis Serve, unpublished Ph.D. thesis, Virginia Polytechnic Institute and State University, 1978.

22. **McWhirter, N. and Matthews, M. F.,** *Guinness Book of Records,* Guinness Superlatives, London, 1966.

23. **Plagenhoef, S.,** Tennis racquet testing related to "tennis elbow", in *Proc. Natl. Symp. Racquet Sports,* Groppel, J. L., Ed., Univerisity of Illinois, Champaign, 1979, 291.

24. **Owens, M. S. and Lee, H. Y.,** A determination of velocities and angles of projection for the tennis serve, *Res. Q.,* 40, 750, 1969.

25. **Golenko, V. A.,** A study of the kinematic structure of the tennis serve, *Theory Pract. Phys. Cult.,* 3, 35, 1973. Edited in Yessis' *Review of Soviet Physical Education and Sport,* 9, 971, 1974.

26. **Borg, B.,** Learn to play the Bjorn Borg way, *Tennis Austral.,* 69, May 1982.

27. **Rand, K. T., Hyer, M. W., and Williams, M. H.,** A dynamic test for comparison of rebound characteristics of three brands of tennis balls, in *Proc. Natl. Symp. Racquet Sports,* Groppel, J. L., Ed., University of Illinois, Champaign, 1979, 240.

28. **Vogy, M. A.,** The Effect of Grip and Wrist Strengthening Exercises on Tennis Playing Ability, unpublished Ph.D. thesis, University of North Carolina, 1961.

29. **Komi, P. V., and Bosco, C.,** Utilization of stored elastic energy in leg extensor muscles by men and women, *Med. Sci. Sport,* 10, 261, 1978.

30. **Fish, D.,** Footwork, *JOPERD,* May, 27, 1983.

31. **Abernethy, B. and Russell, D. G.,** Skill in tennis: considerations for talent identification and skill development, *Austral. J. Sports Sci.,* 3, 3, 1983.

32. **Glencross, D. J. and Cibich, B. J.,** A decision analysis of games skills, *Aust. J. Sports Med.,* 9, 72, 1977.

33. **Pecore, L. D.,** A cinematographic analysis of the one-handed backhand drive as used by skilled and unskilled performers, in *Proc. Natl. Symp. Racquet Sports,* Groppel, J. L., Ed., University of Illinois, Champaign, 1979, 253.

34. **Van Gheluwe, B.,** A Three Dimensional Analysis of the Tennis Forehand, Unpublished Manuscript, Vrije Universiteit, Brussels, Belgium, 1983.

35. **Hensley, L. D.,** Analysis of stroking errors committed in championship tennis competition, in *Proc. Natl. Symp. Racquet Sports,* Groppel, J. L., Ed., University of Illinois, Champaign, 1979, 225.

36. **Tilmanis, G. A.,** *Advanced Tennis for Coaches, Teachers and Players,* Australian and New Zealand Book Co., Sydney, 1975.

37. **Groppel. J. L., Dillman, C. J., and Lardner, T. J.,** Derivation and validation of equations of motion to predict ball spin upon impact in tennis, *J. Sports Sci.,* 1, 111, 1983.

38. **Blievernicht, J. G.,** Accuracy in the tennis forehand drive: cinematographic analysis, *Res. Q.,* 39, 776, 1968.

39. **Hobart, D. J.,** A Cinematographic Analysis of the Tennis Backhand Using Three Different Levels of Skill, Master's thesis University of Maryland, Baltimore, 1967.

40. **Holcomb, D. L.,** A Cinematographical Analysis of the Tennis Forehand, Backhand and American Twist Strokes, Unpublished Master's thesis, Florida State University, Tallahassee, 1963.

41. **Young, G.,** An Analysis of Selected Mechanical Factors and Accuracy in Tennis Strokes as Related to Ball Velocity and Skill Level, Unpublished Ph.D. thesis, Temple University, Philadelphia, 1970.

42. **Anderson, J. P.,** An Electromyographic Study of Ballistic Movement in the Tennis Forehand Drive, Unpublished Ph. D. thesis, University of Minnesota, Minneapolis, 1970.

43. **Pruitt, M. J.,** A Survey of Selected Anthromometric Measurements of Undergraduate College Women with Special Reference to the Teaching of Specific Physical Skills and the Design and Construction of Athletic Equipment, Unpublished Ph.D.thesis, Texas Women's University, Denton, 1968.

44. **Groppel, J. L.,** A Kinematic Analysis of the Tennis One-Handed and Two-Handed Backhand Drives of Highly Skilled Female Competitors, Unpublished Ph.D. thesis, Florida State University, Tallahassee, 1978.

45. **Groppel, J. L.,** A Kinematics Analysis of Topspin and Backspin Techniques in the Tennis Forehand Drive, Unpublished Master's thesis, University of Illinois, Champaign, 1975.

46. **Elliott, B. C.,** Tennis: the influence of grip firmness on reaction impulse and rebound velocity, *Med. Sci. Sports Exercise,* 14, 348, 1982.

47. **Schroeder, K., Groppel, J. L., Perry, J. L., and Milner, E. K.,** A comparison of performance changes in novice tennis players when learning either a one-handed or two-handed backhand drive, in *Proc. Natl. Symp. Racquet Sports,* Groppel, J. L., Ed., University of Illinois, Champaign, 1979, 165.

48. **Rhinehardt, P. T.,** A Comparison of the Accuracy of the One-Handed and Two-Handed Backhand Tennis Strokes, Unpublished Master's thesis, Springfield College, Springfield, Mass., 1975.

49. **Turner, J. M.,** An Analysis of Tennis Volley Techniques, Unpublished Master's thesis, San Diego State College, San Diego, Calif., 1966.

50. **Knuttgen, H. G.,** The Effects of Varying Tennis Racket Dimensions on Stroke Performance, Unpublished Ph.D. thesis, Ohio State University, Columbus, 1959.

51. **Ward, T. and Groppel, J. L.,** Sport implement selection: can it be based upon anthropometric indicators?, *Mot. Skills Theor. Pract.,* 4, 103, 1980.

52. **Elliott, B.,** Tennis racquet selection: a factor in early skill development, *Aust. J. Sports Sci.,* 1, 23, 1981.

53. **Hewitt, J.,** Revision of the Dyer backboard tennis test, *Res. Q.,* 36, 153, 1965.

54. **Nash, G.,** How flexible is your tennis racket?, *World Tennis,* 16, 52, 1968.

55. **Nash, G.,** How flexible is your metal racket?, *World Tennis,* 20, 80, 1972.

56. **Seetharaman, A. N.,** A Comparative Study of the Aluminium and Wood Tennis Rackets, Unpublished Master's thesis, Springfield College, Springfield, Mass., 1969.

57. **Hegmann, E. H.,** A Comparative Study of Aluminium and Steel Tennis Rackets, Unpublished Master's thesis, Springfield College, Springfield, Mass., 1970.

58. **Brody, H.,** Physics of the tennis racket, *Am. J. Phys.,* 47, 482, 1979.

59. **Brody, H.,** Physics of the tennis racket. II "Sweet spot", *Am. J. Phys.,* 49, 816, 1981.

60. **Racket Almanac,** *World Tennis,* December, 42, 1984.

61. **Fisher, A.,** Super racket — is this the shape of things to come in tennis?, *Pop. Sci.,* 210, 44, 1977.

62. **Blanksby, B. A., Ellis, R. and Elliott, B. C.,** Performance characteristics of regular-sized and over-sized tennis racquets, *ACHPER,* 86, 21, 1979.

63. **Gruetter, D. E. and Davis, T. M.,** Oversized vs standard racquets: does it really make a difference?, *Res. Q. Exercise Sport,* 56, 31, 1985.

64. **Brody, H.,** The moment of inertia of a tennis racket, *Phys. Teacher,* April, 213, 1985.

65. **Elliott, B. C., Blanksby, B. A., and Ellis, R.,** Vibration and rebound velocity characteristics of conventional and oversized tennis rackets, *Res. Q. Exercise Sport,* 51, 609, 1980.

66. **Sykes, K., Scott, A. E., and Kellet, D. W.,** The centre of percussion and its implication for sport, *Res. Pap. Phys. Educ. (Carnegie School Phys. Educ.),* October, 36, 1971.

67. **Groppel, J.,** Gut reactions, *World Tennis,* November, 28, 1983.

68. **Ellis, R., Elliott, B., and Blanksby, B.,** The effect of string type and tension in jumbo and regular sized tennis racquets, *Sports Coach,* 2, 32, 1978.

69. **Bosworth, W.,** What? String tighter for more control?, *World Tennis,* 18, May, 1981.

70. **Pouzzner, J. G.,** A Comparison of the Resilience of a Nylon and Gut-Strung Racket, Unpublished Master's thesis, Springfield College, Springfield, Mass., 1969.

71. **Nelson, R.,** Can an exotic new racket improve your game, *Scholastic Coach,* 46, 46, 1976.

72. **Baker, J. A. and Wilson, B. D.,** The effect of tennis racket stiffness and string tension on ball velocity after impact, *Res. Q.,* 49, 255, 1978.

73. **Elliott, B. C.,** The influence of tennis racket flexibility and string tension on rebound velocity following a dynamic impact, *Res. Q. Exercise Sport,* 53, 277, 1982.

74. **Putnam, C. A. and Baker, J. A.,** Spin imparted to a tennis ball during impact with conventionally and diagonally strung rackets, *Res. Q. Exercise Sport,* 55, 261, 1984.

75. **Brody, H.,** That's how the ball bounces, *Phys. Teacher,* November, 494, 1984.

76. **Nigg, B.,** Measurement and magnitude of loads in selected sports, in *Biomechanical Assessment of Sports Protective Equipment,* University of Waterloo Press, Waterloo, Can., 1983, 1.

77. **Nigg, B.,** The load on the lower extremities in selected sports activities, in *Collected Papers on Sports Biomechancis,* Wood, G. A., Ed., University of Western Australia Press, Perth, 1983, 62.
78. **Leuthi, S. M. and Nigg, B. M.,** The influence of different shoe constructions on discomfort and pain in tennis, *Biomechanics IX-B,* Winter, D. A., Norman, R. W., Wells, R. P., Hayes, K. C., and Patla, A. E., Eds., Human Kinetics Publishers, Champaign, Ill., 1983. 149.
79. **Horan, J. G.,** Feet won't fail you now, *World Tennis,* May, 38, 1985.
80. **Hatze, H.,** Forces and duration of impact and grip tightness during the tennis stroke, *Med. Sci. Sports Exercise,* 8, 88, 1976.
81. **Watanabe, T., Ikegami, Y., and Miyashita, M.,** Tennis: the effect of grip firmness on ball velocity after impact, *Med. Sci. Sports,* 11, 359, 1979.
82. **Baker, J. A. and Putnam, C. A.,** Tennis racket and ball responses during impact under clamped and freestanding conditions, *Res. Q.,* 50, 164, 1979.
83. **Grabiner, M. D., Groppel, J. L., and Campbell, K. R.,** Resultant tennis ball velocity as a function of off-center impact and grip firmness, *Med. Sci. Sports Exercise,* 15, 542, 1983.
84. **Missavage, R. J. and Baker, J. A. W.,** Theoretical modeling of grip firmness during ball-racket impact, *Res. Q. Exercise Sports,* 55, 254, 1984.
85. **Liu, Y. K.,** Mechanical analysis of racket and ball during impact, *Med. Sci. Sports Exercise,* 15, 388, 1983.
86. **Brannigan, M. and Adali, S.,** Mathematical modeling and simulation of a tennis racket, *Med. Sci. Sports Exercise,* 13, 44, 1981.
87. **Ohmichi, H., Miyashita, M., and Mizuno, T.,** Bending forces acting on the racquet during the tennis stroke, in *Science in Racquet Sports,* Terauds, J., Ed., Academic Publishers, Del Mar, Calif., 1979.
88. **Kacelson, M., Zaizev, B., and Petrov, B.,** Analysis of the force experienced by the tennis player at the moment of the impact of the tennis racket on the ball, *All Union Sci. Res. Exp. Inst. Consumer Prod. Mach. Constr.* (translated from Russian),
89. **Kane, T. R., Hayes, W. C., and Priest, J. D.,** Experimental determination of forces exerted in tennis play, *Biomechanics IV,* Nelson R. C., and Morehouse, C. A., Eds., University Park Press, Baltimore, 1974, 284.
90. **Fritz, M. and Hartmann, C.,** Accelerations and forces in a tennis racket during swing phase and impact, in *Funktionelle Morphologie, Ruhr-Universiität, Bochum,* W. Germany, Unpublished Manuscript, 1979.
91. **McLaughlin, T. M. and Miller, N. R.,** Techniques for the evaluation of loads on the forearm prior to impact in tennis strokes, in *Proc. Intl. Conf. Medical Devices and Sports Equipment,* San Francisco, August 1980, 63.
92. **Brody, H.,** *Science Made Practical for the Tennis Teacher,* USPTR Instructional Series, Vol. 6, 1985.
93. **Van Gheluwe, B. and Hebbelinck, M.,** Muscle actions and ground reaction forces in tennis, *Intl. J. Sports Biom.,* 2, 88, 1986.

Chapter 9

MECHANICS OF CYCLING

Dirk J. Pons and Christopher L. Vaughan

TABLE OF CONTENTS

I. INTRODUCTION

Bicycles are ubiquitous machines, used throughout the world for locomotion, exercise, sport, and research. Consequently, an understanding of the biomechanics of cycling should be important to those involved with cyclists. Hull and Jorge[1] wrote in 1985 that particular reasons for studying cycling biomechanics were

1.   The reduction of knee injuries caused by cycling
2.   The use of stationary ergometers for therapy
3.   Improved performance in cycling competitions

Despite the apparent importance of cycling and the decades that bicycles have been in existence, Faria and Cavanagh[2] felt compelled to write in their book on cycling that: ''Science has a long way to go to catch up with some of the empirical data collected on a 'trial error' basis by the cycling fraternity.'' While this might still be true of some aspects of cycling, there have since been noteworthy advances in the biomechanical study of cycling. These are reviewed here.

II. KINETICS OF CYCLING

A. Muscle Activity

The electromyogram (EMG) during cycling on a sports bicycle or an ergometer has been documented by many researchers, among them Ericson et al.,[3] Hull and Jorge,[1] Faria and Cavanagh,[2] Desipres,[4] and Houtz and Fischer.[5] One of the most detailed of these studies is that of Ericson et al.[3] They measured surface EMG, produced a linear envelope, and normalized the signal to the EMG recorded during an isometric maximum voluntary contraction. A diagram of the important leg muscles in cycling is illustrated in Figure 1, while the results of Ericson et al.[3] are shown in Figure 2.

The importance of a muscle in the cycling movement may be seen in the ratio of its peak EMG to that of the isometric maximum voluntary contraction. These values are shown in Table 1. From these results it is apparent that the muscles most used in cycling are the vastii, gastrocnemius lateralis, and soleus. The rectus femoris does not appear to be of great functional importance.

By way of comparison, the EMG recorded by other researchers for some of the muscles of the leg are shown in Figure 3. The convention used in studies of normal cycling is to define the vertical position of the crank as zero crank angle, with counterclockwise rotation taken as positive. The crank angles at specific events are shown, with an accuracy of $\pm 5°$. Unfilled regions of EMG bars denote lesser muscle activity. The cycling EMG results from Desipres[4] are with seat heights of 105 and 95% of the symphysis pubis height.

From these diagrams, it is apparent that there are large differences in the cycling EMG

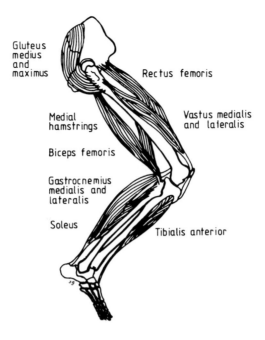

FIGURE 1. The major leg muscles used during cycling.

recorded by the various researchers. These differences may be due to subject variability, different postures, and the differences in signal processing (raw EMG, integrated EMG and EMG envelope have been used). Furthermore, those researchers who showed EMG as an on/off bar may have differed in the cut-off level that they chose.

There is scope for further work on the EMG of cycling. Many muscles (such as the adductors, ilio-psoas and the calf muscles) have been neglected in EMG studies. Just as the nonsagittal pedal loads (once assumed negligible) were found to be significant, it is conceivable that muscles presently considered unimportant might actually perform important functions in cycling. To study the finer, deeper muscles it will probably be necessary to use intramuscular electrodes.

On the matter of recording crank angle during EMG studies, it is pertinent to point out that many researchers have assumed that pedal speed is constant throughout the crank cycle, and hence have used only a single marker on the crank. This assumption appears to be at least partly true,[4] but until further study has been done it will not be known what, if any, information is being lost. If the crank velocity is not constant then the crank acceleration will not be either, and this might have significant effects on biomechanical analyses of the cycling motion.

B. Pedal Forces

Hoes et al.[6] were among the first to measure pedal forces. They strain-gauged a crank and pedal so as to measure crank torque and normal pedal forces. Since then there have been numerous studies using pedal dynamometers. Most of these have followed the same course as Soden and Adeyefa[7] in measuring only the normal and tangential pedal forces, and assuming that the other components were negligible. The most significant recent work in the measurement of pedal force has been performed by Hull and Davis.[8] One of the most important results of their study was that the nonsagittal forces are of significant magnitude.

Hull and Davis constructed a pedal dynamometer that measured all six load components. Their results are shown in Figure 4. For ease of interpretation of these results, their coordinate system is illustrated in Figure 5. Note that the M_z and M_x moments are of significant

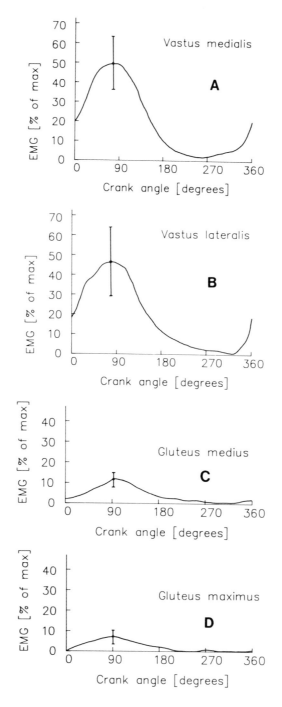

FIGURE 2A-D.   The EMG activity of all the leg muscles as a function of the crank angle. These curves are based on the data of Ericson et al.[3] The vertical position is defined as zero crank angle.

magnitude. The positive M_x moment signifies that the force was applied on the outside of the pedal. Further research on the foot-pedal interface, by the same authors,[10] showed that this lateral moment was highly variable. They attributed this to the variability in the positioning of the foot on the pedal, even when fastening systems were used. The M_z and M_x moments must be resisted by the ankle and knee; Hull and Davis suggested that these

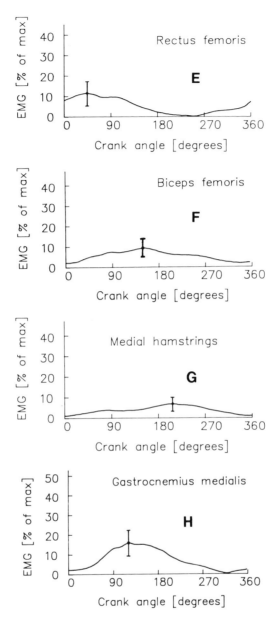

FIGURE 2E-H.

moments might be responsible for overuse injuries in cyclists. The moment M_y is small but not zero, because it balances the shear force F_x which is offset from the pedal spindle, so that the resultant moment about the spindle is zero. Pedal forces much greater than those shown here, are also possible; Soden and Adeyefa[7] measured pedal forces of up to three times body weight at starting.

It is only the tangential pedal force that makes a useful contribution to the motion. The measure of the usefulness of sagittal pedal force has been called the effectiveness[9,10] and is the magnitude of the tangential force divided by the magnitude of the resultant sagittal force.

While it is the effective force that drives the vehicle forward, it is the resultant force, the vector sum of the effective and the (ineffective) radial forces, that the rider generates. The

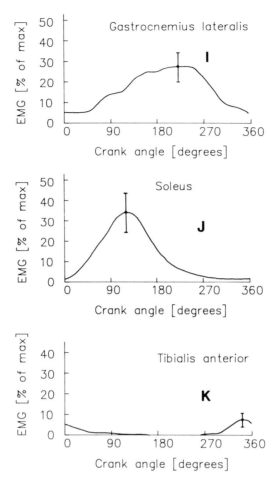

FIGURE 2I-K.

normal and tangential crack forces are shown in Figure 6. Note that the normal force is larger than the tangential force.

The tangential force, applied at the radius of the crank, generates a torque which is transmitted through the gears to the wheel. Since the effective force varies through the pedal cycle the torque does, too. Studies have shown that part of the torque curve may be negative, that is, the bicycle does work on the rider,[7,9] but the sum from the two legs is greater than zero and provides a net propulsive force. A typical torque curve is shown in Figure 7.

Not only is the torque curve unsteady, but it has been shown by Dal Monte et al.[11] that the pedal forces are variable from cycle to cycle, and asymmetrical in that one leg may do more work than the other, although the asymmetry may vary from day to day.[2] However, Faria and Cavanagh[2] could not relate this effect to limb dominance. Kunstlinger et al.[12] found that experienced cyclists exerted lower peak forces at all work loads than did non-cyclists and suggested that this may have been due to greater involvement of slow-twitch muscle fibers.

Hull and Jorge[1] are the only researchers to have elucidated some of the relationships between EMG and pedal loading, and their results are worthy of further study. From pedal-loading data they determined the moments at each joint. These total moments were then separated into kinematic moments (i.e., moments that originate in the acceleration of masses) and static moments (i.e., moments that generate the pedal forces). They then related these moments to the surface EMG. The moments are shown in Figure 8.

Table 1
PEAK EMG AS A
PERCENTAGE OF AN
ISOMETRIC MAXIMUM
VOLUNTARY CONTRACTION
(MVC), FOR VARIOUS
MUSCLES

Muscle	MVC (%)
Gluteus maximus	7
Gluteus medius	11
Rectus femoris	12
Vastus medialis	54
Vastus lateralis	50
Biceps femoris	12
Medial hamstrings	10
Gastrocnemius medialis	19
Gastrocnemius lateralis	32
Soleus	37
Tibialis anterior	9

Note: Power is 120 W, speed is 60 rpm, seat height is middle, and the foot is positioned with the metatarsal heads over the pedal spindle.

Data adapted from Ericson et al.[3]

Hip moments were found to depend on the angular acceleration of the thigh because of its large inertia. The value of the hip moment depended on the normal pedal force and the moment of the resultant pedal force about the hip. While the magnitudes of the static and kinematic hip moments were always greater than zero, their sum was not, and showed a change in polarity.

Static knee moments were found to be dependent on the tangential pedal force. Increases in torque were found to come from increases in the normal rather than the tangential force. However, significant negative tangential shear was generated as power output increased, and this appeared to be a characteristic of a consistent pedaling style. Higher speeds caused greater segment accelerations and larger kinematic joint moments. In the case of the hip, the increased kinematic moment served to decrease the total hip moment, suggesting that there might be an optimum speed at which this moment was at a minimum. Redfield and Hull[13] demonstrated that the minimum was approximately 105 rpm. Kinematic ankle moments were low because of the low inertia of the foot and the static moments followed the normal pedal force.

Redfield and Hull[14] modeled the bicycle-rider system as a planar five-bar linkage with pedal forces and pedal dynamics as input. Maintaining a constant bicycle power, they used mathematical optimization techniques to obtain an optimal pedal-force profile. They minimized two cost functions: one based on joint moments and the other on muscle stresses. They found that the muscle stress cost function was a good predictor of joint moments and that the predicted muscle activity correlated well with EMG data. They further postulated that pedaling effectiveness was a complex function of the pedal force vector orientation and muscle mechanics.

Another use for a pedal dynamometer is to train cyclists to pedal more effectively. This has been done by Davis and Hull,[10] and the results are shown in Figure 9.

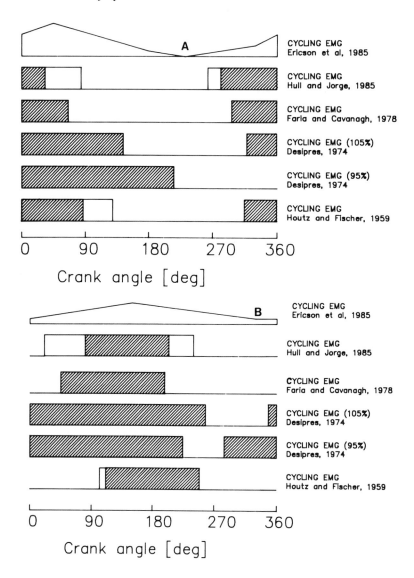

FIGURE 3.   A comparison of the EMG data from various authors [1-5] for four major muscle groups, (A) the rectus femoris; (B) hamstrings; (C) gastrocnemius; and (D) gluteus maximus. Unfilled regions of EMG bars denote lesser muscle activity, while the data of Desipres[4] are for seat heights of 105 and 95% of the symphysis pubis height.

C. Role of Individual Muscles

Based on the results of Hull and Jorge[1] and Ericson et al.,[3] the role of individual leg muscles (shown in Figures 1 to 3) in the cycling motion, appears to be as follows: the rectusfemoris, a flexor of the hip and extensor of the knee, is active during the power phase of cycling, when the hip is being extended. However, it also contributes to the motion at the knee at this time. The rectus femoris generates a tangential pedal force and a kinematic moment.

The hamstrings oppose knee extension, being flexors of the knee, but also contribute to the motion of the hip joint at the same time. The hamstrings show greatest activity at the bottom of the stroke, when their effectiveness as protectors of the knee is reduced because of their small moment arm about that joint. The hamstrings also generate hip- and knee moments, generate pedal force, and drive the leg linkages.

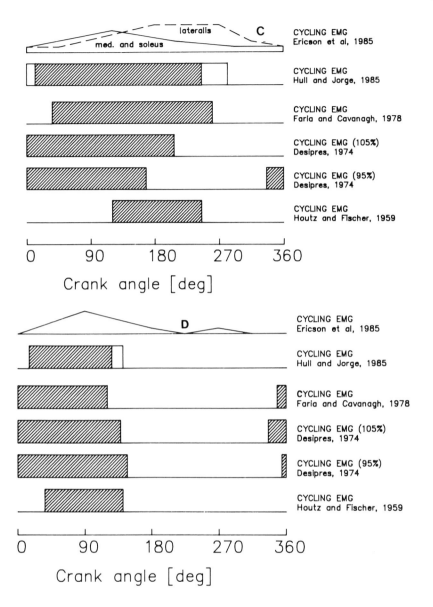

FIGURE 3,C and D.

The tibialis anterior muscle is active when there is little ankle moment; it flexes the ankle during the upstroke in preparation of the next thrust.

The gastrocnemii only generate force to balance the ankle moment generated during the thrust phase; they produce no kinematic moment. Ericson et al.[3] suggested that the gastrocnemii push the pedals through the bottom-dead-center, thereby preparing the opposite foot for its thrust. The gastrocnemius lateralis is more active when the metatarsal heads, rather than the instep of the foot, are placed on the pedal spindle, but the gastrocnemius medialis exhibits no such phenomenon. The muscles are also more active when the seat is raised.[15] The gastrocnemii receive significant support from the other calf muscles.

The gluteus maximus produces normal pedal force, aided by the inertia of the leg,[1] while the vasti muscles generate the knee moment which sustains the tangential pedal force.

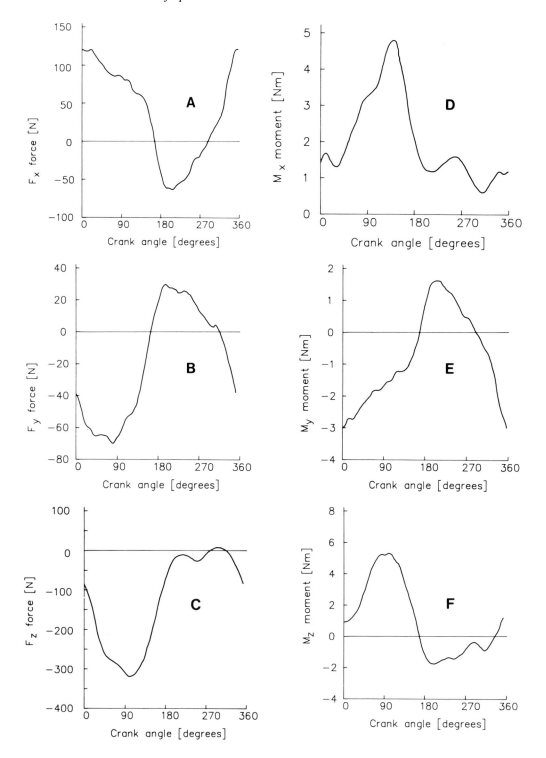

FIGURE 4A-F.   The six components of pedal loading at 180 W and 80 rpm (Adapted from Hull and Davis[8]).

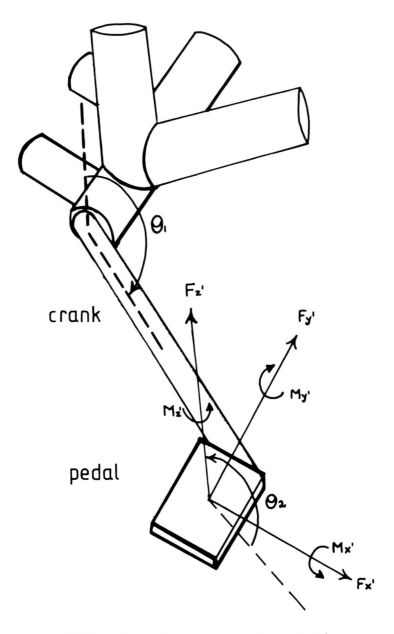

FIGURE 5.   The coordinate system used by Hull and Davis.[8]

D. Handlebar Forces

Biomechanical studies of cycling have invariably neglected the forces that the hands may exert; the only exception appears to be the study of Soden and Adeyefa.[7] They measured large pedal forces (up to three times body weight) which they ascribed to the cyclist pulling on the handlebars. The pedal forces could not be accounted for by acceleration of the rider, since during the power stroke, the body actually accelerated downwards, reducing the pedal forces. They calculated the vertical forces in the hands to be as follows:

- At starting: 1.08 times body weight in one hand and 0.44 in the other
- When climbing a hill: 0.36 and 0.27 times body weight
- Steady cycling: 0.11 and 0.17 times body weight

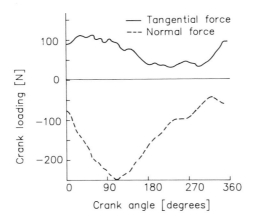

FIGURE 6.   Normal and tangential crank forces.[1]

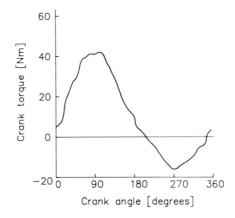

FIGURE 7.   The crank torque as a function of crank angle.[1]

The unequal forces prevented overbalancing due to offset pedal loads. Note that at starting, the forces on the handlebars were of the order of body weight.

Thus, it has been found that the hands generate significant forces during cycling. Further work needs to be done on this aspect of cycling. It will probably be necessary to strain-gauge the handlebars in order to measure real loading. It is possible that improvements in handlebar design could stem from such work.

E. Retarding Forces

1. Rolling Resistance

The rolling resistance is inversely proportional to the wheel diameter.[16] Rolling resistance depends on the type of tire too; the worst may take three times the energy of the best.[2] Generally, the larger-cross-section tires give a larger resistance. For example, Dill et al.[17] found that a 28 × 2 1/8″ tire required an oxygen consumption from the rider 0.19 ℓ/min more than did a 27 × 1 1/4″ tire. The inflation pressure of the tire is also important, higher pressures result in less rolling resistance.[16] Yet another determinant of rolling resistance is the ground surface. The resistance on tar is 5% greater than on concrete,[2] and linoleum gives a speed 0.28 m/sec faster than is possible on tar for the same conditions.[18]

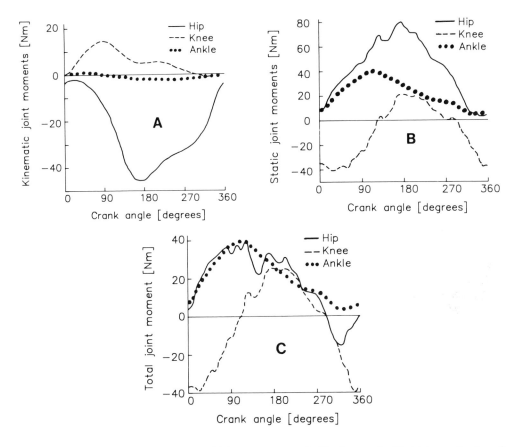

FIGURE 8A-C.   Kinematic, static, and total joint movements at the hip, knee, and ankle joints as a function of crank angle.[1]

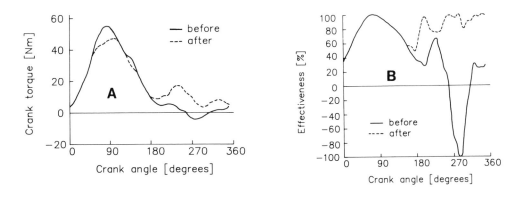

FIGURE 9A, B.   Crank torque and effectiveness before and after recommending changes of style to the cyclist.[8]

2. Aerodynamic Drag

At high speeds, most of the energy produced by the cyclist is expended against the drag force of the air. The equation for the drag force is

$$F = 0.5\ C_d A \rho v^2 \tag{1}$$

where F is the drag force, C_d the drag coefficient, A the area exposed, ρ the density of the air, and v the air velocity.

Davies[18] found that the drag force was

$$F = 0.0175 \ v^2 \tag{2}$$

where the units for v were meters per second.

His values for projected area and drag coefficient were 0.5 and 0.56 m², respectively. His work was based on 15 subjects riding their own bicycles on a motor-driven treadmill in a wind tunnel. Of all studies on cycling, these conditions perhaps most closely simulate actual conditions likely to be encountered by a cyclist. di Prampero et al.[19] found the drag term to be $0.19 \ v^2$. By comparison, the drag for a wheelchair is $F = 0.4 \ v^2$ for velocities greater than 4 m/sec, established by Brubaker and McLaurin.[20]

One way to reduce the drag is to reduce the area. The simplest method is to crouch down over the handlebars. By this means the frontal area is reduced from 0.50 m² for an upright posture, to 0.42 m² for touring (hands on the top of the handlebars), to 0.34 m² in the fully crouched racing posture, a 30% overall reduction.[2] Further reductions in frontal area are achieved by reclining the rider, as on recumbent bicycles.

Other attempts to reduce drag have concentrated on the reduction of the drag coefficient, since even small modifications can reduce the drag considerably. Wearing smooth, tight-fitting racing clothing reduces the drag by 30% compared to pants and a jacket, while a plastic sheet between the frame members and on the wheels reduces the drag by nearly 50%. Fairings reduce the drag further, although they are susceptible to cross winds.

On the subject of area, Nonweiler[21] reported that size and posture of rider (once in the racing position) have little effect on the projected area and, hence, on the drag. However, Faria and Cavanagh[2] advocate the use of wind tunnels to fine-tune a competitive cyclist's posture. They achieved 5% reductions in drag in this way. Brooks and Hibbs[22] have made the point that the area term in the drag equation is the frontal area when the body is a bluff one (like a motor car), causing drag by flow separation, but in the case of a streamlined vehicle (as some bicycles are) the drag is due to skin friction, and surface area is a better value for the area term.

3. Mass

The lifting of the legs against gravity and the maintenance of angular velocity require at least some of the energy output of the cyclist. This has been estimated to be from 5 to 27% of the work output by Kaneko and Yamazaki[23] and Faria and Cavanagh.[2]

The mass and the moment of inertia of the bicycle and rider do not affect the physiologically measured response to work or the subjective rating of effort[24] when moving on a level surface. However, the mass is crucial when it comes to hills. Neglected air resistance and the speed up a hill, are limited by the down-slope component of the weight, as follows:

$$\text{speed} = \frac{\text{available power}}{\text{weight} \times \sin(\text{angle of slope})} \tag{3}$$

This halving of the weight results in a doubling of the speed. However, robustness and lightness are difficult to achieve together, and the best solution is to have the lightest machine that will perform under the expected conditions.[2]

4. Friction

The friction in the machinery of a bicycle accounts for less than 5% of the total force.[2] The gearing itself is 98 to 99% efficient,[25] although it might not be quite so good when worn or dirty. Kyle and Caiozzo[26] found that bicycle ergometer losses increase with power output, being approximately 3.8% for a 300 W output.

Table 2
HIP AND KNEE ANGLES AS A FUNCTION
OF SEAT HEIGHT

Joint	Seat height (cm)	Flexion (°)	Extension (°)	Range (°)
Hip	62.2	62	37	25
	53.3	76	42	34
Knee	62.2	103	48	55
	53.3	117	62	55

Note: Seat height was measured from the center of the chain wheel. We see that hip motion decreases with increasing seat height. Values shown are in degrees.

Modified from Houtz, S. J. and Fischer, F.[5]

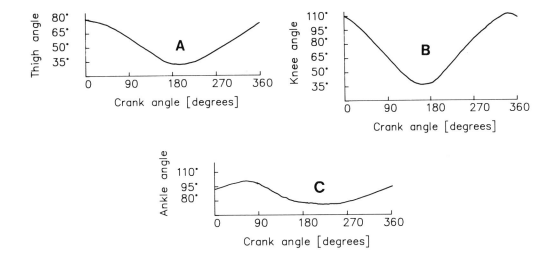

FIGURE 10A-C. Thigh, knee, and ankle angles as a function of crank angle.

III. KINEMATICS OF CYCLING

A. Joint Angles

Houtz and Fischer[5] determined joint motion during cycling. The ankle was found to move through its complete range of motion. The knee did not move through complete extension, nor did the hip fully extend. Its flexion was found to be limited to 90°. At top-dead center the hip internally rotates and adducts. The results of the study are shown in Table 2, while the sagittal plane kinematics of Faria and Cavanagh are presented in Figure 10.

Foot angle is a sinusoid function with frequency equal to the pedal speed.[1] The foot-pedal position has a great effect on the kinetics of cycling. Placement of the pedal under the ankle results in reduced joint motion. Toe-clips place the foot in the correct position, with the metatarsal heads over the pedal. Segmental angular acceleration data[1] are presented in Figure 11.

B. Pedal Speed

Pedal speed affects oxygen consumption and the magnitude of the integrated EMG.[27] The pedal speed that allows the lowest rate of oxygen consumption on stationary ergometers in

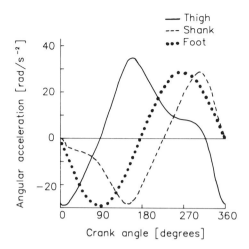

FIGURE 11.   Angular acceleration data for the three leg segments as a function of crank angle.[1]

the laboratory is approximately 60 rpm.[28] Subsequently, Coast and Welch[29] found that the optimum speed was dependent on power. They gave it as

$$w_{opt} = 0.125 \, P + 4.05 \tag{4}$$

where P was the power in watts, between 100 and 300 W, and ω_{opt} was the speed in rpm at which oxygen uptake and heart rate were lowest.

Patterson et al.[24] found that cyclists were unable to direct the pedal forces optimally as pedal speeds increased. However, racing cyclists prefer faster pedal speeds, up to 140 rpm.[30] For anaerobic exercise, the maximum power output can be produced even at 140 rpm.[26] Apart from the need to generate more power at any cost, another possible reason for these higher speeds other than the physiological optimum, may be that the forces are lower for a given power output, and hence the onset of fatigue is delayed. This is probably a result of the force-velocity curve for muscles.[28] The force-velocity curve exhibits a flattening out for high pedal speeds, which Sjogaard[28] suggests may be due to storage and subsequent release of negative work, or to prestretching.

C. Foot Motion and Crank Length

Several types of propulsive motion have been used in the past in human-propelled vehicles. Of these, cycling has perhaps been the most common, but by no means the only motion. In cycling, the feet move in a circular path; other motions may be elliptical or, as in rowing, linear.

The question of which is the better motion between rowing and cycling was investigated by Harrison[31] and the results are worth some careful examination, even though only five subjects were studied. In essence, Harrison found that cycling produced more power than did conventional moving-seat rowing. He attributed this to the loss of kinetic energy imparted to the trunk during rowing. This led him to build a rowing ergometer that allowed the kinetic energy of the limbs to be fed back into the device. He called this type of rowing "forced rowing", because it had a fixed period with which the subject had to synchronize. After 5 min of work, the power outputs by cycling, and free and forced rowing all tended towards 350 W, but for short-duration work there was a large disparity, the most power being generated by forced rowing with the seat fixed, then forced rowing with the feet fixed, then cycling, and lastly free rowing with either seat or feet fixed. Unfortunately, the forced-rowing arrangement is impractical on a moving vehicle, and cycling thus appears to be the next best motion.

The case between circular and elliptical motion is not so clear-cut. Harrison suggested that a constant foot-velocity motion should allow the greatest release of power. Cycling does not have such a motion despite the circular path, because the forces exerted by the leg on the pedal vary along the pedal path. Harrison reasoned that an elliptical foot motion, with the major axis vertical, should allow constant foot velocity during cycling. However, an approximately constant velocity motion that he devised produced no measurable increase in power output.

In passing, it is worth noting that an elliptical chainwheel (not to be confused with an elliptical foot motion) has not been conclusively shown to be either superior or inferior to the conventional round chainwheel. Harrison found that his five subjects preferred an elliptical chainwheel for producing large torques (heavy loads and low speed) as it enabled a steadier speed to be maintained. Kyle and Caiozzo[26] tested several different cam-shaped sprockets and found that the conventional round shape performed as well as any other.

An optimum crank length should exist since longer cranks mean more leg movement (a disadvantage) as well as smaller foot forces (an advantage). According to Inbar et al.,[32] the optimum crank length for short-term power output in cycling was 0.157 of the leg length. This conclusion was based on data for 13 male subjects. They also found a 1% power loss for a 50-mm deviation in crank length from the optimum. Gross and Bennett[33] found that a crank length of 0.20 of the symphysis pubis height allowed minimum exertion during cycling. A standard crank length of 171 mm was too long for 60% of adult males and almost all adult females.

D. Steering and Stability

Balancing and steering of a bicycle are closely related. Steering is achieved either by turning the front wheel or by leaning the bicycle. Leaning the bicycle at speed naturally turns the wheel in towards the lean. This effect may also be achieved by briefly turning the wheel in the opposite direction to that intended. This causes the bicycle to lean towards, and thus steer in, the desired direction[34].

A comprehensive description of the stability of the bicycle is given by Jones.[35] He found that the bicycle was balanced as follows:

1. The rider steered into the direction of a fall and so moved in a curved path of radius such as to provide sufficient centrifugal force to prevent the fall. The handlebars had to be in front of the steering axis so that the centrifugal force on the hands of the cyclist turned the wheel out of the curve rather than sharply into it.[36]

2. The front wheel precessed about the steering axis and generated a gyroscopic force which corrected it when the bicycle tilted. However, this force was normally insufficient to stabilize a laden bicycle at low speeds.

3. A stable bicycle was one where the steering geometry was such that the center of mass (CM) of the front wheel fell when the bicycle was tilted. This lowering of potential energy provided a force which turned the wheel into the curve and thereby increased the centrifugal force.

4. The bicycle had geometric caster stability which provided self-righting in the event of a perturbation in the course. The requirement of the steering geometry was that the steering axis had to intersect the ground in front of the point of wheel-ground contact. (A tricycle may have a different steering geometry, because it is free of the constraint of two wheeled stability.)

IV. WORK, ENERGY, AND POWER

A. Energy and Power

Power output depends on the duration of the exertion; large powers can be generated for brief periods, e.g., 1500 W for 6 sec.[26] According to Faria and Cavanagh,[2] the power that a cyclist produces in a sprint is 1500 W (using anaerobic metabolism), in an endurance situation 370 W, and at comfortable pedaling 75 W. They also made the point that such power outputs are somewhere between those of a kitchen mixer and a 50-cc motorcycle. The world record for ergometer exercise is 455 W for 1 hr, held by Merckx in 1975.[26] Instantaneous power in a single pedal stroke has been measured at 3100 W by Kyle and Caiozzo.[26]

It has been shown by Croisand and Boileau[37] that oxygen consumption, $\dot{V}_{O2}$, is not a function of power so much as of the constituents of power, namely, pedal rate and brake load.

B. Effectiveness

The effectiveness (a measure of the useful force produced at the pedals) of cycling has been found to increase as the load increases.[10] They calculated that a factor of 1.8-fold increase in pedal force resulted in a 2.4-fold increase in power. However, air drag increases as the third power of velocity and, thus, a 2.4-fold increase in power results in only a 1.34-fold increase in speed. Thus, increasing the pedal force by a factor of 1.8 increases the speed by a factor of only 1.34.

C. Efficiency

The efficiency is not the same as the effectiveness; they correlate only weakly.[9] Efficiency refers to the efficiency of the human body and the machine to do work. Care must be excised as researchers define efficiency in different ways. (For example, the resting caloric requirement may or may not be subtracted from the total caloric requirement.) Efficiency is defined in various ways, of which the best, according to Gaesser and Brooks,[38] is the Delta Efficiency:

$$n = \frac{\text{change in work output}}{\text{change in metabolic energy used}} \tag{5}$$

La Fortune and Cavanagh[9] also used this definition of efficiency. Other researchers define efficiency as work done divided by energy used. The choice of which efficiency to use is an important one, because the delta efficiency has been found to decrease with pedal speed (35 to 25%) and with load (32 to 15%),[38] while the other efficiency increases with load and pedal speed.

For cycling, the efficiency is typically 0.25.[39] By comparison, the efficiency for running is 0.39[40] although there too, the definition is equivocal, and for handrim wheelchair propulsion it is 0.06 to 0.1.[20] Efficiency decreases with speed and load, probably as inefficient fast-twitch muscle fibers are recruited.[38]

V. EFFECTS OF CYCLING POSTURE

A. Seat Height

A change of seat height changes the joint angles and puts muscles on different parts of their length-tension curves. The result is that a lower seat causes higher muscle forces and greater rate of oxygen consumption. The seat height that results in the minimum $\dot{V}_{O2}$ is 109% of the inside leg measurement[2] or of the symphysis pubis height.[41] A seat height of 100% of the greater tronchanteric height has also been used.[1] Seat height is defined as the maximum distance from the pedal to the top of the seat along the seat-support frame. There is minimum movement of the ankle at this optimal seat height.[41] Through ignorance, most recreational cyclists have their seat considerably lower than the optimal.

In their research, Houtz and Fischer[5] found that the muscle activity during cycling was unchanged with seat height. This has since been found to be erroneous; muscle activity, particularly of the gastrocnemius, depends on the seat height and the position of the foot on the pedal. The cause of the erroneous conclusion of Houtz and Fischer[5] is probably based on the fact that they had their subjects place the instep of the foot on the pedal, and they might not have explored the full range of saddle heights. Ericson et al.[3] found increased activity in only the gluteus medius, medial hamstrings, and gastrocnemius medialis with increased seat height. This clearly points to the importance of accurately controlling experimental parameters during cycling studies.

B. Hand Position

Faria et al.[42] found that the dropped-bar cycling posture was superior to the top-bar posture on the basis of 1.08 greater $\dot{V}_{O2max}$, 17% greater work output, 28.5% greater specific work output, and 8% greater $\dot{V}_e$. They suggested that possible mechanisms for these effects could be enhanced ventilation due to reduced weight on the chest, and larger muscle mass involvement for the dropped-bar posture.

C. The Toe-Straps Debate

During the backstroke, there is a force opposing the motion. This is due to the passive leg being lifted by the active one. In an attempt to eliminate this retarding force, competitive cyclists make use of "toe straps" and "cleats". These are devices which fix the foot to the pedal so that the leg can be used to lift the pedal instead of push down on it. In practice, some researchers[2,6] have found that even experienced cyclists fail to pull at the pedals, while others[3,7] have found that they do. For example, at 906 (a high load) at 130 rpm, Soden and Adeyefa[7] measured a pull on the pedal of 100 N, and on a different subject, at starting, 460 N. Ericson et al.[3] found greater EMG in the rectus femoris, biceps femoris, and tibialis anterior when toe-straps were used, an indication that these muscles were pulling the pedal up.

It may be that cyclists do take advantage of toe-straps and cleats when the load is greater. Cleats are certainly not useless, since they enable the application of greater tangential (shear) forces to the pedal, and, by holding the feet on the pedals, perhaps permit higher pedaling speeds, too.

The toe-straps issue is perhaps largely a statistical one. For example, Moffat and Sparling[43] found no statistically significant difference in mean $\dot{V}_{O2max}$ or performance time between toe-strap and no-toe-strap conditions. However, there was some difference; $\dot{V}_{O2max}$ was 62.4 mℓ/kg·min for toe straps and 60.4 mℓ/·min without. While these results may indeed be statistically insignificant at the 0.05 probability level, in practice this may be sufficient difference to give one cyclist an edge over another.

La Fortune and Cavanagh[9] also found that cleats allowed some decrease in oxygen consumption, and they suggested that this could be due to the cleats altering the load-sharing scheme of the muscles. In a way, this is confirmed by Ericson et al.[3] who found that positioning the anterior part of the foot over the pedal spindle significantly reduced the activity in the gluteus medius and rectus femoris, and increased the activity of the soleus. Use of toe clips was associated with greater activity in the rectus femoris, biceps femoris, and tibialis anterior muscles, along with decreased activity in vastus medialis, vastus lateralis, and soleus.

These advantages of cleats and toe-clips are evident in the torque and efficiency plots of Figure 12. By improving the effectiveness, cleats allow a decrease in muscle loads and, hence, a decrease in muscle fatigue. Hull and Davis[8] used pedal forces to instruct the subject in ways of improving the effectiveness of his cycling. By shifting the forces to more useful orientations in this way, they obtained improvements of 24% in effectiveness.

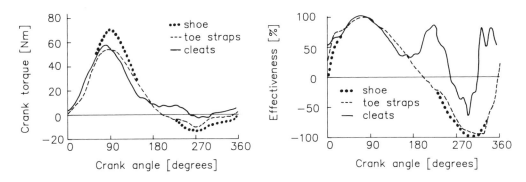

FIGURE 12.   Crank torque and effectiveness for different types of foot-pedal interfaces.[8]

D. Comparison of Sitting and Supine Postures

The most important advance in cycling in the last 10 years has probably been the development of recumbent bicycles. A reclined posture may be either prone (face downwards) or supine (face upwards). Both postures have been used in high-speed human-powered vehicles where the reduction of aerodynamic drag by the reduction of frontal area is necessary. A study on six subjects by Kyle and Caiozzo[26] showed that the supine posture was superior to the prone, since a 5% greater power output was possible (for tests of 1 min and longer). The study also showed that the supine posture allowed the production of nearly the same power output (97%) as did the standard cycling posture. The prone position had no advantage in power output.

An interesting study was performed by Stenberg et al.[44] on leg and arm cycling in sitting and supine postures using normal subjects. They found that, for leg work;

- Oxygen consumption was lower for supine than sitting (5 vs. 4ℓ/min)
- Pulmonary ventilation was lower for supine than sitting
- Heart rate was slower for supine than sitting
- Stroke volume was greater for supine than sitting
- Blood pressure was greater for supine than sitting
- Cardiac output at high work loads was slightly lower for supine than sitting, but higher for supine at small loads

It therefore appears that a supine recumbent posture is superior to sitting and prone recumbent postures.

VI. MODELING AND SIMULATION

A. Equations of Motion for a Cyclist

The force opposing the motion of a bicycle may be predicted from measurements of the rolling resistance and aerodynamic drag. One such expression, from di Prampero et al.,[18] is

$$F = 0.045 \, M + 0.041 \, A\rho v^2/T \tag{6}$$

where F is in Newtons, M is mass in kilograms, v is the air speed in meters per second, A is body surface area in square meters, ρ is air pressure in torr, v is air speed in meters per second, and T is temperature in degrees Kelvin. di Prampero et al.[19] substituted values for a cyclist on a conventional racing bicycle, in the fully crouched position, and obtained

$$F = 3.2 + 0.19\ v^2 \tag{7}$$

The first term is the rolling resistance, and the second the drag. These are not necessarily the true values; other experimenters have measured substantially different values, as described earlier. An expression for power may be obtained by multiplying the force by velocity, hence:

$$P = 0.045\ M\dot{s} + 0.041\ A\rho v^2\dot{s}/T \tag{8}$$

where P is power in watts, and $\dot{s}$ is ground speed in meters per second. Taking the slope into account yields

$$P = 0.045\ M\dot{s} + 0.041\ A\rho v^2\dot{s}/T + 9.8\ M\dot{s}\ \sin(\theta) \tag{9}$$

where θ is the angle of the slope in radians. Using this last equation the speed of a free-wheel downhill descent may be calculated.

Power can also be measured indirectly in terms of the oxygen consumption. The conversion from watts to oxygen consumption usually assumes a respiratory quotient of 0.96, that 1 mℓ O_2 equals 20.9 J,[18] and that the muscle efficiency is 0.25. Thus, the equations derived by measuring the work output can be converted to oxygen consumption:

$$\dot{V}_{O_2} = 0.0086\ M\dot{s} + 0.0078\ A\rho v^2\dot{s}/T + 1.87\ M\dot{s}\ \sin(\theta)$$

or, more simply

$$\dot{V}_{O_2} = 0.61\ \dot{s} + 0.014\ \rho v^2\dot{s}/T \tag{10}$$

The energy expended decreases with altitude, since the drag force decreases with pressure. This implies that it is easier to pedal at higher altitudes. However, the maximum rate of oxygen consumption also decreases with altitude. Knowing an individual cyclist's $\dot{V}_{O_{2max}}$ and its dependence on pressure, the altitude for the best performance can be calculated. This works out to be approximately 3000 m. Since the surface area, A, depends on body mass to the 0.66 power, heavier people require less $\dot{V}_{O_2}$ per unit mass than lighter people. This difference could be as much as 15%.[19]

B. Modeling the Leg

In cycling, the foot is constrained to move on a given path, but the motion of the individual segments is nonetheless indeterminant, since the leg is (at least) a three-bar linkage and the hip usually moves, too.[2] Nordeen and Cavanagh[45] simulated the kinematics of the leg during cycling, but, in order to do so, they had to simplify the system. They did this by asssuming that the hip moved in a fixed way and that the leg could be approximated by a two-chain linkage. The most comprehensive model of the leg during cycling has been developed by Hull and Jorge.[1] They modeled it as a five-bar linkage, incorporating segment masses and moments of inertia. This model was used to determine the static and kinetic contributions of the muscles, and more recently has been used by Redfield and Hull[14] in an optimization study.

VII. BIOMECHANICAL COMPARISON OF CYCLING AND OTHER FORMS OF LOCOMOTION

A. Comparison of Cycling with Walking and Running

EMG measured during walking by Ericson et al.[3] has shown that there is a much greater activity in the vastus medialis, vastus lateralis, and gastrocnemius lateralis muscles during cycling than there is during walking. Muscles that are used more in walking than in cycling include the gastrocnemius medialis and the tibialis anterior.

The power output of cyclists is comparable to that of runners, but since the non-drag component of the retarding force is less, the cyclist travels two and a half times further than the runner for the same energy expenditure.[18] However, in terms of rate of oxygen consumption per unit time, cycling and running are compatible. Furthermore, $\dot{V}_{O_{2max}}$ is greater for running than for cycling.[43]

A physiological comparison between running and cycling was made by Koyal et al.[46] The most important result from this study was that minute ventilation, $\dot{V}_e$, was greater for cycling than for running (70 vs. 50 ℓ/min at a $\dot{V}_{O_2}$ of 2 ℓ/min). This was accomplished by a greater tidal volume. Elevated $\dot{V}_e$ during cycling was found to be a consequence of the smaller muscles mass involved, which resulted in a higher metabolic rate, acidosis, and respiratory compensation. This was demonstrated by the lower pH, higher lactate, and lower HCO_3^- concentrations for cycling.

B. Comparison of Leg and Leg-Arm Cycling Work

The maximum rate at which oxygen can be utilized ($\dot{V}_{O_{2max}}$) during arm work alone is approximately 70% that of leg work[47] Hence, the power output of arm work is less than that of leg work. Astrand et al.[47] found that blood lactate concentration was lower, heart rate was seven beats/minute lower, and blood pressure 20 to 25 mm Hg higher for arm work than leg work. The results of Stenberg et al.[44] showed that $\dot{V}_{O_2}$ is the same for leg cycling and combined leg-arm cycling. Nonetheless, the power output has been found to be 17% greater for the latter[26] and, indeed, combined leg-arm work has been used to an advantage in high-speed human-powered vehicles. Furthermore, it has been found that an intermittent exercise strategy, using the legs alone for 30 sec and then the legs and arms for 30 sec produces a greater power output than does continues leg-arm work.[26]

C. Cycling as a Means of Transport

A measure of the propulsion efficiency of a vehicle is the combination of mass and aerodynamic drag in the lift/drag ratio (or weight-to-drag), proportional to velocity/specific power.[22] Cyclists have larger lift-to-drag ratios than pedestrians, motor cars, or airplanes and, hence, require less energy to move a unit weight. However, contrary to popular belief, the bicycle is not the most efficient means of transport in terms of energy/distance/weight.[22] Many other forms of transport are more efficient.

The cost of transport, i.e., the energy used to move a unit distance, is, for cycling:

$$C_r = 0.0083 \, M + 0.0078 \, A\rho v^2/T + 1.87 \, M \sin(\theta) \tag{11}$$

Comparing the transport costs for various other human activities:

$$C_{cycling} = 0.6 + 0.037 \, v^2$$

$$C_{skating} = 3.5 + 0.038 \, v^2$$

$$C_{running} = 13.3 + 0.034 \, v^2 \tag{12}$$

At a given speed the energy used to overcome drag (the v^2 term) is approximately constant for the different means of locomotion. The speeds attainable thus depend almost solely on the non-drag component. Cycling is a more efficient means of carrying load than is walking, as shown by Myo-Thein et al.[48] They found that the extra power per unit load was 2.55 W for walking and 1.12 W for cycling.

VIII. CYCLING INJURIES AND THE USE OF CYCLING IN REHABILITATION

A. Cycling Injuries

During normal cycling, the core temperature has been found to rise to 38.5°C by Brown and Banister.[49] The risk of heat stroke is increased with temperatures much higher than this.

The ulnar nerve in the palm may be compressed during cycling, perhaps leading to permanent paralysis.[2] The solution is to use padded handlebars and change the grip frequently. The knee is vulnerable to chondromalacia patella and capsular strains during cycling. Such injuries may be due to poor foot placement.[2]

B. Cycling for Therapy

While cycling ergometers are often used by cardiologists to load the cardiovascular system, cycling has had limited use for therapy. Houtz and Fischer[5] suggested that a stationary bicycle be used as an apparatus to increase the range of motion of the hip, knee, and ankle joints and to strengthten the muscles of patients with orthopedic disabilities. McLeod and Blackburn[15] found that the seat height controlled the forces in the knee ligaments and proposed the use of cycling, on stationary and moving devices, as a means of applying controlled forces to these structures to enhance their recovery.

A study by Ericson et al.[3] showed that the exercising of selective leg muscles should be possible by a suitable choice of cycling workload, pedal speed, saddle height, foot position, and foot-pedal attachment, as shown in Table 3. For example, soleus could be exercised by putting the metatarsal heads (rather than the instep of the foot) over the pedal, and avoiding the use of toe-clips. Cycling should be particularly good for strengthening the vasti, since the EMG recorded from these muscles during cycling is some four times greater than during walking.[3] However, there has been no known use of such strategies for therapy.

C. Cycling as an Alternative Form of Locomotion for the Disabled

A study by Smith et al.[50] showed that an arm crank is a less strenuous method of locomotion than handrim propulsion of wheelchairs. They based this conclusion on measurements of oxygen consumption, ventilation rate, and heart rate. Various hand-cranked wheelchairs have been developed and these may be superior to handrim propulsion. Electrical stimulation of paralyzed leg muscles to power a wheelchair has also been investigated,[51-53] and this technology holds potential for the rehabilitation of paraplegics.

An interesting finding of several of these studies, was the poor correlation between EMG recorded from able-bodied subjects on the device and the optimal stimulation sequence for paraplegics. Perhaps the reason for this was the necessity to compensate for muscles that are active during normal cycling, but inactive under stimulation. Further investigation of this phenomenon seems warranted.

IX. TECHNIQUES FOR STUDYING THE BIOMECHANICS OF CYCLING

Mechanical-power output should be measured in any exercise test, and a device that does this is called an ergometer. A friction belt on a flywheel is commonly used to measure and dissipate the power, although electric generators and eddy current devices may also be used.

Table 3
EFFECTS OF VARIOUS CYCLING PARAMETERS ON EMG[3]

	Effect on EMG	
Cycling parameter	**Increases**	**Decreases**
Increase in workload	Vastus medialis	
	Vastus lateralis	
	Gastrocnemius medialis	
	Gastrocnemius lateralis	
	Soleus	
Increase in pedal speed	Gluteus maximus	
	Gluteus medius	
	Medial hamstrings	
	Gastrocnemius medialis	
Increase in saddle height	Medial hamstrings	
	Gastrocnemius medialis	
Metatarsal heads rather than in-step over pedal	Soleus	Gluteus medius
		Rectus femoris
		Vastus medialis
Use of toe-clips	Rectus femoris	Vastus medialis
	Biceps femoris	Vastus lateralis
		Soleus

Power is a useful abscissa against which $\dot{V}_{O_2}$, heart rate, and other such physiological variables are frequently plotted. Von Dobelin[54] described the design of an ergometer over three decades ago which is still in widespread use today.

The ergometer has a flywheel and calibrated brake, but it is substantially different from a normal racing bicycle in construction. It is difficult to simulate ordinary bicycle loads, especially the aerodynamic loads which increase with the square of the velocity. The inertia of a bicycle ergometer is usually substantially less than that of a real bicycle.[55] Therefore, the results obtained from a bicycle ergometer must be treated with some circumspection. Short-term (anaerobic) power measurements have been made using an inertia flywheel ergometer.[26] Such a device does not have any brake; the resistance is purely in accelerating the flywheel.

A treadmill is a useful device, especially when used inside a wind tunnel, as the conditions are then most near real cycling and actual bicycles may then be used. Treadmills may be inclined to give a drag force.[26] Friction rollers are of limited use as the load is not quantified, nor is air drag simulated. However, they do require that the rider balance as during normal cycling.

Cinematography has been used to determine joint motion by replaying single frames and measuring the change in movement of various anatomical landmarks. With the new video equipment interfaced to computers and automatic marker detection this method need not be as tedious as the traditional film techniques. Forces and torques have been measured using strain-gauges glued to the crank and pedals.[6-8] Various mathematical models have been developed to describe the cycling motion.[14,45]

Standard EMG techniques have been used to determine the activity of various muscles. By way of example, Hull and Jorge[1] used a sample frequency of 2000 Hz per channel (which is more than adequate), normalized the EMG to the maximum for that muscle, and used a 50% cut-off level.

Wind tunnels move the air past the cyclist rather than have the researchers chase after the cycle, and have been used to study the effects of wind speed. Without a wind tunnel it is very difficult to simulate accurately the drag on a cyclist. The best type of wind tunnel is one that has a moving ground plane so as to eliminate the boundary layer.

Various physiological measurements are possible. Perhaps the most useful of these is the maximum rate of oxygen consumption, $\dot{V}_{O_2}$, because it reflects the energy consumption. Heart rate is invariably measured, and usually with an electrocardiogram (Stoboy et al.,[56] Koyal et al.,[46] and others). In the study of Stenberg et al.,[44] cardiac output and stroke volume were measured by the dye dilution technique, although this is an invasive method not without certain risks. Blood pressure can be measured with a sphygnomanometer or using catheters. The position of the catheter has been observed to affect the results.[47]

The O_2 and CO_2 partial pressures may be determined by spirometry, and the oxygen uptake, $\dot{V}_{O_2}$, may also be calculated. Maximum oxygen uptake can be determined by exercising the subject until his maximum power output is reached[57] or by extrapolating on the plot of $\dot{V}_{O_2}$ against heart rate.

Pulmonary (or minute) ventilation, $\dot{V}_e$, is another quantity frequently measured. The ratio $\dot{V}_e/\dot{V}_{O_2}$ has been used in some studies.[58] Respiratory quotient (or Exchange Ratio), $R = \dot{V}_{CO_2}/\dot{V}_{O_2}$, indicates the nature of the metabolic processes.

In many studies, no measure of metabolism is undertaken other than the respiratory quotient. Body temperature has been measured by Koyal et al.,[46] although their purpose was to compensate for the effect that temperature has on pH and blood gas concentrations (errors of 3 mmHg and -0.005 pH due to a 0.5°C rise in temperature). Measurement has been made of pH, $[HCO^-_3]$, P_{CO_2} and Pa_{CO_2} using brachial and femoral catheters.[46,47] However, many metabolic parameters may be monitored without resorting to such highly invasive techniques: for example, blood lactate concentration by blood sampling.[47]

X. CONCLUSIONS

The mechanics of normal cycling have been investigated by numerous researchers. However, the use of cycling devices in rehabilitation has not progressed very greatly in the last few decades, apart from the ubiquitous use of bicycle ergometers for research purposes and general fitness training. The advantages of cycling over other forms of human-powered locomotion include the lower energy transport cost, the exertion of controllable loads on the musculo-skeletal system, the limited number of degrees of freedom of the cycling motion, and the inherent stability of a cycling machine. These advantages have not been exploited to the fullest in the rehabilitation field and we suggest that this would be a fertile area for future research efforts.

REFERENCES

1. **Hull, M. L. and Jorge, M.,** A method for biomechanical analysis of bicycle pedalling, *J. Biomech.*, 18, 631, 1985.
2. **Faria I. and Cavanagh, P.,** *The Physiology and Biomechanics of Cycling,* John Wiley & Sons, New York, 1978.
3. **Ericson, M. O., Nisell, R., Arbroelius, U. P., and Ekholm, J.,** Muscular activity during ergometer cycling, *Scand. J. Rehabil. Med.,* 17, 1985.
4. **Disipres, M.,** An electromyographic study of competitive cycling conditions simulated on a treadmill, in *Biomechanics IV,* Nelson, R. C. and Morehouse, C. A., Eds., University Park Press, Baltimore, 1974, 349.
5. **Houtz, S. J. and Fischer, F.,** Analysis of muscle action and joint excursion during exercise on a stationary bicycle, *J. Bone J,. Surg.,* 41, 123, 1959.

6. **Hoes, M., Binkhorst, R., Smeekes-Kuyl, A., and Vissers, A.,** Measurement of forces exerted on pedal and crank during work on bicycle ergometer at different loads, *Intle. Z. Angew. Physiol. Einschl. Arbeitsphysiol.,* 26, 33 1968.

7. **Soden, P. and Adeyefa, B.,** Forces applied to a bicycle during normal cycling, *J. Biomech.,* 12, 527, 1979.

8. **Hull, M. L. and Davis, B. R.,** Measurement of pedal loading in bicycling. I. Instrumentation, *J. Biomech.,* 14, 843, 1981.

9. **La Fortune, M. and Cavanagh, P.,** Effectiveness and efficiency during riding, in *Biomechanics VIII-B,* Matsui, H. and Kobayashi, K., Eds., Human Kinetics Publishers, Champaign, Ill., 1983, 928.

10. **Davis, R. R. and Hull M. L.,** Measurement of pedal loading in bicycling. II. Analysis and results, *J. Biomech.,* 14, 857, 1981.

11. **Dal Monte, A., Manoni, A., and Fucci, S.,** Biomechanical study of competitive cycling, in *Biomechanics III,* Cerquiglini, S., Venerando, A., and Wartenweiler, J., Eds., University Park Press, Baltimore, 1973, 434.

12. **Kunstlinger, U., Luwid, H.-G., and Stegemann, J.,** Force kinetics and oxygen consumption during bicycle ergometer work in racing cyclists and reference group, *Eur. J. Appl. Physiol.,* 54, 59, 1985.

13. **Redfield, R. and Hull, M. L.,** On the relation between joint moments and pedalling rates at constant power in bicycling, *J. Biomech.,* 19, 317, 1986.

14. **Redfield R. and Hull, M. L.,** Prediction of pedal forces in bicycling using optimization methods, *J. Biomech.,* 19, 523, 1986.

15. **Mcleod, W. and Blackburn, T.,** Biomechanics of knee rehabilitation with cycling, *Am. J. Sports Med.,* 8, 175, 1980.

16. **Whitt, F. R. and Wilson, D. G.,** *Bicycling Science: Ergnmics and Mechanics,* MIT Press, Cambridge, 1974.

17. **Dill, D., Seed, J., and Marzulli, F.,** Energy expenditure in bicycle riding, *J. Appl. Physiol.,* 7, 320, 1954.

18. **Davies, C.,** Effect of air resistance on the metabolic cost and perfomance of cycling, *Eur. J. Appl. Physiol. Occup. Physiol.,* 45, 245, 1980.

19. **di Prampero, P., Cortili, G., Mognoni, P., and Saibene, F.,** Equation of motion of a cyclist, *J. Appl. Physiol.,* 47, 201, 1979.

20. **Brubaker, C. and McLaurin, C. A.,** Ergonomics of wheelchair propulsion, in *Wheelchair III,* Golbranson, F. L. and Wirta, R. W., Eds., Rehabilitation Engineering Society of North America, San Diego, 1982, 22.

21. **Nonweiler, T.** The work production of man: studies on racing cyclists, *J. Physiol.,* 141, 8, 1958.

22. **Brooks, A. N. and Hibbs, B.,** Some observations on the energy consumption of human powered vehicles, in *Proc. 1st Human Powered Vehicle Scientific Symp.,* Abbot, A. V., Ed., International Human Powered Vehicle Association, Anaheim, Calif., 1981, 42.

23. **Kaneko, M. and Yamazaki, T.,** Internal mechanical work due to velocity changes of the limb in working on a bicycle ergometer, in *Biomechanics VI-A,* Asmussen, E. and Jorgensen, K., Eds., University Park Press, Baltimore, 1978, 86.

24. **Patterson, R. P. Pearson, J. L., and Fisher S. V.,** The influence of flywheel weight and pedalling frequency on the biomechanics and physiological responses to bicycle exercise, *Ergonomics,* 26, 659, 1983.

25. **Wilson, D. G.,** Research needs for human powered vehicles, in *Proc. 1st Human Powered Vehicle Scientific Symp.,* Abbot, A. V., Ed., International Human Powered Vehicle Association, Anaheim, Calif., 1981, 130.

26. **Kyle, C. R. and Caiozzo, V. J.,** Experiments in human ergometry, *Proc. 1st Human Powered Vehicle Scientific Symp.,* Abbot, A. V., Ed., International Human Powered Vehicle Association, Anaheim, Calif., 1981, 65.

27. **Goto, S., Toyoshim, S., and Hoshikawa, T.,** Study of the integrated EMG of leg muscles during pedalling at various loads, frequency, and equivalent power, in *Biomechanics V-A,* Komi, P., Ed., University Park Press, Baltimore, 1976, 246.

28. **Sjogaard, G.,** Force-velocity curve for bicycle work, in *Biomechanics VI-A,* Asmussen, E. and Jorgensen, K., Eds., University Park Press, Baltimore, 1978, 93.

29. **Coast, Welch,** Linear increase in optimal pedal rate with increased power output in cycle ergometry, *Eur. Appl. Physiol.,* 54, 339, 1985.

30. **Kroon, H.,** The optimal pedaling rate, *Bike Technol.,* 2, 1, 1983.

31. **Harrison, J. Y.,** Maximizing human power output by suitable selection of motion cycle and load, *Hum. Factors,* 12, 315, 1970.

32. **Inbar, O., Dotan, R., Trousil, T., and Dvir, Z.,** The effect of bicycle crank-length variation upon power performance, *Ergonomics,* 26, 1139, 1983.

33. **Gross, V. J. and Bennett, C. A.,** *Proc. 6th Congr. Intl. Ergonomics Assoc.,* University of Maryland, College Park, 1976, 415.

34. **Schwandt, D. F.,** Design development of arm-powered bicycles for the disabled, SAE Technical Paper Series, No. 840023, Society of Automotive Engineers, Warrendale, Palo Alto, 1984.
35. **Jones, D. E. H.,** The stability of the bicycle, *Phys. Today,* 23, 34, 1970.
36. **Warner, B., Hager, L. C., and Allen, J. S.,** The evolution of a hand-powered tricycle, *Bike Technol.,* 2, 10, 1983.
37. **Croisant, P. T. and Boileau, R. A.,** Effect of pedal rate, brake load and power on metabolic responses to bicycle ergometer work, *Ergonomics,* 27, 691, 1984.
38. **Gaesser, G. and Brooks, G.,** Muscular efficiency during steady state exercise: effects of speed and work rate. *J. Appl. Physiol.,* 38, 1132, 1975.
39. **Pugh, L. G.,** The relation of oxygen intake and speed in competition cycling and comparative observations on the bicycle ergometer, *J. Physiol.,* 241, 795, 1974.
40. **Zacks, R.,** The mechanical efficiencies of running and bicycling against a horizontal impeding force, *Intle. Z. Angew. Physiol. Einschl. Arbeitsphysiol.,* 31, 249, 1973.
41. **Hamley, E. J. and Thomas, V.,** Physiological and postural factors in the calibration of the bicycle ergometer, *J. Physiol.,* 191, 55, 1967.
42. **Faria, I., Dix, C., and Frazer, C.,** Effects of body position during cycling on heart rate, pulmonary ventilation, oxygen uptake and work output, *J. Sports Med. Phys. Fitness,* 18, 49, 1978.
43. **Moffat, R. S. and Sparling, P. B.,** Effect of toeclips during bicycle ergometry on VO_{2max}, *Res. Q. Exercise Sport,* 56, 54, 1985.
44. **Stenberg, J., Astrand, P. O., Ekblom, B., Royce, J., and Saltin, B.,** Hemodynamic response to work with different muscle groups, sitting and supine, *J. Appl. Physiol.,* 22, 61, 1967.
45. **Nordeen, K. and Cavanagh, P.,** Simulation of lower limb kinematics during cycling, in *Biomechanics V-B,* Komi, P. V., Ed., University Park Press, Baltimore, 1976, 26.
46. **Koyal, S. N., Whipp, B. J., Huntsman, D., Bray, G. A., and Wasserman, K.,** Ventilatory responses to the metabolic acidosis of treadmill and cycle ergometry, *J. Appl. Physiol.,* 40, 864, 1976.
47. **Astrand, P. O., Ekblom, B., Messin, R., Saltin, B., and Stenberg, J.,** Intra-arterial blood pressure during exercise with different muscle groups, *J. Appl. Physiol.,* 29, 253, 1965.
48. **Myo-Thein, Lammert, O., and Garby, L.,** Effect of trunk load on the energy expenditure of treadmill walking and ergometer cycling, *Eur. J. Appl. Physiol.,* 54, 122, 1985.
49. **Brown, S. L. and Banister, E. W.,** Thermoregulation during prolonged actual and laboratory-simulated bicycling, *Eur. J. Appl. Physiol.,* 54, 125, 1985.
50. **Smith, P., Glaser, R., Petrofsky, J., Underwood, P., Smith, G., and Richard, J.,** Armcrank vs handrim wheelchair propulsion: metabolic and cardio-pulmonary responses, *Arch. Phys. Med. Rehabil.,* 64, 249, 1983.
51. **Glaser, R. M., Gruner, J. A., Frinberg, S. D., and Collins, S. R.,** Locomotion via paralyzed leg muscles: feasibility study for a leg-propelled vehicle, *J. Rehabil. Res. Dev.,* 20, 87, 1983.
52. **Petrofsky, J. S., Heaton, H. H., and Phillips, C. A.,** Outdoor bicycle for exercise in paraplegics and quadriplegics, *J. Biomed. Eng.,* 5, 229, 1983.
53. **Pons, D. J., Vaughan, C. L., Jaros, G. G., and Popp, H. M.,** Design of a cycling device for use with functional neuromuscular stimulation, in 2nd Intl. Workshop on Functional Electrostimulation, Vienna, Austria, 1986.
54. **Von Dobelin, W.,** A simple bicycle ergometer, *J. Appl. Physiol.,* 7, 222, 1954.
55. **Van Valkenburgh, P.,** Human power research methodology, in *Proc. 1st Human Powered Vehicle Scientific Symp.,* Abbot, A. V., Ed., International Human Powered Vehicle Association, Anaheim, Calif., 1981, 95.
56. **Stoboy, H., Rich, B. W., and Lee, M.,** Workload and energy expenditure during wheelchair propelling, *Paraplegia,* 8, 223, 1971.
57. **Zwiren, L. and Bar-Or, O.,** Responses to exercise of paraplegics who differ in conditioning level, *Med. Sci. Sports,* 7, 94, 1975.

INDEX